Praise for *Living PCOS Free*

This is a much-needed book that should have been written many years ago. It addresses an important and often neglected women's health problem in clear and reader-friendly language. Nitu and Rohini have a holistic approach to health which empowers women. It is excellent.

Dr Adeola Olaitan, MD FRCOG,
Consultant Gynaecologist and Gynae Oncologist

Educate, energise and empower your hormonal health for *Living PCOS Free* with the transformative knowledge, delectable recipes and 21-day plan found in this book!

Dr Will Bulsiewicz, Gastroenterologist and
New York Times Bestselling Author of Fiber Fueled

Living PCOS Free is the companion that every person with PCOS (and their providers) need in order to fill the gaps we currently have in PCOS management. The authors form a dynamic duo of multi-dimensional expertise that is matched by their inclusive, compassionate approach to making sustainable lifestyle changes.

Dr Dylan Cutler, PhD, Holistic Health Content Creator

One can only hope this book reaches as many people living with PCOS as possible. A critically important resource packed with evidence-based lifestyle advice and tools to help those suffering from this debilitating condition resume control of their health and restore their quality of life.

Simon Hill, Nutritionist, Author and Host of *The Proof Podcast*

A wonderfully thorough, inclusive and compassionate resource for anyone living with PCOS - I'll be recommending it to patients and colleagues alike!

Dr Hannah Short, GP Specialist in Menopause & Premenstrual Disorders

This wonderful book gives you the tools by which to live a healthier life. Although aimed at those with PCOS, it is relevant to all who want to dramatically reduce their risk of chronic illness. After all, the same healthy habits support us all to thrive. Written from decades of personal and clinical experience, Nitu and Rohini share what they know will work as it has done for their countless patients and themselves. The 21-day plan, which includes healthy and delicious plant-based recipes, is a true gift to support you to regain your health, vitality and hormonal health.

Dr Shireen Kassam, Consultant Haematologist, Lifestyle Medicine Physician, Author and Founder of Plant-Based Health Professionals UK

This book covers the complex condition of PCOS in an accessible way while also discussing the latest research and evidence-base. Nitu and Rohini are a mother-daughter duo clearly striving to write with compassion and are inclusive in their language. A rich and comprehensive must-read for those affected by PCOS, their loved ones and health professionals interested in lifestyle medicine.

Dr Linda Karlberg, NHS Junior Doctor and Host of WIDLIMS podcast

The two authors – one an experienced ObGyn and the other a health professional who has confronted PCOS herself – have created a masterwork on the condition. They present clear explanations and hopeful, effective strategies to optimise the body's function on every level, despite PCOS. But, as they state in their Conclusion, "... this isn't just a book about PCOS. The nutrition and lifestyle approaches we have detailed ...are the building blocks for living a long and healthy life". Indeed, they are – and in this welcoming and authoritative book, you will find guidance for healthy eating, delicious recipes galore, and guidance for lifestyle practices that will bring balance and health into anyone's life. It's hard to ask more of a book on PCOS! I will recommend it to my patients.

Dr Michael Klaper, MD, Primary Care Physician and Director of the Moving Medicine Forward Initiative

An insightful, sensitive, wonderful book that deep dives into all aspects of PCOS and healing from it, giving the reader a 360 view of the problem. It will be extremely useful when put into practice.

Dr Sheela Nambiar MD, ObGyn, Lifestyle Medicine Physician & Fitness Consultant; President of the Indian Society of Lifestyle Medicine (ISLM)

When I was diagnosed with PCOS at the tender age of 11, it was life-changing. Finally, I had an answer for why I felt how I felt. That was just the start though, then it led to more questions, questions no doctor could really answer for me. This sparked a 20-year independent research crusade that has cost thousands, just to try to understand the condition that plagued me, a little better. If *Living PCOS Free* had been available then, it would have transformed the way I felt. It is why I am glad it has been written in such an easy and accessible way. No one should have to be diagnosed with a lifelong condition without knowledge. Knowledge is power and that is why this book is so powerful for all of us living with PCOS.

Elisha Deol, patient living with PCOS

LIVING PCOS FREE

How to regain your hormonal health with Polycystic Ovary Syndrome

**Dr Nitu Bajekal MD DNB FRCOG Obs Gyn,
Dip IBLM 'The Plant-Based Gynae'**
with
**Rohini Bajekal, Nutritionist MA Oxon,
MSc, Dip IBLM**

with a Foreword by **Brenda Davis RD**

BOOKS

Hammersmith Health Books
London, UK

First published in 2022 by Hammersmith Health Books – an imprint of
Hammersmith Books Limited
4/4A Bloomsbury Square, London WC1A 2RP, UK
www.hammersmithbooks.co.uk

Reprinted 2022

The information contained in this book is for educational purposes only.
It is the result of the study and the experience of the authors. Whilst the
information and advice offered are believed to be true and accurate at the
time of going to press, neither the authors nor the publisher can accept
any legal responsibility or liability for any errors or omissions that may
have been made or for any adverse effects which may occur as a result of
following the recommendations given herein. Always consult a qualified
medical practitioner if you have any concerns regarding your health.

British Library Cataloguing in Publication Data: A CIP record of this book
is available from the British Library.

Print ISBN 978-1-78161-213-2
Ebook ISBN 978-1-78161-214-9

Commissioning editor: Georgina Bentliff
Designed and typeset by: Julie Bennett of Bespoke Publishing Ltd, UK
Cover design by: Madeline Meckiffe
Index: Dr Laurence Errington
Illustrations by Tech-Set Ltd
Photograph of the authors by Kate Lindeman
Production: Deborah Wehner of Moatvale Press, UK
Printed and bound by: TJ Books, Padstow, Cornwall, UK

Contents

Contents

Contents

To everyone living with PCOS

Being inclusive

There are health issues that affect people assigned female at birth (AFAB), including some who identify as non-binary, intersex or transgender. This book is written for all people with polycystic ovary syndrome (PCOS) and is meant to include each and every one of you with this condition, however you choose to identify. We will use the terms woman/women but wish to include anyone who identifies as a woman or has female reproductive organs, irrespective of gender. This book is also for those who have loved ones with PCOS in their lives.

Advisory note:
The advice in this book is not meant to be taken as individualised medical guidance. It is a guide for you to learn more about the condition of PCOS. This book is about using plant-based nutrition and lifestyle approaches so you are better equipped to make changes to manage your PCOS, under the appropriate medical advice from your own trusted doctor.

Dr Nitu Bajekal, MD DNB FRCOG Obs Gyn, Dip IBLM
Rohini Bajekal, Nutritionist, MA Oxon, MSc, Dip IBLM

Foreword

It was on a Holistic Holiday cruise that I became acquainted with the Bajekal family. I was smitten. They seemed to me what every family strives to be – connected, loving and joyful. When Dr Nitu Bajekal shared her plans to write a book on PCOS, I was elated. I could not imagine a more competent person to tackle this topic. Dr Bajekal has extensive experience, both professional and personal, but beyond that, she is a gifted and compassionate communicator. To add to the integrity of the manuscript, she engaged a brilliant plant-based nutrition expert, her own dear daughter, Rohini Bajekal.

As a registered dietitian and author/coauthor of 13 books on plant-based nutrition, I understand the personal and professional commitment that is required to write a book that is evidence-based, innovative and relevant. I have been privy to many exciting book-writing dreams that failed to materialise. But I had a good feeling about this one, so when the manuscript landed on my desk, it felt like a gift… to me, to my colleagues, and to all those who are touched, directly or indirectly, by PCOS.

PCOS affects about 10% of women worldwide. The world's number one killer, heart disease, affects about 6% of women. Yet if you ask almost anyone if they know a woman with heart disease, chances are their answer will be yes. If you ask that same person if they know a woman with PCOS, chances are their answer will be no. This is not because they do not know anyone living with PCOS, but rather that those they know often suffer in silence. They may be unaware that their symptoms are linked to the condition or have been unfairly dismissed. In some cases, women go years without an accurate diagnosis, and those who have received a diagnosis are often uncomfortable about sharing that diagnosis with family and friends.

I will always remember my first experience working with a client who had PCOS. The year was 1998. The client was a 29-year-old woman named Sally. Sally had many of the usual tell-tale signs – irregular menstrual cycles, acne and even a little dark facial hair. But the most devastating for her was infertility. She and her husband had been trying to get pregnant for almost three years. Sally wondered if fine-tuning her diet could help. When she came to me, PCOS was barely on my radar. I was grateful for the opportunity to learn more about this syndrome but was taken aback by the lack of information around diet and lifestyle. Knowing that insulin resistance was part of the equation, I decided to ask Sally if she would be willing to experiment with a nutrient-dense, whole-food, plant-based diet, and other simple lifestyle changes, such as daily exercise and stress management. Sally agreed, saying that she was willing to try almost anything. She was a quick learner, following the protocol to a tee. I was gobsmacked by the outcome. Within six months, Sally's skin had cleared, her menstrual cycles had become regular and her facial hair was diminishing. Before the end of the year, she was pregnant. I was convinced that this was no mere coincidence, but I had no solid proof. While I kept my finger on the pulse of the PCOS literature, it took over two decades before the resource the world needed was written.

Living PCOS Free is not just another book – it is a game-changer. This is the book that needs to be read by every person who lives with PCOS, who treats PCOS patients, or who is concerned about someone with PCOS. I love everything about *Living PCOS Free* – its scope, its content and its capacity to make a real difference in tens of thousands of lives. This book is inclusive, culturally sensitive, astonishingly comprehensive and entirely evidence-based.

It is beautifully organised, with four distinct parts. Part One takes you on a deep dive into the details of PCOS and the workings of the female reproductive system. It explores the causes of the disease, its common signs and symptoms, the particulars regarding diagnosis and the condition's unique impacts on adolescents and different ethnic groups. Part Two provides the information you need to make lifestyle choices that are effective in treating PCOS. In this section, you will become acquainted with Lifestyle Medicine – a vital partner of conventional medicine. You will learn about the Six Pillars of Lifestyle Medicine and why each pillar is critical to health. An entire chapter is dedicated to the first pillar which is nutrition.

Part Three addresses the symptoms of PCOS and how best to manage them, including many lesser-known symptoms such as depression, sleep disturbances and eating disorders. It also examines the impact that PCOS has on menopause. In Part Four, Rohini steps in with the 21-Day PCOS Programme. This section offers a blueprint for navigating the wonderful world of plant-based nutrition and Lifestyle Medicine. It answers many pressing nutrition questions and delivers solid lifestyle guidance. It also provides practical shopping strategies, a 21-day meal and lifestyle plan, and a set of delicious plant-based recipes.

Throughout the book, there are Case Studies that bring real life experiences into the conversation, Myth Busters that tackle controversial issues and misconceptions and PCOS Pointers that summarise the key points of each section.

If you have picked up this book because you or someone you love is suffering from PCOS, you can rest assured that you are in very capable hands. This is the resource that will free you from the grips of this distressing condition. *Living PCOS Free* brilliantly, thoughtfully and compassionately provides a simple approach to a complex problem. Read it. Embrace it. Share it.

Brenda Davis, RD

Plant-based pioneer, author, speaker

About the Authors

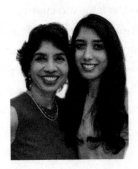

Dr Nitu Bajekal, MD is a Senior Consultant Obstetrician and Gynaecologist in the UK with over 35 years of clinical experience in women's health. Her special interests include, PCOS, menopause, endometriosis, period problems, precancer, complex vulval problems and lifestyle medicine.

She is a Fellow of the Royal College of Obstetricians and Gynaecologists in the UK and recipient of the Indian President's Gold Medal. An experienced keyhole and robotic surgeon, she applies a holistic approach, offering a range of appropriate treatment options in each case.

In 2018, she became one of the first board-certified Lifestyle Medicine Physicians in the UK and has written the women's health module for the first plant-based nutrition course at a UK university.

Dr Bajekal is passionate about education, providing reliable medical and lifestyle information for the general public, doctors, workplaces and schools.

www.nitubajekal.com

Rohini Bajekal is a nutritionist and a board-certified Lifestyle Medicine Professional. She provides evidence-based nutrition and lifestyle advice to her clients around the world and has previously worked in India and Singapore.

A keen recipe developer, Rohini is passionate about making delicious and nourishing plant-based meals. In her spare time, she volunteers as a cookery teacher at Made in Hackney, the UK's only eco-community cookery school and charity.

Rohini is the communications lead at Plant-Based Health Professionals UK, an organisation that provides education around whole-food plant-based nutrition for the prevention and management of chronic diseases. She also provides expertise around South Asian diets as part of the Dietitian and Nutritionist Advisory Committee at Diet ID.

www.rohinibajekal.com

Acknowledgements

Dr Nitu Bajekal

For years, I dreamt of writing a book, but it always seemed like something other people could do, not me. A busy career and family life meant it took a pandemic for me to finally write my first draft.

Thank you to Georgina, the publisher of Hammersmith Health Books and our wonderful editor. When we first spoke, you immediately understood what we wanted to convey. I can't thank you enough for your thoughtful edits and your guidance throughout the publication process. As first-time authors, we couldn't have asked for anyone more supportive. The entire team has been brilliant, especially Madeline Meckiffe who gave life to our vision for the book cover, and Julie Bennett and Daniel Baty for the medical illustrations and typesetting. Thank you to Hayley Smith and Caroline Burgess-Pike at Eden Green PR for getting us such amazing opportunities to publicise our work.

A special thank you to our hero, Brenda Davis, for reading the proof and writing such a wonderful foreword. We are truly honoured.

My original idea had been to write a general book on women's health issues but it was on the advice of Rohini, my daughter and co-author, that I should use my expertise in specific health conditions, that I decided to focus on PCOS. This was an area in which my experience has helped many patients and it was a topic close to both our hearts as Rohini herself has the condition. Rohini wanted others to benefit from my knowledge just as she felt she had. Thank you, dear Rohini, for patiently reading, editing and rereading countless versions, and always pointing out when I used too much medical jargon. This book would not be here without you.

Thank you to Linda Karlberg, now a medical doctor, for her incredibly helpful comments and input.

Thank you to some of our dear friends in the plant-based world for their support: Dr Michael Klaper, Dr Shireen Kassam, Dr Gemma Newman, Dr Sheela Nambiar, Dr Alan Desmond, Dr Hannah Short, Klaus Mitchell, Robbie Lochie, Dr Dylan Cutler, Drs Ayesha and Dean Sherzai, Dr Will Bulsiewicz and Simon Hill. I so admire your work and am grateful for this community.

To my soulmate of 40 years, Rajiv. I love how you would enthusiastically say, 'I never knew that' or 'I wish I had known that!' after reading every chapter. It kept me going and was the best motivation to finish the book. Thank you for your continued love and belief in me and for fuelling me with delicious plant-based meals throughout the pandemic.

A very big hug and thank you to Naina, our wonderful younger daughter. You were firm yet so encouraging, making me think beyond the ordinary. You took the time out of your schedule as a busy editor in your day job to read my work in your scarce free time. I love you. To Siddhant, my son-in-law, I am so grateful to you for helping me refine the message and think about all aspects of the book.

I would also like to acknowledge Dr Adeola Olaitan, my extended family, especially Simon Tinsley, my friends and my book club group, for your positive encouragement throughout the process. I feel so blessed.

To my adorable dogs, Kappu and Tippu, who waited patiently near my feet for their walks, while I finished a paragraph. While watching them chase squirrels in the woods during lockdown, I was able to think of my next chapter.

To my beloved parents, Vimala and Venkataraman, my fantastic parents-in-law, Manorama and Atmaram, and to Gontu, our first dog. You are always in my heart.

I am grateful to so many people for making this book happen but most of all to you, my dear readers. If you are living with PCOS or have a loved one with the condition, I hope this book helps you. I also want to express my gratitude to each and every one of my patients over the last 35 years of my practice as an Obstetrician and Gynaecologist. Without the experience of caring for you, this book would never have seen the light of day.

Rohini Bajekal

Writing a book about a condition you're living with is both harder than I thought and a far more rewarding experience than I could have ever imagined. It has been a privilege to share this experience with my mother, Dr Nitu Bajekal.

This book would not have been possible without our phenomenal publisher, Georgina Bentliff, and her team at Hammersmith Health Books. Your keen insight and editorial support made this book eminently more readable and accessible.

A heartful thank you to Dr Shireen Kassam for your continued support and mentorship, as well as the entire team at Plant-Based Health Professionals UK and MAD Ideas.

Thank you to Dr Gemma Newman for sharing your wisdom and encouraging me from day one. To Dr Dylan Cutler, thank you for creating such an inclusive community for those of us living with PCOS and for your generous support.

To my family and dearest friends, thank you for being by my side and for being so excited for me. A big hug to my sister Naina for your expertise and editing skills, honest feedback and bravery. To say I'm proud of you is an understatement. To my father, Rajiv, for being so kind and reliable, and for the best sprouted porridge deliveries. I would also like to express my gratitude to my mother-in-law, Mamta, and my sisters-in-law, Nivedita and Niharika, for your emotional support and encouragement.

Elisha Deol, thank you being so enthusiastic about the manuscript and for sharing your PCOS story with me all those years ago. To Catherine Lough, not only did you make the time to read the draft but you also suggested immensely helpful changes. Thank you for your friendship over the last two decades.

To my partner-in-life, Siddhant. Thank you for making me feel special and loved every day, and for your brilliant advice around the structure of our book. You helped me unravel so many thoughts while writing, kept me grounded and made me laugh when I took myself too seriously.

Lastly, thank you to my mother. I'm so lucky to have a parent, co-author and friend in you. You are a constant source of strength and inspiration. It makes me so happy that others will benefit from your wisdom in these pages, as I have throughout my life.

Preface

When your periods stop
Dr Nitu's story

The early morning winter air rushed toward my face as I wound down the car window. It was an ordinary day in the year 2000 and I was on my way to work at the hospital. All of a sudden, I felt an intense sensation of heat and a creeping wave of fear wash over me. I was having a hot flush and a panic attack at the same time. Unknown to me, I was going through premature ovarian insufficiency, a condition where the ovaries stop working properly.

I had an almost academic detachment to begin with, but as I joined the dots, I became rather upset. I couldn't shake the indignation that this simply couldn't be happening to me, a fit and healthy woman who was only 38 years old. My menstrual cycle had always run like clockwork. This was the last thing I could have expected.

It's getting hotter

The start to the new millennium was notable for me, as this was the year that my periods started to hop, skip and fade away, accompanied by frequent hot flushes, panic attacks and a low mood that was sometimes difficult to shake. I was used to being in control as a doctor. This loss of control over my body and not knowing where to turn had a profound effect on me.

Premature ovarian insufficiency (POI) affects one in 100 women under the age of 40. It is now the globally preferred description over previously used terms for the same condition such as 'premature ovarian failure' or 'premature menopause'. Menopause is when the eggs in a woman's ovaries are depleted enough for menstrual cycles to stop completely, with no periods for more than 12 months. The average age of menopause is around 51 years all over the world. My periods had stopped much earlier and, as in most cases of premature ovarian insufficiency, there was no obvious reason why. There can be an autoimmune link in some cases, where the body's natural defence system can't tell the difference between our own cells and foreign cells. The body then mistakenly attacks normal cells in various organs. There does not appear to be any robust connection between POI and PCOS.

I had specialised in Obstetrics and Gynaecology and was considering medical hormone replacement therapy. Like most doctors, I did not receive any nutrition education during my medical training in India and in the UK. I had no idea where to access reliable lifestyle information that could help me. This meant I had to find out everything for myself.

The ostrich effect

I did what many people do in stressful situations. I buried my head in the sand. Doctors do tend to be the worst patients and I was no exception. I put my symptoms down to stress. At the time, I was applying for consultant posts, while holding down an extremely busy job not to mention caring for our young family with a limited support network in England. I was being bullied at work and I was unsure if it was all in my head, a not-uncommon assumption by many women in toxic work environments. By the time I turned 40, I had not had a period for over a year. This was not a fun birthday present.

Looking back, my advice to my younger self (and to anyone in a similar situation) would be to seek specialist medical advice. Qualified help is increasingly available on both medical and lifestyle fronts, with impressive recent developments in the latter.

The role of lifestyle

My experience of premature ovarian insufficiency ignited my interest in the power of lifestyle changes, not just for myself but also for my patients and loved ones. I consider myself a highly committed doctor, putting my patients' interests first. However, in many situations, I noted that nothing seemed to work until my patients turned their diet and lifestyle around. I saw first-hand the devastation created by lifestyle-related chronic diseases such as type 2 diabetes, not just for my patients but also for their families. After extensive research, I came to understand the critical role played by plant-based nutrition and lifestyle interventions alongside conventional medicine. It seemed that many of my patients grappling with these illnesses would benefit from lifestyle changes. I now regularly see amazing improvements in my patients' health, improvements that seemed out of reach in my clinical practice a few years ago. Simply put, lifestyle was much more important than I had previously realised.

I have always been deeply passionate about all areas of women's health. I felt I would not be fulfilling my primary role as a doctor if

I did not share more widely the knowledge I had gained over the years about lifestyle and nutrition. I wanted these evidence-based lifestyle and nutrition interventions to be available to people of all ages and from all walks of life.

In 2018, I studied and passed an international examination to become one of the first board-certified Lifestyle Medicine physicians in the UK. I now use this expertise alongside decades of gynaecological experience to guide and advise my patients, doctors and the public.

> Looking back, it seems almost fortuitous that I became menopausal all those years ago. I didn't know then that this event would shape the course of the rest of my life. That over the course of the next decade, it would spark my interest in the power of plants and the significant role that lifestyle factors play in women's health. It would make me who I am today. Most importantly, it has given me my life's purpose – to make a positive impact in so many more people's lives than ever before.

Dr Nitu MD, The Plant-Based Gynae
(For a longer version of my story visit www.nitubajekal.com)

Introduction

Dear Reader,

You may have picked up this book because you have already been diagnosed with polycystic ovary syndrome (PCOS), or you may be wondering if you have it. Perhaps you have a loved one living with the condition, or you're simply interested in learning more about reproductive health? You may be trying to manage the symptoms of endometriosis, fibroids, infertility, menopause or painful or heavy periods. Whatever the reason, I hope what we have to say will help you and your loved ones. We have added a glossary to explain some of the key medical terms commonly used in the book (page 385).

As a senior Consultant Obstetrician and Gynaecologist and Board-Certified Lifestyle Medicine Physician, with over 35 years of clinical experience looking after thousands of women, I understand the importance of treating people holistically rather than focusing on a single issue or symptom.

No one knows your body better than you

Many of us struggle to listen to the cues our body gives us. It's easy to feel overloaded by external stimuli and a dizzying amount of advice about how to lead a better life. In reality, no one knows your body better than you do. And the good news is that it's never too late to get to know your body better.

It's easy to underestimate how intimately the mind is connected to the physical body and ignore the signals the body sends throughout the day. Your body may be stressed, bloated, tired or weak, with your brain pleading with you: 'Slow down. It's okay to take a day off. You don't have to say yes to everything. You will not miss out if you turn your phone off for a few hours.'

But you may not hear your body crying for help, because somewhere along the way you have forgotten how to trust yourself. By reading this book, you have taken the time to educate and empower yourself. Now is as good a time as any to strengthen your relationship with your body and enjoy your life to the fullest.

How can you find a solution for your PCOS, if you don't have a diagnosis to start with?

Let's talk about polycystic ovary syndrome, also known as PCOS, PCOD and polycystic ovarian syndrome. PCOS is the most common endocrine (hormone)[1,2] disorder worldwide, affecting at least one in 10 women of reproductive age.[3, 4, 5] The true incidence of PCOS is likely to be higher as it depends on how carefully doctors look for the condition, the criteria used to define it and how often women are encouraged to seek help for their symptoms. Unfortunately, the vast majority of those who have PCOS never get a diagnosis.[5, 6]

PCOS is a complex hormonal condition that affects the way the ovaries function. Hormonal imbalances in PCOS appear to be triggered through a number of mechanisms, the most important of which seems to be insulin resistance.

The most commonly recognised reproductive, metabolic and psychological symptoms of PCOS, some better known than others, are:

- Menstrual irregularities
- Excessive hair growth on face and body
- Adult acne

- Infertility
- Pregnancy complications
- Acanthosis nigricans
- Anxiety
- Depression
- Disordered eating
- Excess weight gain
- Body image issues
- Sleep disturbances

The social stigma associated with many PCOS symptoms means people with PCOS often struggle to talk about it openly or to seek the help they deserve. PCOS is the commonest cause of infertility in women and the condition has other far-reaching consequences. The long-term consequences of living with it include increased risk of type 2 diabetes, womb (endometrial) cancer,[7] likely increased heart disease risk and even catching COVID-19 infection,[7a] adding a significant toll for those living with PCOS. In addition, the enormous physical, mental and financial burden from managing symptoms of PCOS can cause distress and chronic stress for those affected.

PCOS typically starts in the teenage years but usually doesn't get diagnosed until much later, if at all. The condition also has an impact on how we experience the menopause. Through a combination of both causation and correlation, PCOS appears to be more common in certain groups, such as those with fertility issues and/ or excess weight and in certain ethnic groups.

The PCOS epidemic

There has been a persistent upward trend in the prevalence of PCOS, with the proportion of women with the condition increasing in the last decade. These were the findings of a detailed 2020 review of 27 surveys that met strict inclusion criteria with data extracted from over 32,000 participants.[3] Despite these alarming numbers, PCOS is not yet perceived as an important health problem globally. With nearly three-quarters of women with the condition remaining undiagnosed,[5] there is an urgent need to address this silent epidemic.

According to an economic meta-analysis published in 2021 in the *Journal of Clinical Endocrinology & Metabolism*, PCOS accounts for an estimated $8 billion in healthcare costs annually in the USA alone. The estimate includes the direct costs of treating long-term metabolic health conditions related to PCOS, such as type 2 diabetes, as well as pregnancy-related costs. Understanding and managing the condition better can help improve the quality of life for those living with PCOS while reducing the economic burden.[7b]

There is evidence to suggest that while the condition of PCOS is nothing new, it may have been less severe in previous generations. There were even benefits to women who were affected, such as greater resilience, a rearing advantage for their children, and a reduction in the risk of dying during pregnancy and up to a year after giving birth.[8, 9]

PCOS affects men too

Although hormonal imbalance is common in PCOS,[10] the condition does not just affect women. New genetic research, published in a 2021 study of more than 175,000 men in the UK, suggests they too can develop characteristics of PCOS. Men who had a high genetic risk score for PCOS within their families had increased risks of male-pattern baldness as well as excess weight, type 2 diabetes and cardiovascular disease, all risks seen in PCOS too. Although this has long been suspected, there is now evidence to suggest the primary cause of PCOS may not be linked to the ovaries.[11]

Genes are not our destiny

It is true that PCOS runs in families, but it is also a condition that is heavily influenced by our lifestyle. The effect of the food we eat on our minds and bodies is greatly underestimated. Our sleep, exercise, stress levels, use of drugs, tobacco and alcohol, along with the relationship we have with our community and our environment, have a far greater impact than many of us would like to believe. It therefore makes sense to use nutrition and lifestyle changes to help manage PCOS alongside, or instead of, conventional medical treatment.

It has been my experience that most of my patients significantly overestimate the impact of their genetics on their health, while underestimating the impact of their lifestyle.

A cure for PCOS?

While there is no known cure for PCOS, there is good news. We can make changes in our lifestyles to successfully prevent, manage and treat the condition and its long-term effects.

Educate, energise, empower

Many patients feel disempowered when only medications, supplements or surgery are recommended as treatment. We want to show you how lifestyle interventions and conventional medicine can complement each other and energise you to turn around your PCOS. Patients often believe they have to choose between one or the other. This couldn't be further from the truth. In reality, an evidence-based approach to both conventional medicine and lifestyle is an incredibly powerful combination.

It can also be particularly hard to navigate widespread misinformation about reproductive health. We will bust myths throughout the book based on the latest scientific evidence. We want to educate and empower every reader to make informed health choices about PCOS.

The blame game

There is a tendency for women to be blamed or to blame themselves when it comes to health conditions. This is a documented result of societal stigma, unreliable advice and pervasive and/or inaccurate myths. We also know that health is a privilege in our current world, one that is not available to everyone. This could be due to a lack of access to healthcare, housing, healthy food or one of the many other inequalities present in society. It is therefore impossible to ignore the social determinants of health which negatively affect people living with PCOS.[12, 13]

Medication shaming: While we want to help you treat the root cause of PCOS, there is no defeat in taking medications. PCOS and other health conditions affect everyone differently and sometimes medications are needed to improve quality of life. You are not letting yourself down by being on medications. It is important not to demonise medications or surgery as this creates fear, shame and stigma, all of which we wish to avoid in conversations around PCOS. Perfection is a myth; do the best you can within your limitations.

Remember that you are not to blame for your PCOS. This is a complex condition we are still learning more about. Wherever you are in your life right now, we hope to empower you with knowledge around PCOS as well as offering practical advice on *Living PCOS Free*. Our intention is to share guidance, and never to shame anyone about their body or choices.

PCOS 101

The first three parts of this book will teach you everything you might want to know about PCOS. You will learn about the symptoms and signs to look out for, and when to seek medical help. Whether it is acne or anxiety, missed periods or infertility, excessive hair growth or unwanted weight gain, we will explain the symptom using straight-forward language and advise you on how you can take control. We also use composite case studies drawn from real-life experience, although we have removed all identifiable information. Please do not be fazed by the more science-heavy chapters (Chapters 1, 2 and 3) as you can always return to them later.

Helping your PCOS with lifestyle

As a surgeon and gynaecologist, I understand the critical role medications and surgery have in treating health conditions. As a trained Lifestyle Medicine doctor, I also see the power of nutrition and lifestyle in helping manage and treat these conditions.

With tried-and-tested tools, you will learn how you can make a positive difference for yourself. As well as focusing on the science of plant-based nutrition, you will learn the importance of managing the six pillars of lifestyle. We explain how nutrition, stress and sleep can affect your hormones, the benefit of regular exercise for hormonal health, the effect of risky substances on PCOS symptoms and the importance of maintaining positive social relationships for mental health. Each pillar has an important part to play.

The 21-Day PCOS Programme

The final and fourth part of this book is co-written with my daughter, Rohini, a nutritionist and a board-certified Lifestyle Medicine Professional. It begins with her own story of living with PCOS.

Our focus in this part is on helping you successfully transition to a plant-based way of eating without a focus on miserable calorie counting. We clear up the myths and confusion around soya – a food that has so many benefits for reproductive health and PCOS. You will learn about the anti-inflammatory nature of plant foods (such as fruit, vegetables, beans, herbs, spices and whole grains) and how they have positive effects on reducing heavy flow and pain associated with periods.

You will also learn to incorporate daily affirmations and physical movement. The motivational and achievable three-week programme includes tips to reduce stress, improve sleep and prioritise self-care. We provide tips on shopping for nutritious and budget-friendly plant-based foods along with home-cooked recipes bursting with flavour, with oil-free and gluten-free options. It is our hope that you will emerge fully equipped with the tools to transform your health.

Trusted resources

This is an important cautionary note. Please don't take medical advice from well-meaning friends, YouTube videos or social media influencers as medical truth. Quick fixes rarely exist and my advice is always to follow evidence-based health resources (see page 381).

Communication matters

Your treating doctor should have an overall view of your condition so that they can guide and refer you to other specialists if needed, to manage the various symptoms of PCOS. If possible, request or choose health professionals who have expertise in helping people with PCOS. This can make a significant difference to the overall outcome and your satisfaction. Most importantly, you must feel actively involved in all decisions regarding your health.

If you do not feel listened to, try to advocate for yourself and find a healthcare professional who is understanding. Regardless of the perceived severity of your condition, your doctor should always take your symptoms seriously if you are concerned.[5] Insist that regular communication is maintained among all those responsible for your care as fragmented care can result in conflicting advice and confusion.

Choosing words carefully

My advice to you is to tell your health professional what terminology you prefer when they refer to excess weight and to be aware that 'overweight', 'obese' and 'obesity' are medical terms when used correctly. I recommend health professionals consider the words they use as people often find these medical terms offensive and hurtful. I will be using the words 'excess weight' instead of 'overweight' or 'obese' unless there is a medical reason to use these words as part of some studies.

Using terms like 'male hormone' to describe testosterone can be stigmatising for many patients with PCOS. It is also simply medically inaccurate as testosterone, progesterone and oestrogen are sex hormones found in all genders in varying amounts at different stages of life, as I explain in Chapter 1.

Living PCOS free

If you recognise your symptoms as possible PCOS, our advice is to seek the help of a qualified and trusted health professional as soon as possible to manage your condition. We hope this book will help you take a step in the right direction, give you the confidence to address your symptoms through evidence-based recommendations and empower you to seek the right medical advice. By increasing education and awareness around the condition, we want to help you find out if you might have PCOS and get the professional help you need. Our hope is that anyone with PCOS will benefit from reading this, as will anyone who wishes to support loved ones or patients with the condition. We hope the book resonates with you and helps transform your life to go from surviving to thriving with PCOS, *Living PCOS Free.*

Dr Nitu Bajekal with **Rohini Bajekal**

Part One

Understanding polycystic ovary syndrome

1

Periods: A vital sign
Know your body

Case study: Sarah

Sarah, a 22-year-old university student, had come to see me in my clinic for an unrelated problem. During the consultation, she recalled multiple missed or delayed periods since having started them at the age of 12. She was not on any form of hormonal contraception that would have explained her missing periods.

'It's not just me, Doctor. My friends also think it's normal to not have a period every month,' said Sarah.

In addition to her infrequent periods, she had some of the other symptoms of PCOS, such as acne and anxiety. She had never heard of the condition and was keen to learn more.

It's not unusual for there to be confusion about periods and the menstrual cycle. Did you know there are over 5000 slang words to describe periods, including 'time of the month', 'Aunt Flo', 'The Blob' and 'Code Red'? I grew up in India where periods were referred to as the 'monthly'. I encourage you to use whatever word you want but talk about periods freely and without stigma. The more we talk about them, the sooner we can break down barriers and myths surrounding menstruation. This chapter is for anyone who wants to understand periods better.

Avoiding medical jargon

Doctors do seem to love tongue-twisters. Menometrorrhagia, oligomenorrhoea, menorrhagia and dysmenorrhoea are just some of the ones we use in my specialty – Gynaecology. Most doctors have no prior knowledge of Greek or Latin and I remember this terminology being almost comically difficult to master when I trained in medical school.

Thankfully, doctors are now making a concerted effort to reduce medical jargon so patients may understand us better. Simply using uncomplicated words such as 'painful periods' rather than 'dysmenorrhoea', or 'infrequent menstrual cycles' instead of 'oligomenorrhoea', makes it so much easier for everyone to understand medical conditions without getting confused, put off or scared.

It is, however, important to know a few of the medical and scientific terms so you may understand both PCOS and your doctor better. I tell my patients that knowledge is power, as it means you can be a better advocate for yourself or your loved one and be involved at every step of your care. Ask your doctor to explain in simple language if you do not understand what is being said. I find diagrams are often helpful for my patients.

I will do my best not to use too many of these technical words in this book. When I do, I will explain what they mean in the text as well as in the glossary.

Periods: the fifth vital sign

If you are ever admitted to the hospital, a nurse will measure your body temperature, breathing rate, pulse rate and blood pressure. Vital from the Latin word *vita*, or 'life', means necessary to life. These four important indicators of general wellbeing are known as 'vital signs'. All doctors and nurses are taught how to take these measurements early in their career. Health practitioners should consider menstruation/periods to be an important health indicator on the same level as these four vital signs. In fact, this was the expert committee opinion put forward by the American College of Obstetricians and Gynecologists and supported by the American Academy of Pediatrics (AAP) in 2006 and endorsed again in 2015, which stated that menstrual periods should be the 'fifth vital sign'.[1] Every clinical appointment involving people with periods should prioritise conversations about periods. For example, if you went into hospital with anything from a broken arm to appendicitis to depression, you should be asked about your menstrual cycles, and not just if you could be pregnant before having a surgical procedure.

Bone health and menstrual health are intricately linked as are mental health and periods, or fatigue, anaemia and menstrual flow. Our periods tell us about more than just our reproductive wellbeing. This is particularly true with PCOS as it is an endocrine (hormone) condition.

An endocrine disorder

The endocrine system involves glands and organs in your body that make hormones. These hormones (chemical messengers) are released directly into the bloodstream, so they can travel to tissues and organs to control many important functions in the body, including growth and reproduction. Examples of endocrine disorders are PCOS, type 2 diabetes and those involving the thyroid and/or adrenal glands.

The egg baskets

An ovary has an oval shape and is usually the size of a large grape. The main function of ovaries is the production of hormones and eggs.

Women and AFAB people (those assigned female at birth) are born with two ovaries, with thousands more eggs in those ovaries than will ever be needed. No new eggs will ever be developed beyond those present at birth and most eggs will die without reaching maturity. This natural process of egg loss occurs throughout life, including before someone is even born. It is underway before puberty and even while on birth control, until the number of eggs drops to a critical level and periods permanently stop. This is called the menopause.

You can function perfectly well with just one ovary.

Periods

It is quite common to be confused about your menstrual cycle and the different hormones involved. However, it is helpful to understand the changes that happen to your body so you know when things go wrong. You may also find the diagrams (Figures 1-2) on pages 18 and 20 helpful.

All organisms on Earth have evolved to reproduce, and humans are no different. Every month a menstruating person's body typically goes through a series of finely tuned changes in anticipation of a pregnancy.

The average menstrual cycle comes around every 24-35 days and is divided into two halves – the follicular phase followed by the luteal phase. Natural variations in periods occur throughout life.

In the first, **follicular phase**, rising levels of the hormone oestrogen select one out of many immature follicles, small egg-containing sacs filled with fluid that are found in the ovary, to grow and release an egg (ovulation). The lining of the womb (uterus) now starts to thicken in preparation for a pregnancy.

In the second, **luteal phase**, the hormone progesterone is produced to help the womb prepare for the implantation of a fertilised egg – in other words, to carry a pregnancy. If pregnancy does not occur, the egg is reabsorbed into the body. The levels of oestrogen and progesterone then start to fall. This causes blood and tissue from the inner lining of the womb to be shed through the vagina in what we call a period.

Periods in non-human animals

An interesting fact from nature is that most other female mammals don't bleed outwardly in the way we humans do. Fascinatingly, in dogs, cows and cats, the womb lining is almost completely reabsorbed with hardly any noticeable blood loss. Humans, however, along with a number of primates such as chimpanzees, have visible periods. Tinier mammals, like some bats and the elephant shrew, are also known to menstruate outwardly.

Understanding your menstrual cycle

Figure 1: *The menstrual cycle hormones and phases*

1 Menstrual Phase
This is when the womb lining (endometrium of the uterus) is shed if a pregnancy has not occurred, with a normal period lasting 7 days or less.

2 Follicular Phase
This starts with the onset of menstruation and ends with ovulation. Under the influence of hormones (FSH), a few ovarian follicles are selected within the ovary and one of the follicles becomes dominant. The egg within it starts to reach maturity as the follicle size increases. Oestrogen levels start to rise, and the womb lining now starts to thicken and rebuild.

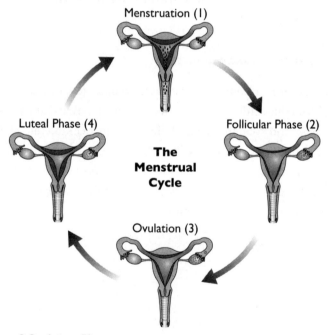

Menstruation (1)

Luteal Phase (4)

The Menstrual Cycle

Follicular Phase (2)

Ovulation (3)

3 Ovulatory Phase
A hormonal surge (LH) 24-36 hours before, triggers the release of the mature egg from the dominant follicle (ovulation). The egg travels down the fallopian tube and lives for about 24 hours if it is not fertilised.

4 Luteal Phase
This phase lasts from the start of ovulation to the first day of the period. Progesterone levels start to increase and work along with oestrogen to thicken the womb lining even further in preparation for a pregnancy.

The menstrual cycle is controlled by hormones released by our brain. We can measure the levels of these hormones in our blood by performing blood tests.

Hormones that control the development of puberty as well as ovarian function are released by the pea-sized pituitary gland that sits at the base of the brain. These hormones travel in the bloodstream to exert their action far away on the reproductive organs deep in the pelvis.

The two pituitary reproductive hormones are **follicular stimulating hormone (FSH)** and **luteinising hormone (LH)**. FSH is responsible for stimulating egg follicle development in the ovaries and for causing the levels of oestrogen to rise. LH helps in maturing the egg and provides the hormonal trigger needed to release the egg from the ovary to cause ovulation.

The master switch

FSH and LH are in turn controlled by **GNRHs (gonadotrophin releasing hormones)**, which are hormones released by the hypothalamus, a tiny hormone controller in your brain. Imagine a master switch which allows hormones to be turned on and off.

A lot of complex messages are sent to and from the brain and pelvis. This is why stress and sleep can affect your periods (see Chapter 21).

The function of sex hormones

Oestrogen, progesterone and testosterone are the main sex hormones produced by the ovaries. Contrary to popular belief, testosterone is not just a male hormone. All three hormones are produced, mainly by the ovaries in women, sharing a common pathway involving cholesterol, a waxy fatty substance which acts as the building block for these hormones (see Figure 2). Our liver

Figure 2: *How our sex hormones work together*

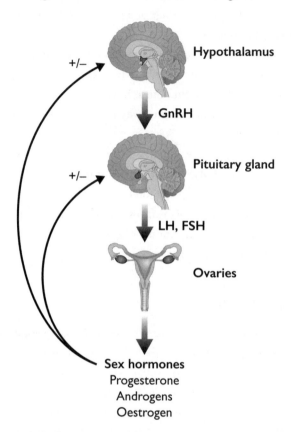

produces all the cholesterol our body needs and we do not actually need any extra cholesterol from our food.

The levels of these three hormones fluctuate throughout the menstrual cycle and during a woman's life. Men also produce all three sex hormones – oestrogen, progesterone and testosterone – mostly from their testes, but in differing amounts and at different stages of their lives.

In women, oestrogen is particularly needed for puberty to occur, with the development of breasts and changes in fat distribution in hips, legs and breasts. Progesterone and oestrogen are necessary to prepare the uterus for menstruation. Testosterone is needed to maintain normal metabolic function, muscle and bone strength, urogenital health, mood and memory.

Androgens

Androgens are a group of hormones which influence the growth of the reproductive organs in all genders. They also have a role in bone growth and libido. The most well-known of all is testosterone, which is often used interchangeably with the term 'androgens', although there are several other androgens (dihydrotestosterone, dehydroepiandrosterone etc.) but you don't really need to know about them.

We need androgens to make oestrogen

Few people realise that all oestrogen is derived from androgens. In simple terms, without testosterone there can be no oestrogen. In women, about half of all androgens are produced in the ovaries, the majority of which get converted into oestrogen, the main female sex hormone. The rest of the androgens are produced by the adrenal glands, two little but important glands sitting on top of the kidneys. The adrenals also produce hormones like cortisol and adrenaline that regulate our metabolism and other vital functions. A small number of androgens are also produced by our fat cells and in the skin.

The first period

'Menarche' is the term used for the first menstrual cycle, when periods begin. This usually happens between the ages of 10 and 16, with most starting between 12 and 13 years of age across well-nourished populations in higher income countries.[2, 3] A couple of years before periods start, there are signs of puberty, such as underarm and pubic hair, vaginal discharge, acne, increased sweating and breast development. Parents or carers should check in with their family doctor if there are early or delayed signs of puberty or if their child's periods have not started by the age of 15, even if it is just for reassurance.

A lifetime of periods

Nowadays, those living in economically developed countries generally have far more periods in a lifetime than their ancestors did. In previous centuries, women started having children soon after the onset of menstruation and were either pregnant or breastfeeding (exclusive breastfeeding usually suppresses menstruation) for most of their much shorter lives. Many died in childbirth and those who were fortunate enough to reach menopause had a handful of periods.

You can now expect to have between 350 and 500 cycles in your lifetime, depending on how many children you have, whether you breastfeed, if you take hormonal contraception, as well as the age when you start and finish your periods. This change, in addition to the stresses of modern-day living, has had an impact on the numbers of women suffering from painful or heavy periods. These stresses include a more sedentary lifestyle and food choices which have made the condition of PCOS more prevalent.

Infrequent periods

If your periods go missing for more than three months, it's helpful to see your doctor, as this may be a sign of PCOS or another medical condition and should not be ignored. Missed or delayed periods can occur naturally for a short while around puberty and when approaching menopause. We explore some of the reasons why irregular or absent periods may occur in Chapter 14.

Periods while on hormonal contraception

It is perfectly fine not to bleed if you are taking hormones. You may be on the progesterone-only pill, coil, injection or implant, in which case you typically would not bleed regularly. If you are on the combined oral contraceptive pill (COCP), you can choose to have a break every few months rather than every month, as these are withdrawal bleeds rather than true 'periods'. It is to your advantage not to bleed every month while on hormonal contraception, allowing you more control of your menstrual cycles, especially if your periods are heavy and/or painful, contributing to your iron-deficiency anaemia or associated with mood fluctuations. The idea that it is healthy to have a withdrawal bleed while taking hormonal contraception is entirely a myth.

Know your body

Most women I speak to wish they had a better understanding of the different organs in the reproductive system. One study found that one in 10 women in the UK were unable to correctly label a diagram of a woman's reproductive system. Nearly one in four misidentified the vagina and nearly 50% were unable to properly recognise the neck of the womb (cervix).[4] Take the time to understand your body so you can be a strong advocate for yourself. Figure 3 gives you the key information.

Figure 3: *External and internal diagrams of the female organs*

Female Reproductive System

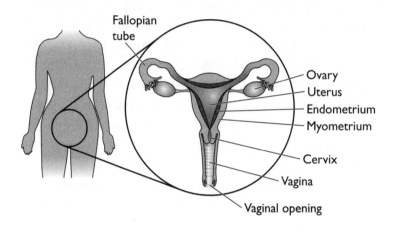

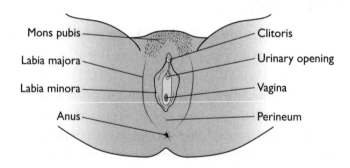

Case study outcome: Sarah

After our discussion, Sarah felt empowered to learn more about her body and its functions. She asked me several questions about the menstrual cycle and began to keep track of her monthly cycle using her diary. This knowledge helped her to understand the link between her infrequent periods and PCOS. She now understood the importance of having regular periods as a sign of health, and that it's natural not to bleed every month if on hormonal contraception.

The PCOS Myth Buster

Myth: A period is needed to detoxify the body and get rid of excess blood.
The facts: Centuries of misconceptions and taboos that periods are unclean, with toxins to be flushed out, were perpetuated by early research and are still believed by many today. A period is not a way of the body flushing out toxins or a way to get rid of excess blood. Menstrual flow consists mostly of the lining of the womb mixed with blood, vaginal secretions and cervical mucus.

Myth: The vulva is the same as the vagina
The facts: These terms often cause confusion but relate to very different parts of the body. The vulva is part of the external female organs on the outside of the body, from the top of the mound or *mons pubis* down to the top of the anal opening, and includes the outer and inner lips called the labia, the clitoris, the vaginal opening and the perineum. The vagina is the muscular tube that connects the uterus to the vulva. Knowing these different functions can help you be more in control of your body.

PCOS pointers

- Take the time to know and understand your body.
- The menstrual cycle is controlled by hormones released by the brain.
- Oestrogen, progesterone and testosterone are the three main sex hormones produced by all genders in varying amounts.
- Menarche is the first ever menstrual cycle, usually between the ages of 12 and 13.
- For most women, periods come every 24 to 35 days until the menopause.
- Women can have 350-500 periods in their lifetime.
- Missed or infrequent periods can be a sign of PCOS.
- It is fine not to have periods if you are on hormonal contraception.
- Knowing your body can help you be more in control.

2

Demystifying PCOS
Understanding the condition

Case study: Siobhan

Siobhan, a 26-year-old payroll assistant, asked me: 'Do you think I have PCOS? I got scared when I looked online but I seem to have some of the symptoms. I am hoping you can help me.' Siobhan was keen to take charge of her own health but, like many people her age, relied on the internet for information on health.

Knowledge is power

Taking the time to read these next few chapters will help you to understand PCOS better and will give you the confidence to talk to your own doctor to get more information. You can then hopefully get the care you or a loved one needs and deserves. Misinformation understandably causes confusion and unnecessary fear. It is really important to refer to reliable health resources. Our wish is for everyone with PCOS to have access to the right resources, tests, and treatment.

PCOS explained

PCOS is a hormonal disorder which affects how the ovaries function but is not just a gynaecological issue. It is a complex endocrine condition with a wide range of metabolic, reproductive and psychological symptoms. These symptoms seem to be triggered by a number of mechanisms which can cause an imbalance of hormones (hormonal dysregulation), such as insulin, luteinising hormone, testosterone and oestrogen.

How widespread is PCOS?

PCOS should be an urgent public health issue. It is the most common endocrine (hormonal) condition to affect women of reproductive age and yet most people have never heard of it. Experts say eight to 13 out of every 100 women have the condition,[1] but the true prevalence can range from 2.2 to 26%,[2, 3, 4, 5] with up to seven out of 10 affected with PCOS remaining undiagnosed.[1, 4, 6]

Evidence suggests the highest prevalence of PCOS is among certain ethnic groups, such as Black and Middle Eastern women, followed by Caucasian women, with the lowest prevalence in Chinese women.[7]

In certain high-risk groups, the prevalence and complications of PCOS are even higher. This includes those with subfertility, excess weight, type 1 or type 2 diabetes or a history of gestational diabetes mellitus, those on anti-seizure medication and those with first-degree relatives with PCOS.[1, 8, 9, 10, 11]

Up to 80% of people with PCOS may have excess body weight,[12] but some researchers suggest that these figures may be an overestimate;[13] those who are distressed about weight gain may be more likely to seek medical advice than those with PCOS who are of healthy body weight.

The cause of PCOS

Polycystic ovary syndrome is still a poorly understood condition and the exact cause is unknown. Insulin resistance, a condition in which our cells become resistant to the action of the hormone insulin, appears to be the main mechanism in causing PCOS and many of its symptoms.

The second mechanism that can cause PCOS and its symptoms, even in the absence of insulin resistance, is thought to be through excess body weight. There is an accompanying excess of oestrogen produced by the increased fat within the cells (intracellular fat) when there is weight gain. I explain this in more detail in the androgen excess and body weight chapters, Chapters 6 and 7.

While excess body weight is a common cause of insulin resistance, lean people with PCOS can also be insulin resistant. I discuss insulin resistance in more detail later in a dedicated chapter (Chapter 5).

PCOS often runs in families. There appears to be a strong genetic predisposition involving several genes, often expressed as type 2 diabetes and/or premature hair loss, or male-pattern baldness in male relatives.[14, 15] New genetic research suggests that men too can develop characteristics of PCOS, as discussed in Chapter 1, indicating for the first time that the primary cause of the condition may not be linked to the ovaries after all and making it first and foremost an endocrine condition which also happens to affect ovarian function.

PCOS is affected by lifestyle

We now know that behavioural and environmental factors play a critical part in influencing the genes we inherit from our biological parents.[2, 16, 17] This is from our increasing knowledge of 'epigenetics', which is the study of how our behaviours (what we eat and how physically active we are, for example) and our environment (our mother's nutrition when we were in the womb, pollution etc.) can cause changes that affect the way our genes work. Unlike genetic changes, epigenetic changes are reversible and do not change our gene (DNA) sequence, but they can change how our body reads a DNA sequence.

When our outside environment and changes within our body come together to influence the genes we have inherited, a situation may be created which allows the condition of PCOS to develop. How we live our lives can have a huge impact on PCOS, either harming our health or helping it. This is why PCOS is considered by experts to be a lifestyle-related condition. This is good news as it means we can influence our internal and external environment to change which of our genes are expressed, switching them on or off to create disease or health.

PCOS has many similarities to metabolic syndrome, type 2 diabetes and heart disease. These are chronic lifestyle diseases which you most likely have heard of or even know someone living with one of them. These illnesses respond really well to lifestyle approaches and can often be prevented, if changes are brought in early enough, or at least managed with fewer medical or surgical interventions.

We cannot change the genes we are born with but we can certainly change the way our genes are expressed to work in our favour rather than against us. That is what this book is going to teach you.

A misleading name

The 'cysts' that give the name to the condition polycystic ovary syndrome are not really cysts at all. The medical definition of a 'cyst' is a fluid or semi-solid collection in the ovary or another part of the body. The so-called 'cysts' in PCOS are, in fact, multiple tiny egg follicles in the ovary that do not reach maturity and often have a typical 'string of pearls' appearance when seen on an ultrasound scan.

Polycystic ovary syndrome is therefore an unfortunate choice of name for a hormonal condition influenced by our lifestyle and genetics. In fact, experts have debated whether the condition should be renamed as metabolic reproductive syndrome but it has been agreed this would probably cause more confusion.[18]

PCOS or PCOD?

Polycystic ovary syndrome (PCOS) is used interchangeably with polycystic ovarian disease (PCOD) in some parts of the world. There is absolutely no difference, just a matter of terminology. PCOS is considered a syndrome rather than a disease as it has more than one possible cause and a variety of clinical symptoms.

Case study outcome: Siobhan

Siobhan did the right thing by seeking medical advice for her symptoms. Her medical history and blood tests confirmed the diagnosis of PCOS. Since then she has focused on taking on board medical advice while listening to her own body as she works to manage her condition. Since our consultation, she has felt confident about how to access reliable and accurate medical information on the internet and understood the importance of individualised care.

The PCOS Myth Buster

Myth: You can reverse PCOS.

The facts: Unfortunately, the short answer is that there is no known cure for PCOS. The condition doesn't go away permanently in most situations, as so much depends on our environment and our genetics. The long answer, however, is not so clear cut, hence the reason for writing this book. Can you control PCOS and live healthily? Absolutely. While there may be no cure for this hormonal disorder, there is plenty of hope and help available to make it possible to live a full and meaningful life with PCOS, by bringing in the nutrition and other lifestyle changes we discuss throughout the book. The first step is knowing what to look out for if you think you might have PCOS, and in the next chapter, we discuss the key things to be aware of.

PCOS POINTERS

- PCOS is more than just a gynaecological condition.
- PCOS is the most common endocrine (hormone) condition, affecting at least one in 10 women and AFAB people of reproductive age.
- PCOS manifests with a range of reproductive, metabolic and psychological symptoms.
- PCOS affects ovarian hormone function.
- The exact cause of PCOS is unknown.
- Insulin resistance appears to be the main mechanism involved in PCOS.
- The 'cysts' of PCOS are not true cysts but immature egg follicles in the ovary.
- PCOS runs in families.
- There is a higher risk of PCOS if there's a family history of PCOS, type 2 diabetes and/or male-pattern baldness.
- PCOS symptoms are often influenced by lifestyle.
- While there is no cure for PCOS, it can be managed successfully with lifestyle changes alongside medical treatment as needed.

3

PCOS: What to look out for
Signs and symptoms

One of the difficulties with PCOS is that it can manifest in a number of ways. As a result, you may end up seeing healthcare professionals from different specialties for symptoms ranging from the commonest and most well-known – for example, irregular menstrual cycles, acne and excess hair growth – to lesser-known ones – such as disordered eating or sleep disturbances. The dots may never get joined up to make a proper diagnosis of PCOS. This can lead to fragmented and disjointed medical advice and treatment, often leaving women frustrated with themselves and distrusting the healthcare system.[1] It is not all in your head.

It's important to remember that you may not have all the symptoms and signs of PCOS, even if you have the condition. However, it is good to be aware of all the possibilities to look out for. The box on the next page lists some of the main symptoms and signs people with PCOS may notice.

Symptoms of PCOS

Infrequent periods or missed periods (oligomenorrhoea/
   amenorrhea)

Excess facial/body hair (hirsutism)

Adult acne, often cystic and painful

Acanthosis nigricans (darkened skin: behind the neck,
   underarms, groin)

Weight gain

Scalp hair loss (alopecia)

Fertility problems

Pregnancy complications (miscarriage, gestational diabetes)

Disordered eating

Psychological issues (depression, anxiety and mood disorders)

Sleep disturbances

Excessive daytime sleepiness

Breathing problems (sleep apnoea, snoring)

Sexual and relationship dysfunction

PCOS is a diagnosis of exclusion, meaning other more uncommon or serious conditions should be ruled out by your doctor (see Chapter 6).[2]

The onset of PCOS

PCOS typically starts around puberty (known as adolescent PCOS), but as irregular periods and acne are common at the start of menarche (first period) for many teenagers without the condition, symptoms are often overlooked until much later.

PCOS mostly affects those of reproductive age (from the start of your first period until menopause).

Chapter 3

PCOS is about more than just fertility

The narrative we often hear and what the conversation focuses on almost always has to do with fertility. PCOS, however, affects people in many additional ways, with different symptoms at different life stages. We now know that there are long-term effects of PCOS which last beyond the menopause, with increased risks of type 2 diabetes, metabolic syndrome and womb cancer, and possible increased risk of heart disease (see Chapter 23). This is about looking after your health now and in the future, particularly due to the higher risk of these chronic lifestyle diseases.

Family history of PCOS

There is a strong familial link with PCOS.[2, 3, 4] If your mother and/or sister(s) have the condition, or if there are family members with type 2 diabetes, there appears to be an increased risk of PCOS. There also seems to be a link between women who have PCOS and premature hair loss in male members of the family.[5, 6] Studies of twins and of first-degree relatives of those with PCOS confirm these links.[7, 8]

Genes, however, certainly do not equal destiny. As the researcher George Bray famously said, 'Genes load the gun but the environment pulls the trigger.'[9] This realisation can be extremely empowering. In other words, we can modify our outcomes and minimise many lifestyle conditions by making certain lifestyle changes.

The PCOS Myth Buster

Myth: The cysts on my polycystic ovaries are causing me pain.
The facts: Pain is not a feature of PCOS. Tiny 'cysts' may be seen in one or both ovaries on a pelvic ultrasound scan

---

in those with PCOS. These are not true cysts but immature egg follicles which do not grow to any significant size and do not cause pain. There may be other coincidental causes of pain in PCOS, such as painful periods, pelvic infections, endometriosis or a symptomatic ovarian cyst, and treatment for these will depend on the underlying cause. If you are having persistent pain, it is really important that you seek medical advice and do not assume it is because of PCOS.

PCOS POINTERS

- As PCOS is a syndrome that can manifest in a number of ways, health professionals may not 'join the dots' but offer treatment for individual symptoms.
- PCOS is not just about fertility and can cause issues after as well as before the menopause, impacting one's quality of life.
- The symptoms of PCOS are diverse and many are not well recognised.
- PCOS often starts in adolescence when symptoms like acne and irregular periods can be mistaken for 'normal' issues at this age.
- There is a hereditary link, with increased risk where close family members have PCOS or type 2 diabetes, but remember, genes do not equal destiny.

4

Solving the PCOS puzzle
Diagnosis of PCOS

Receiving the right care for PCOS begins with getting the right diagnosis. The diagnosis of PCOS in adults involves a detailed medical history taken by your doctor, biochemical tests and a pelvic ultrasound scan, where indicated. The correct interpretation of symptoms and tests is important to prevent under-diagnosis in order to receive early support. On the flipside, assigning someone the label of PCOS could result in unwanted psychological distress in vulnerable people, so it is equally important to avoid over-diagnosis.[1]

Diagnosing PCOS

In 2003, international experts from all over the world met in Rotterdam for a PCOS consensus workshop. They agreed that for the diagnosis of PCOS in adults, any two out of three key criteria had to be met ('ovulatory dysfunction', 'hyperandrogenism' and/ or 'polycystic morphology' on ultrasound: see Box on page 40). A single diagnostic criterion was considered insufficient for an accurate diagnosis. For example, if ovaries appear polycystic on a pelvic ultrasound scan but there are none of the other criteria, this is not

PCOS. This was once again endorsed by new International PCOS Guidelines in 2018.[3] I explain each of these criteria in more detail below.

2003 Rotterdam PCOS criteria: Any two out of three have to be met to diagnose adult PCOS

1. Ovulatory dysfunction (delayed or missed periods)
2. Hyperandrogenism (clinical signs e.g. acne, excess hair growth, or lab evidence of excess androgen hormones)
3. Polycystic ovary morphology (appearance) in one or both ovaries on ultrasound.

Ovulatory dysfunction (delayed or missed periods)

If a woman has delayed or missed periods (irregular menstrual cycles), this is a sign of infrequent or absent ovulation (also called 'oligo-' or 'an-ovulation') and is known by the overall term, ovulatory dysfunction. It means that the ovaries are not currently releasing eggs on a regular basis.

Hyperandrogenism

An excess of androgens in the body, a group of hormones that includes testosterone, is known as hyperandrogenism. This may manifest with signs of excessive facial and body hair ('hirsutism'), acne and/or female-pattern scalp hair loss ('alopecia'), or with laboratory biochemical evidence of androgen excess by carrying out specific blood tests.

Polycystic ovary morphology (appearance)

On an ultrasound scan, certain criteria have to be met to label an ovary as 'polycystic'. Ovaries are said to show 'polycystic ovary morphology' (PCOM) if the criteria are met for a specific number and size of follicles and/or have increased overall volume. When seen on a scan, the tiny egg follicles may have a 'string of pearls' or rosary-like appearance just below the surface of the ovary. Both ovaries do not have to show these changes; if a single ovary fits the criteria described above, it is enough to call it polycystic.

Figure 4: *Polycystic ovary morphology*

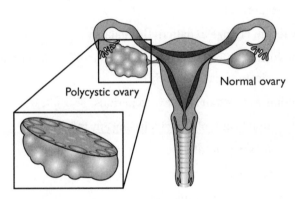

Adolescent PCOS

For those within eight years of first starting their periods, the latest international guidelines recommend that both hyperandrogenism and ovulatory dysfunction must be present when diagnosing PCOS, as ultrasound is not recommended in this group. Ultrasound is generally unreliable in this age group, as even teenagers without PCOS normally have multiple small cysts on their ovaries ('multifollicular' ovaries) at this life stage. However, an ultrasound scan can sometimes be useful to rule out other conditions, such as ovarian cysts that may need treatment.

Getting the most out of your medical appointment

When you are seeking a diagnosis, being as prepared as possible can save valuable time which may be used to have other discussions with your doctor. Knowing the answers to many of these commonly asked questions greatly helps your treating doctor to give the right advice:

- Important dates (your first and most recent menstrual period).
- Menstrual flow (light, average, heavy, in your opinion).
- Duration (number of days your periods last).
- Frequency (number of days from the first day of your period and the next period).
- Any recent change in pattern (irregularity).
- Pain during period (how many days, when does it start and finish, medications taken to help).
- Bleeding after sex or in between periods.
- Your sexual health history, including any infections.
- If you find sex painful.
- Current and past contraception use.
- Cervical smear screening history.
- Bring previous medical notes if available.
- It is also helpful to have details of your past or present medical or surgical history, bowel and urinary habits, medications and supplements, any allergies including drug allergies, and relevant family history, including of PCOS and/or type 2 diabetes, to complete the picture.

I often suggest to my patients that they write their symptoms down before attending a doctor's appointment, as it can be daunting to remember it all. It is not unusual for your mind to go blank. If you do remember something of importance later, it is good to send that information to your healthcare professional. If you have concerns regarding your mental health, stress, sleep pattern, smoking, alcohol or other substance use, bring this to the attention of your doctor too, as many of the under-recognised symptoms associated with PCOS include anxiety, disordered eating and disturbed sleep, as I explain in later chapters.

Your doctor may carry out a general physical examination as this is helpful to assess both acne and excessive hair growth. You may also have your blood pressure and body height and weight measured, but you can always decline being weighed as it sometimes can be triggering, especially if you have a history of disordered eating.

An internal pelvic examination is not needed to diagnose PCOS but may be helpful in some circumstances depending on your answers to the above questions. It is only appropriate if you are sexually active and give verbal consent. For support, I recommend asking for a chaperone for any examination, even if seeing a female health professional.

Blood tests your doctor may request to help diagnose and manage PCOS

Blood tests when PCOS is suspected

To calculate the free androgen index (FAI) for hyperandrogenism
- Total testosterone
- Sex hormone binding globulin (SHBG)

To rule out other causes of missed periods
- Follicle stimulating hormone (FSH)
- Luteinising hormone (LH)
- Prolactin

To investigate iron-deficiency anaemia
- Full blood count
- Ferritin (iron stores)

To investigate health problems associated with PCOS
- Thyroid function tests
- Tests for diabetes
- Cholesterol/lipid profile

Blood tests (see Box above) are not essential to diagnose PCOS if you fulfil the Rotterdam criteria, but they are helpful to rule out other possible causes that can mimic PCOS and also to serve as a baseline to compare with future tests. If you are on the Pill (combined oral contraceptive pill or COCP), hormone levels are not helpful for diagnosis as they are usually suppressed. In some situations, it may be best to come off the Pill and check hormones eight to 12 weeks after stopping.

If there is any possibility of pregnancy, you will need a pregnancy test. Once that has been checked, you may be asked to have a few blood tests to check for signs of androgen excess. The usual blood tests requested in the UK are for total testosterone and sex hormone binding globulin (SHBG) from which the 'free androgen index' (FAI) is calculated to assess the amount of physiologically active testosterone present. Hormone levels such as FSH, LH and prolactin are also often tested but are more to rule out other conditions that may cause missed periods.

Further hormone tests or more detailed scans may be requested on an individual basis by your doctor if there is concern that you may have other medical conditions or if your initial blood tests are abnormal. I discuss this in the androgen excess chapter.

As one in five women worldwide are deficient in iron due to heavy periods, you should have a full blood count, including your haemoglobin and ferritin levels (iron stores) being checked. There is an increased incidence of thyroid problems in those with PCOS, so getting your thyroid checked is a good idea.

A blood test may be used to test for diabetes and lipid (cholesterol) levels, especially if you have a family history or if you have excess weight. Tests for insulin resistance are not yet routinely recommended in the UK for PCOS but can be calculated from fasting insulin and fasting glucose levels using certain commercially available tests, if your doctor thinks it will benefit you. Anti- Müllerian hormone (AMH), a hormone produced by ovarian follicles, is used to predict ovarian reserve and function and future fertility in those without PCOS. Studies show AMH is often increased by two- to three-fold in PCOS.[3a] However, it is not standardised enough to be recommended at this stage to be used in isolation for diagnosing PCOS or to be used routinely to predict fertility in those with PCOS.

Ultrasound in PCOS

Not all women with PCOS show changes in their ovaries on an ultrasound scan. Ultrasound is not necessary for the diagnosis of PCOS, if irregular periods and clinical or laboratory evidence of androgen excess are present, but it provides a more complete description of the condition.

Ultrasound uses high frequency sound waves and a pelvic ultrasound scan is used to examine the internal reproductive organs, including your ovaries. It is not a painful procedure and is done as an external scan where gel is applied on the tummy to look at pelvic organs (transabdominal scan), or as a transvaginal scan, when a narrow probe is inserted into the vagina as the images tend to be better. The latter should only be carried out if you are sexually active and are comfortable with having an internal scan. You may request a female sonographer if you prefer.

Other recommended tests

Most other tests are not needed routinely to diagnose PCOS. An MRI scan of the pelvis or a keyhole procedure (laparoscopy) when carried out to check for other conditions may sometimes demonstrate polycystic ovaries. Diagnosis still depends on fulfilling the recommended Rotterdam criteria discussed above. The need for further testing for fertility, gestational diabetes, specialised sleep tests and psychological assessments is decided on an individual basis.

The PCOS Myth Buster

Myth: There are four different types of PCOS
The facts: It is best to think of PCOS as a syndrome with a number of symptoms that deserve individual attention. You may, however, have heard that there are four different types of PCOS. This is due to a clustering of symptoms ('phenotypes') used in medical research on the condition. However, these phenotypes do not have much bearing upon the medical advice we would give to patients, and I would advise you not to look at the condition in this way. This advice is in line with the International Guidelines on the condition, which state it is likely to be more confusing than helpful.[3]

PCOS POINTERS: PCOS diagnosis

- There are three Rotterdam criteria used to diagnose PCOS.
- These are signs of anovulation (missed or delayed periods), signs or blood test evidence of androgen excess and PCO appearance on ultrasound.
- Any two out of these three criteria must be met to diagnose adult PCOS.
- If ovaries appear polycystic on ultrasound but there are none of the other criteria, this is not PCOS.
- Signs of both anovulation and androgen excess must be present to diagnose PCOS in a teenager. Ultrasound appearance is not a criterion in adolescents.
- A detailed medical history is important.
- You may need to be tested for diabetes, anaemia and thyroid problems.
- Specialised tests should be decided on an individual basis.

5

The missing link
Insulin resistance in PCOS

As we have established so far, while we may not know the exact cause of PCOS, we do know insulin resistance is one of the key underlying drivers of the condition. It is responsible for many of its symptoms. Understanding insulin resistance is critical to understanding PCOS and helping you manage your condition better.

Insulin resistance

Insulin is a hormone produced by a gland called the pancreas, located behind the stomach. Our body cannot function without insulin. It acts as a key, letting the glucose (sugar) that has been broken down from the food we eat into our cells to be used as energy. Insulin also signals to the liver to store extra blood sugar in the easily accessible form glycogen for later use.

When tissues at the cell level persistently fail to respond to insulin, a state of insulin resistance develops. The body now has to produce even more insulin to move the same amount of glucose into the cells.

This reduced sensitivity of the tissues and failure to respond to normal levels of insulin causes levels of glucose to rise in the bloodstream as it cannot get into the cells. The pancreas then responds by producing even more insulin to try and clear this blood sugar backlog.

Insulin resistance is a main driver of PCOS

These increased levels of insulin in the bloodstream appear to be the main mechanism for many of the symptoms in people with PCOS who are also in the excess weight range. As many as 70-80% of those with a body mass index (BMI – see page 71) of more than 30 (clinically obese) and 20–25% of lean (BMI less than 25) women with PCOS exhibit these characteristics.[1]

The higher blood levels of insulin associated with insulin resistance have both direct and indirect effects on the levels of androgen hormones (such as testosterone), raised levels of which can cause symptoms such as acne and increased hair growth often seen in those with PCOS.

Directly, insulin mimics the action of a hormone called insulin-like growth factor 1 (IGF-1) that is structurally similar to insulin and is produced mainly by the liver. Insulin binds to the insulin and IGF-1 receptors on the ovary, directly stimulating the ovaries to produce androgens. This in turn disrupts the balance of the hormone system, known as the hypothalamic-pituitary-ovarian (HPA) axis (see Figure 5.1).[1]

Indirectly, high levels of insulin reduce the production of a liver protein called sex hormone binding globulin (SHBG) that normally attaches itself to androgens. Lower levels of SHBG in the bloodstream lead to higher circulating levels of free, or biologically active, testosterone, worsening androgen excess symptoms of acne or excess hair growth.

Insulin resistance itself can also lead to weight gain, which can worsen PCOS symptoms as excess body fat causes the body's tissues to become less responsive to insulin (more insulin resistant) leading to even more insulin production, creating a vicious cycle. [2]

The cause of insulin resistance

While we are not entirely sure what causes insulin resistance, here are some possible reasons for it to develop:

Genetics have a significant role. The familial nature of PCOS and its close relation to type 2 diabetes has led to the examination for possible gene and chromosomal defects in this condition.[3] Approximately half of those with PCOS were found to have unique changes in the insulin receptor that may result in both insulin resistance and androgen excess. There also may be a reduction in insulin secretion in those with a family history of type 2 diabetes.[4]

Excess weight (especially around the waist) and being physically inactive also increase the risk of being insulin resistant. There are several mechanisms such as chronic inflammation,[5] oxidative stress and lipotoxicity (the destructive effect of excess fat on the way glucose gets broken down; this is how excess body fat can contribute to insulin resistance). However, you do not have to have excess weight to have insulin resistance, although it is much more common in that scenario. Several studies have found that gut health disturbance (gut microbiome dysbiosis) may be an important factor in rapid progression of insulin resistance in type 2 diabetes.

Excess unhealthy fats: Dietary fat, especially high levels of unhealthy fats (found in fried foods, animal derived foods such as sausages and red meat and tropical oils such as coconut oil) found in a standard western diet, keeps fat in the bloodstream constantly, leading to increased insulin resistance. This is particularly problematic for someone with PCOS. In the 1920s, Dr

Harvey Shirley showed how a high-fat diet makes people insulin resistant in just a few meals. Circulating insulin produced by the pancreas cannot do its job of unlocking the receptors on the cells to help move blood sugar into the tissues as fat collects within the cells (intramyocellular lipid) blocking up the receptors. Whether this fat is from carrying excess fat within our tummy (visceral fat) or unhealthy fats from our diet, this sets up a vicious cycle of needing more insulin to be produced, with the tissues progressively becoming less sensitive to its action, until ultimately they become resistant to the action of insulin. Insulin resistance and rising blood sugars are the end result. This is one of the reasons why a diet rich in whole plant foods which are naturally low in unhealthy fats works so well in treating insulin resistance.

Endocrine disrupting chemicals (EDCs) may contribute to insulin resistance and could be a risk factor for PCOS. These substances may have the ability to alter the way hormones are produced in the body. For example, studies have found amounts of the endocrine disrupter bisphenol A (BPA) to be higher in those with PCOS compared with those without the condition, and these higher BPA levels correlated with the degree of androgen excess and insulin resistance. BPA is an industrial chemical that has been used to make certain plastics and resins since the 1950s. Much more research is needed in this area but, in the meantime, reducing these chemicals in our day-to-day life seems sensible. For example, opt for BPA-free cans and store food in glass rather than plastic.

Signs of insulin resistance

If you gain excess weight, especially around the waist (known as central obesity), or if you notice signs of androgen excess, such as acne or excessive hair growth, then these may be strong clues to suggest you may have insulin resistance.

You may notice thickening and darkening of the skin affecting your underarms, neck, perineal area (between your vaginal opening and anus), knuckles and/or elbows, which may also suggest you have insulin resistance. This is known as *acanthosis nigricans* and has a characteristic thick, velvety appearance.

Testing for insulin resistance

Depending on your clinical symptoms, your doctor may suggest a few simple tests, such as an oral glucose tolerance test (OGTT), to check for impaired blood sugar levels, and HbA1c (a blood test that gives your doctor a snapshot of your sugar control over the previous three months), which may suggest if you have insulin resistance. When corrected for age and BMI, fasting glucose, 2-hour glucose on OGTT and triglycerides were the best predictors and it is recommended these tests are done as a baseline and then every one to three years, based on individual risk.[9] Tests for insulin resistance. are not currently recommended in the UK for PCOS but can be calculated from fasting insulin and fasting glucose levels using certain commercially available tests, if your doctor thinks it will benefit you.

Treating insulin resistance

It is actually possible to reverse insulin resistance, particularly in the early stages. You want your body's cells to become sensitive to the action of insulin again so that glucose gets cleared from your bloodstream and picked up by your cells more efficiently, meaning your pancreas can stop producing so much insulin. By making changes to your lifestyle (see Chapter 11), you can make your tissues more sensitive to insulin and help avoid the longer-term effects of untreated insulin resistance which can cause PCOS, metabolic syndrome and type 2 diabetes.

The foods you eat (Chapter 12) can also help you reverse insulin resistance by normalising your blood sugars, thus dropping your insulin levels.

One of the major advantages of adopting a delicious whole food plant-based diet is that, as it is naturally low in unhealthy dietary fats while being rich in fibre, it helps your tissues to become sensitive to the action of insulin once again with no compromise to your taste buds.

In some cases, losing even small amounts of excess body weight reduces the amount of intracellular fat within the cells, especially in vital organs such as the liver, making them more sensitive to insulin. This in turn lowers insulin levels, reduces insulin resistance and improves SHBG levels, with many noticing an improvement in their PCOS symptoms. Fad diets that promise all kinds of unsubstantiated benefits and quick fixes may result in an initial weight loss if a calorie deficit is achieved. However, eating mostly whole plant foods is healthful and sustainable and helps improve weight loss if desired without miserable calorie counting. Eating fibre-rich plant foods helps the liver to increase the production of SHBG, which may help in further lowering circulating testosterone and oestrogen levels.

Ultra-processed foods high in refined carbohydrates, added sugar and unhealthy fats, should be significantly reduced along with animal-derived foods (red meat, chicken, dairy, eggs) as all these foods have been shown to worsen insulin resistance.

Physical movement and exercise are immensely helpful in improving tissue sensitivity to insulin, especially when undertaken 30 minutes after the start of a meal. This is because initiating exercise during this time window dampens blood sugar swings that typically tend to peak within 90 minutes of eating a meal. Even a short brisk walk after a meal can go a long way to making a difference.

Exercising after a meal, ideally 30 minutes after the start of a meal, is safe and is effective in managing insulin resistance as well as type 2 diabetes. All types of physical activity can help, especially muscle strengthening and aerobic forms of exercise. Exercise also improves SHBG production by the liver, lowering circulating testosterone levels. This in turn often results in improvement in your acne or reducing facial and body hair.

You will find that by ensuring a good sleep routine and managing stress, levels of your stress hormones – such as cortisol – will come down, helping to improve insulin sensitivity also. Similarly, alcohol and smoking can make insulin resistance worse, so staying away from these risky substances when you have insulin resistance is sensible.

Prescribing medications for managing PCOS-related insulin resistance

There was initial widespread enthusiasm in the medical field for the use of insulin-sensitising medications, such as metformin, in PCOS-related insulin resistance and androgen excess, but research findings no longer support this approach. In fact, a systematic review and meta-analysis of published research, looking at all the available data, published in 2020 in the leading journal *Nature* actively recommended lifestyle modifications to women with PCOS over routine use of metformin.[14] Metformin for PCOS is an 'off-label' prescription, which means that where prescribed it is being used for an unapproved indication in a patient population or at an unapproved dosage. There are very few valid reasons for its use, mostly when other first-line medications, such as the combined Pill (COCP) or fertility medications are not appropriate. It is still, however, prescribed very often for PCOS without due consideration of lifestyle changes. There is currently no evidence that the use of these insulin-sensitising drugs confers any long-term benefit.[15]

These medications may also contribute to vitamin B12 deficiency and other mild gastrointestinal side effects.

Treating the root cause of PCOS

By making lifestyle changes, as described in Chapters 11 and 12, your insulin resistance should improve and you may notice significant improvements in your symptoms of androgen excess and the return of your menstrual cycles. This is because you are treating the root cause of your PCOS, all while avoiding negative side effects of medication. Experts agree that lifestyle changes should be the first step before offering medications in the vast majority of those living with PCOS.

The PCOS Myth Buster

Myth: I have been recommended to eat more animal protein to treat my insulin resistance.
The facts: Animal-sourced foods, such as red meat, chicken, eggs and dairy, including highly processed meats, are the main source of excessive amounts of saturated fats and protein in many fad diets as well as in a standard western-style diet. These foods, when eaten regularly in high amounts, may trick you initially into thinking you are seeing an improvement as your blood sugar levels drop. This is because these foods contain very few carbohydrates. However, over time, as fat continues to accumulate within your muscle and other cells, the tissues become even more resistant to the action of the hormone insulin. It becomes a losing battle, failing to treat the insulin resistance that many of these diets high in animal protein and fat promise to do. Frustration sets in and one diet is given up for another

---

to be attempted only to find it too fails to deliver. In fact, there are no long-term studies that support eating high amounts of animal-derived foods. In Chapter 12, I highlight the benefits of eating more whole plant foods to manage insulin resistance and discuss other diets.

PCOS POINTERS

- Insulin resistance (IR) is one of the key underlying drivers of PCOS.
- High insulin levels are responsible for many of the symptoms of PCOS.
- Genetics and excess body weight both have a role in IR.
- It is possible to reverse IR with weight loss, if excess weight is present, especially in the early stages.
- A plant-based diet of whole or minimally-processed plant foods reduces IR.
- High-animal-protein and high-animal-fat/low-carb-diets both make IR worse in the long term.
- All types of physical activity can help to make tissues more sensitive to insulin.
- Consider exercising shortly after a meal for even more benefit.
- Lifestyle changes are more effective than medications and should be adopted first in PCOS.

6

Androgen excess
Hyperandrogenism

Case study: Mina

Mina, a 32-year-old, busy marketing manager had been
diagnosed with PCOS several years before coming to see me
because of her 'terrible skin' and irregular periods. She was
offered the Pill to manage her symptoms and this suited her as
she also needed effective contraception at the time. She had
not really been advised a great deal about her condition and
had just been relieved to see her skin clear up.

Mina came to see me as her periods were once again irregular
after coming off the Pill. She was planning to try to conceive.
During the consultation, she mentioned she was spending
a fortune to get rid of excess facial and body hair as well as
on skincare to manage her acne breakouts and supplements
to prevent recent scalp hair loss. She wanted to know if her
symptoms were connected. She was eager to find answers
and get medical help. It was important to start with improving
Mina's understanding of PCOS.

Androgen excess is responsible for many of the most common and often distressing PCOS symptoms. It can add significant financial costs due to the various cosmetic therapies and medications used to manage symptoms, often without tackling the root cause, creating further stress and anxiety. I discussed what androgens are and their role in Chapter 1. Testosterone is the best known of all androgens and the terms are often used interchangeably.

The symptoms of androgen excess are easily visible to others, making many people with PCOS feel extremely vulnerable to throwaway unhelpful comments and sometimes dangerous advice. My patients tell me that using simple language while addressing the symptoms of androgen excess which also avoids shaming or stigmatising is important (such as 'excess hair growth' instead of 'hirsute'). The medical term for an excess of androgens is 'hyperandrogenism'.

Symptoms of androgen excess

The three clinical symptoms you may notice from having an excess of androgens with PCOS are acne, excessive facial or body hair and hair loss from the scalp. Most people with PCOS tend to have some evidence of androgen excess (either clinical symptoms and/or from blood tests). However, many people with PCOS will not have elevated testosterone blood levels, despite having clinical symptoms of acne or excess hair growth. Interestingly, the reverse can be true as well. Some women with PCOS may have increased blood androgen levels but show none of the clinical signs, although in my experience that is unusual.

The cause of androgen excess in PCOS

In the vast majority of people with PCOS (50-70%), the main mechanism for androgen excess appears to be as a result of insulin resistance. You may be producing more testosterone than normal as higher circulating levels of insulin and insulin-like growth factor (IGF-1) in this situation stimulate the ovaries to increase testosterone production (see Chapter 5).

High levels of insulin also reduce the liver protein, sex hormone binding globulin (SHBG), which binds to testosterone. Lower levels of SHBG mean there is increased free testosterone available to the tissues,[1] causing the androgen-related PCOS symptoms of acne, hair loss and excess facial and body hair growth. This is why it is important to measure both total testosterone and SHBG levels in the blood to calculate what is called the free androgen index (FAI). Both a plant-based diet that is rich in fibre and exercise help to increase levels of SHBG.[1]

Although it is true that excess weight is a risk factor, PCOS also affects two out of 10 people in the healthy body weight range (often referred to as having 'lean PCOS'), who show evidence of insulin resistance and androgen excess. A significant proportion of those with lean PCOS are found in studies using MRI scans to have increased amounts of intra-abdominal fat (fat that is hidden on the inside), which you may have heard referred to as 'skinny fat'.[2]

The second mechanism for androgen excess is when excess fat collects within the tissues (intracellular fat), meaning that even more oestrogen is produced. This increased oestrogen level in the body causes a small but sustained increase of luteinising hormone (LH), causing a negative feedback loop. The brain tells the ovaries to stop producing oestrogen, so androgens build up. Remember, all oestrogen is produced from androgens (page 21).

In addition, the ovaries now spontaneously start producing more testosterone rather than oestrogen in response to these signals from the brain.[3, 4] This in turn suppresses the release of eggs from the ovaries (ovulation). This is why irregular periods usually accompany symptoms of androgen excess. Losing weight often results in a return of menstrual cycles and improvement in acne and excess hair growth. I have seen this repeatedly in my patients.

Androgen sensitivity

There appears to be yet another mechanism by which those with PCOS, especially those carrying no extra fat and with normal testosterone levels, show signs of androgen excess, such as hormonal cystic acne, excessive facial hair growth, oily skin and even scalp hair loss. This is thought to be due to an increased concentration of testosterone within the hair follicles and skin receptors as well as a heightened sensitivity of the skin to the effects of testosterone. The reasons for this are unclear and more research is definitely needed in this area, as it could guide doctors to suggest more targeted treatment.

Serious causes of androgen excess

The commonest cause of androgen excess is PCOS. However, some rarer but serious conditions such as androgen-secreting ovarian tumours or non-classic congenital adrenal hyperplasia (NCCAH), adrenal tumours and Cushing's syndrome cause excess androgen production by the adrenal glands. These need urgent referral to an endocrinologist for specialised tests and treatment. A rapid growth of facial or body hair, a deepening in voice, male pattern balding, recent increase in the size of the clitoris, severe acne, scalp hair loss or increased muscle mass are all possible symptoms of a condition known as 'virilisation' and need urgent medical attention. Thankfully, this is very rare.

Help, this is all too complicated!

Please do not worry if you find this all too difficult to understand. I just want you to remember that if you have excess weight, losing even a small amount can help with the symptoms of androgen excess and insulin resistance. Even if you do not have excess weight and have PCOS, your skin and hair follicles may be excessively sensitive to increased androgens produced locally. It also helps to understand that your androgen (often used interchangeably with testosterone) blood levels may be completely normal but you can still have all the clinical symptoms of androgen excess. You should still be able to follow the advice in this book while seeking medical advice from a trusted health professional.

How to help myself

It is important to advocate for yourself so you get the best treatment. I understand it is easy sometimes to feel overwhelmed in a doctor's office but you must let them know if your symptoms are causing you emotional distress.

You can help by having as much information as possible at the ready to share with your health professional, such as duration and extent of hair loss, previous treatment, supplements you may be taking, any other relevant medical history, recent or chronic illnesses, any recent stressful events, drugs that you may be on, history of dieting, recent pregnancies if applicable, family history and your menstrual history. It is also helpful to make a note of your haircare routine and the products you use on your face and body.

If you think you have other symptoms of PCOS, then you should ask your doctor for further assessment (see Chapter 4).

Before starting any conventional treatment for managing the clinical symptoms of PCOS, ask for your androgen levels to be checked as a baseline (testosterone, SHBG, FAI as a minimum). However, your symptoms may not always correlate with your circulating androgen levels and your blood tests may be normal. This does not mean you do not have PCOS as diagnosis of the condition depends on a number of factors, as described in Chapter 3.

Choose lifestyle modifications always, with or without other treatments

PCOS-related androgen excess symptoms often respond well to dietary changes and exercise. Lifestyle behaviour change should be brought in irrespective of whether you need medication or not. Healthy lifestyle habits reduce both generalised and local inflammation associated with PCOS, even if you do not have weight to lose (lean PCOS).

Following a predominantly plant-based way of eating can usually help improve androgen excess and help with weight loss, where desired, as well as improve insulin resistance.[5]

Medical therapies for managing androgen excess

If you have PCOS and also wish to avoid pregnancy, symptoms of androgen excess can be successfully managed by suppression of androgens with the combined oral contraceptive pill (COCP), which contains both oestrogen and progesterone in varying proportions. Ask your doctor to prescribe a COCP preparation that contains a type of progesterone that does not worsen hair growth (low androgenic potential). If the Pill is not advisable, other drugs that work by blocking androgens, such as spironolactone and cyproterone, can help, but cannot be prescribed if you are actively trying for a pregnancy.

Skincare routines and cosmetic skin and hair treatments can all help to reduce the symptoms of androgen excess, such as acne flare ups and unwanted hair growth. I do want to stress that while conventional treatments are invaluable in helping to improve your skin and hair, to truly tackle your PCOS symptoms, addressing the root cause is important. You can do this by makes changes to what you eat alongside the other lifestyle measures discussed in detail in Chapters 11 and 12.

Getting a specialist referral early from your family doctor can sometimes help you address the individual aspects of androgen excess. For example, you may benefit from seeing a qualified dietitian or nutritionist for medical nutrition therapy, a dermatologist for acne, a qualified hair-loss specialist (trichologist), or a gynaecologist or endocrinologist with a special interest in PCOS.

I suggest being open to using conventional medicine alongside lifestyle and dietary measures as well as cosmetic therapies for the best outcomes. There is a lot of dangerous misinformation out there, especially bashing the Pill, so it is critical that you access reliable and factual health sources based on scientific evidence.

Case study outcome: Mina

Six months later, Mina sat in the chair opposite me in my clinic looking so much more relaxed than on her first visit. She was eating almost completely plant-based and had joined her local running group. Not only had she lost a few pounds, but her periods had come every month for the last four months, her skin had cleared up hugely and she was sleeping better. She had learned to manage her excess hair growth and was amazed at the improvement in her symptoms. Her partner had also benefited from the dietary changes and had seen an improvement in his energy levels and overall wellbeing.

The PCOS Myth Buster

Myth: Testosterone is just a 'male' hormone
The facts: Testosterone is a hormone produced by all genders. It is often referred to wrongly as the 'male' hormone, which reinforces the gender binary and adds to the stigma associated with PCOS, as most women with PCOS have some symptoms of androgen (testosterone) excess, such as acne or excess hair growth. The truth is that all humans produce all three sex hormones – testosterone, oestrogen and progesterone – in different amounts, depending on their gender, age and stage of life.

The PCOS Myth Buster

Myth: Oestrogen dominance is responsible for hormone-related issues
The facts: The term 'oestrogen dominance' has caught on in popularity but needs debunking, as there are all kinds of reasons cited, from your liver or adrenal glands not working to stress being responsible. There are tiny grains of truth in some of these claims but oestrogen dominance is not a medical condition. The implication of being given this diagnosis, usually by those not qualified to make scientific medical diagnoses, is that if a woman is producing too much oestrogen, then the obvious answer is to prescribe progesterone to balance the hormones. This is too simplistic a solution and can be dangerous. There are now dozens of dubious preparations containing unregulated amounts of progesterone and unproven supplements. These can cause erratic bleeding and other longer-term issues, if taken for a

prolonged period without a proper diagnosis. Yes, oestro-gen-dependent conditions, such as fibroids, endometriosis, breast cancer and PCOS, do get worse in the presence of excess weight, a topic I discuss in the next chapter. Our body fat is a storehouse of hormones, and increased fat in the cells results in increased oestrogen being produced. The answer to treating this excess oestrogen is through weight loss and addressing other lifestyle factors, as we discuss in Chapter 12, and not through taking unproven medications.

When indicated, medically supervised use of progesterone medications can be used to induce regular shedding of the lining of the womb. For example, in PCOS, if you do not wish to take the Pill and if you do not have periods for months at a time, doctors may prescribe progesterone every three months in a cyclical fashion to protect your uterus from overgrowth of its lining and subsequent possible endome-trial hyperplasia and womb cancer (see Chapter 23).

PCOS POINTERS

Symptoms that may suggest androgen excess are:
- Acne
- Excessive facial or body hair growth
- Scalp hair loss or thinning.

Causes of androgen excess include:
- Insulin resistance
- Excess body fat
- Local skin and hair androgen sensitivity.

7

One size does not fit all
Body weight and PCOS

Many of my patients with PCOS who have excess weight mention feeling ashamed, judged and blamed. Negative attitudes and weight stigma often start early within the family, then in school, and, sadly, even in the healthcare setting. These often include false perceptions of people in larger bodies as 'lazy, sloppy, unintelligent, unattractive, lacking self-discipline' as reported from studies on bias and discrimination.

Those living with PCOS commonly report long delays in diagnosis and dissatisfaction with their care. Not being taken seriously as a result of weight stigma is part of this problem.

Fighting stigma

Throwaway comments can affect self-worth and damage the trust and overall relationship with your health professional.[4] Doctors in most settings, including those in primary care and even those specialising in 'obesity management', have been found to discriminate against patients with excess weight.[5] Such negative attitudes are common and serious as they adversely affect patient outcomes.[4, 5, 6] This in turn results in mistrust of the healthcare system, increased stress levels and feeling dismissed or judged. Negative experiences can lead to patients avoiding or delaying seeking medical help. Feeling stigmatised can result in a reduced overall quality of care, even when that may not be the intention of the healthcare professional.[5]

Weight is a sensitive issue for some

To nurture a kind and just society, we have to start listening and asking people what language we should be using to talk about them, whether it is to do with their weight, skin colour or preferred gender pronouns. People don't have control over several aspects of their health, including weight to a large extent, for a number of complex socioeconomic reasons as well as a legacy of discrimination that has lasted for generations.

Educating through kindness brings far greater satisfaction and encourages positive behaviour change. Shaming or belittling serves little purpose except to demotivate, amounting to bullying and harassment. It is time to call out language or behaviour that is unacceptable if you see it around you, and at the same time, we should all be putting in the effort to learn more appropriate terminology. We also have to learn to apologise when corrected and be willing to be challenged when we make mistakes. I am still learning how best to use more inclusive language and terminology.

Change how we communicate

While 'overweight, obese and obesity' may be medical terms, people find these terms along with words like 'fat' or 'fatness' 'heaviness' 'large size' and 'excess fat' used by public and healthcare professionals to carry negative and demeaning social connotations and consider them undesirable for describing excess weight. The term 'fat' is being reclaimed by many who urge to use it as a descriptor, rather than a derogatory term but health professionals should refrain from using it unless the patient has requested it.

My advice to you is to tell your health professional what terminology you prefer. Educate those around you that weight is a complex issue, as is PCOS.

BMI: an outdated measure

Body mass index (BMI) is a ratio for weight and height and is still the most widely used measurement to check if a person is of healthy weight. It is easy to measure, inexpensive and strongly correlates with body fat levels. Hundreds of studies show a high BMI predicts higher risk of chronic disease and early death. It is, however, an imperfect measurement of body fat, especially in some ethnic groups, athletes, older people and people assigned female at birth (AFAB). It also does not consider the person's body composition (body fat, muscle, bone or fluid) or where excess weight is distributed, meaning that it must not be relied on alone to predict health outcomes. For example, athletes may be classed as 'obese' according to BMI metrics because they have a higher ratio of muscle to fat and muscle weighs more.

Other measurements can be used, such as waist circumference and waist-to-hip ratio, both measuring extra fat found around the middle. This is an important factor in predicting disease, even independent of BMI. Such measurements are inexpensive to make and show strong correlations with body fat levels but can be difficult to obtain accurately, especially in those of higher weight. Skinfold thickness using calipers to measure the fat beneath the skin and other more complicated methods also exist.

CT and MRI scans are the most accurate but are typically only used for this purpose in research settings.[8] Studies using these scans have found increased intra-abdominal fat content in women with PCOS in the classed as healthy weight range (lean PCOS) when compared with age- and BMI-matched controls.[9, 10]

Excess weight and PCOS

Most studies included in a 2019 systematic review (see the Glossary) could not conclusively determine whether PCOS contributed to excess weight gain or if excess weight caused PCOS.[3, 11] The complex nature and the varied symptoms of PCOS have made it particularly hard to understand the correlation of PCOS with body fat distribution and excess weight. However, excess weight can be an important factor in predicting PCOS and in those who are genetically predisposed to PCOS, insulin resistance can lead to weight gain. Women with PCOS also appear to have higher genetic susceptibility to putting on excess weight.[12]

Weight gain over 10 years among women with PCOS was significantly greater than in unaffected women in a longitudinal community-based study (see Glossary).[13] With PCOS, weight gain starts to escalate from the teenage years, increasing the risk of disordered eating, so early vigilance and intervention by your doctor are important.[12]

Excess weight, especially when around the middle, worsens insulin resistance and many PCOS symptoms.[3] Over time, women may notice a progressive increase in waist-to-hip measurements between 20 years and 45 years.[14] Even in the absence of PCOS, excess weight can cause irregular periods because of increased oestrogen levels which are associated with increased body weight causing hormonal disturbances.

Womb cancer risks are increased in the presence of excess weight, which is the biggest modifiable risk factor for womb cancer, according to Cancer Research UK. In addition, PCOS itself is a risk factor for womb cancer because of very irregular periods resulting from unopposed high oestrogen levels. Insulin resistance and type

2 diabetes, both strongly associated with PCOS, are also known risk factors for womb cancer. As many other cancer risks, including for breast, bowel and ovarian cancer, are increased significantly in the presence of excess weight, seeking help early can help save lives.

Concerns of those with PCOS

Women with PCOS have reported that their excess weight causes them the most distress and concern. Difficulty in losing weight was a common concern, more important than irregular menstrual cycles and subfertility, when patient groups were questioned.[12, 15]

It appears that those with excess weight may be more likely to seek medical help, making it appear that people with PCOS are of higher weight than their peers.[3, 11, 16] All international PCOS guidelines agree that weight reduction by 5 to 10% of total body weight in six months in those with excess weight has shown metabolic, reproductive and psychological benefits. Any diet pattern irrespective of composition, in the presence of healthy food choices, can work as per the latest international guidelines for PCOS.[12]

Long-term weight loss is an extraordinarily complex issue. It involves more than just diet and exercise and requires behaviour change as psychological factors play a critical role. International guidelines for PCOS[12] highlight the need for behavioural strategies, such as goal setting, self-monitoring and establishing routines. Unless behavioural factors are considered and addressed, adherence to lifestyle interventions are destined to fail.

People living with PCOS feel there is inadequate information and support around lifestyle change.[12, 17] Many are confused as to the best way to lose weight and keep it off as that is the hardest thing to do. Most patients I meet with excess weight want to lose some of it. They have been on many diets and after some initial successes are back to square one, feeling even more frustrated and helpless.

A different approach to weight loss

I recommend motivating yourself to adopt healthy lifestyle changes without focusing on weight loss as the only goal. Instead, shift your attention to a way of living that improves your other symptoms of PCOS and also has a positive side effect: one of sustainable and long-lasting weight loss. By optimising hormonal and general health through nutrition and lifestyle changes (see Chapters 11 and 12), your quality of life will improve in both the short-term and the long-term. Changing your mindset and attitude may appear hard and even overwhelming at the start but having seen so many successes, I know it can be done.

Leading authorities on nutrition agree that eating more fruit, vegetables, beans and whole grains is healthful for all populations at all ages and stages of life, both for optimal health and disease prevention.[18] The current scientific evidence, including long-term observational studies, strongly suggests a plant-predominant or plant-exclusive diet offers the most health benefits to people of all backgrounds. None of the fad diets which focus on excluding complex, healthy carbohydrates (animal-based keto, paleo, high-fat low-carbohydrate or high-protein low-carbohydrate diets) have been shown to have any robust data that cover a period longer than a few months, and low-carbohydrate diets can indeed be harmful in the medium to long term (see Chapter 12).[19, 20]

Why weight loss can help in PCOS

It appears that weight loss on its own does help as studies show losing weight with any kind of diet does result in improvement, even if temporarily. Weight loss, especially losing weight around your middle, helps with PCOS symptoms by reducing the amount of fat deposition within the cells; that in turn makes the tissues more sensitive to insulin so less insulin resistant. Weight loss also reduces the amount of excess oestrogen circulating in the body. In other words, weight loss can result in improvement in the symptoms of PCOS by improving insulin resistance, reducing testosterone and oestrogen hormone levels, improving body composition and reducing BMI.[21, 22]

People respond to weight loss differently. More than one third of women with PCOS achieved full recovery following sustained weight loss with mild calorie restriction and physical activity in a small 2011 follow-up study. Others saw significant improvements but not complete resolution with similar amounts of weight reduction.[23] More studies are needed with larger numbers of patients to confirm these findings.

How to help yourself

You deserve to receive proper care and non-judgmental advice at every step of your health journey. Ideally, weight loss or weight maintenance alone should not be your only goal but should be factored into sustainable and long-term lifestyle changes. If you have a history of disordered eating or a current eating disorder, it can help to work with an experienced health professional who can guide you as an individual, understanding that potential triggers such as weigh-ins are unlikely to be appropriate. Your doctor or a local PCOS group may be able to guide you to the right person.

Looking for change

Remember that it is your body and your choice. Not everyone with PCOS wishes to lose weight. It is important for your health professional to identify if your weight affects the way you feel about yourself and if you are dissatisfied with your eating patterns. If that is the case, you should be offered appropriate help and further assessment from a qualified health professional.

Worth at every size

We need to stop assuming someone's health status based on how they look. Not all those who are in smaller bodies are healthy. Weight loss as a way of managing your PCOS is scientifically important but don't worry if you decide you don't want to or cannot focus on that due to a current or past history of disordered eating, or any other issue. It is better to focus on healthy behaviours and the other pillars of lifestyle, such as getting adequate restful sleep, eating more fruit and vegetables and reducing stress (see Chapter 10).

You should also be open to medications and/or weight loss (bariatric) surgery, if needed to help you achieve your goals. There should be no shame in this. You have one life and you want to live it the best way you possibly can.

Goal setting and self-monitoring

It is helpful to seek the support of qualified, empathetic health professionals so you develop good skills to manage your condition. Setting yourself goals, such as doing a 'couch to 5K' or a charity walkathon, can help to motivate you. You may find support groups, both face-to-face and online, that help you through difficult times, allowing you to share common experiences that you may not be able to do as easily with friends or family.[24]

Staying focused on health goals and health-promoting behaviours rather than solely fixating on weight loss can be helpful. Even if you do not have excess weight to lose, lifestyle modifications can improve all aspects of PCOS.

The PCOS Myth Buster

Myth: It is impossible to lose weight if I have PCOS.
The facts: This statement is not true. While it appears to be easier both to gain and to hold on to excess weight for many living with PCOS, weight loss can be successfully achieved and maintained by embracing behaviour, dietary and lifestyle changes. Ideally, choosing a goal that does not fixate only on weight loss tends to bring the biggest rewards. 'I want to get fitter', 'I want to stay healthy to be able to travel,' 'I want to walk my dog without getting breathless' are some goals my patients have chosen and experienced satisfying weight loss as a positive side effect. However, if this does not have the desired effect for you by six months, then your doctor may consider weight loss medications and/or bariatric surgery in appropriate situations, after a thorough and informed discussion with you.[25, 26]

PCOS POINTERS

- The use of inclusive language should be encouraged both in society and by health professionals when discussing body weight.
- It is not clear whether PCOS causes weight gain or vice versa.
- Weight loss, if desired, can significantly improve symptoms of PCOS in people with excess weight.
- Weight loss methods should be sustainable rather than short-term fixes.
- Adopting healthy behaviours rather than focusing on weight loss as a goal can have more achievable results.
- Focus on how your body feels rather than numbers on a scale.

8

Not just teenage angst
Adolescent PCOS

Case study: Megan

Sixteen-year-old Megan came to see me because of her missed periods. She was accompanied by her mother. I always like to check my patients are happy for their carers to be present. Megan was keen for her mother, Sue, to be present throughout the consultations.

Megan's periods had been irregular from the time they had started at the age of 12, coming every couple of months. They could be heavy enough for Megan to miss school on the first few days, but for the last six months Megan had not had her period. As I asked some questions, it became apparent that Megan was very conscious of her darker facial and chest hair as well her acne which mostly seemed to be on her chin and back. She suffered with mood swings, often staying in her room for hours, missing meals and not coming to the dinner table.

Megan said she hated PE in school and Sue suggested it

was perhaps because Megan felt self-conscious about her weight. Megan had never been sexually active and the first thing she said to me was she did not want to take the Pill (COCP) which she had been offered by her family doctor, as she (mistakenly) believed she would put on weight while on it. She appeared fidgety and anxious, not making a lot of eye contact. I realised there was a lot to unpack and I would need to spend extra time with her.

Adolescent PCOS

PCOS starts in the teenage years, although typically, the diagnosis may not be considered by doctors and can often be delayed for years. The predisposition to developing insulin resistance and androgen excess, both hallmarks of PCOS, is thought to start when you are in the womb. Environmental factors such as stress and nutrition play a part in modifying genes from your parents.[1, 2, 3] However, birth weight has not been consistently associated one way or the other with future development of PCOS and more research is needed in this area.[4]

Diagnosing PCOS in teenagers

PCOS as a diagnosis should be considered in any adolescent girl with excessive facial or body hair growth and/or acne that does not respond to simple treatments, along with irregular menstrual cycles, especially if associated with excess weight gain. The diagnosis is one of exclusion, meaning other serious causes need to be ruled out first (see Chapter 6).

To be diagnosed as a teenager with PCOS, the first two of the three diagnostic Rotterdam criteria (see page 40) is a requirement. In other words, both irregular menstrual cycles and evidence of androgen excess from either physical signs (acne or excess hair growth) or laboratory findings from blood tests must be present.

An ultrasound scan is not helpful for the diagnosis of PCOS in teenagers within eight years of them starting their periods. This is because many young people have multi-follicular ovaries at this life stage which can mimic the multiple small follicles seen in PCOS. This can lead to over-diagnosis of PCOS. However, if there is a concern about heavy periods or ovarian cysts, or if considering another diagnosis, then your doctor may suggest an ultrasound scan (see Chapter 4).

Reassess for PCOS if at increased risk

Some teenagers have symptoms of PCOS but do not meet the strict diagnostic criteria mentioned above. They should be considered to be at 'increased risk' of the condition and reviewed again eight years after starting their periods. For example, if you started your periods at 13 and have some PCOS symptoms, you should be reassessed for PCOS around the age of 21. This is especially important to follow through if you had some symptoms of PCOS before starting the Pill for any reason (for your skin, heavy or painful periods or if you needed contraception). You should also ask to be reviewed for PCOS if any of your symptoms persist (see Chapter 3) or if you are gaining significant weight without intending to. The Pill does need to be stopped for approximately two to three months before doing tests to confirm PCOS. Do use effective alternative contraception if you are having penetrative vaginal sex.

At the clinic

You may be feeling rather vulnerable and anxious so do consider asking your parent/carer to accompany you to your appointment. This may also be your first visit to the doctor for an intimate situation. The doctor should put you at ease while taking a detailed medical history and performing a general examination (see Chapter 4). If you are the carer or parent, ask that the doctor takes extra time if needed to put your teenager at ease. No internal examinations should be performed on someone who has never had penetrative vaginal sex.

You are allowed to ask your carer to leave the room if you wish to discuss any confidential issues. This is absolutely fine but do insist there is another chaperone from the clinic present throughout the consultation.

Managing adolescent PCOS

Teenagers with PCOS are at increased risk of anxiety and/or depression and disordered eating. Your doctor may suggest an urgent referral to an age-appropriate eating disorder centre or for psychological support in your local area, where available, if they feel you would benefit. This is based on the information you or your carer has shared with them.

You may be asked to consider having your blood tested to check your hormone levels and if your body weight is outside the range for your age group, for your glucose (sugar) levels to be checked (see Chapter 4). If you are not comfortable, you can decline or ask not to have the number read out to you when you stand on the scale.

Just as for adults with PCOS, lifestyle advice can be very useful for you as a teenager as this will help you manage many of the problems associated with your condition. As you are still growing, focus on consuming a healthy diet with an emphasis on plant foods such as fruit and vegetables, whole grains, beans, nuts and seeds, rather than only on weight loss.

Remember body weight is a complex issue and it is better to have help from a qualified and empathetic dietitian or nutritionist sooner rather than later. Don't hesitate to ask your doctor about this as losing even a small amount of weight healthily can boost your mood and help with regulating your hormones. You may also see an improvement in your acne and excess hair growth as weight loss helps to improve insulin resistance (see Chapter 5). However, do avoid restrictive diets, as these can increase your risk of developing an eating disorder.

Making a few lifestyle changes, both with food and exercise, may be enough to regulate your periods and reduce androgen-excess symptoms, especially acne, whether or not you choose to take hormonal medication. Local methods of hair removal, such as shaving, bleaching, or waxing, can also be very helpful if you wish to manage any excess hair growth on your face or body.

The Pill for teenage PCOS

The combined oral contraceptive (COCP) pill does give the best results if you are distressed by excess hair growth, cystic acne or missed periods, provided there are no contraindications (see Chapter 13). Mood was found to be more affected when taking the Pill in teenagers compared with adults, as was indicated in a large Danish study published in 2016,[7] with depression as a potential side effect of hormonal contraceptive use, higher in those using progestogen-only pills. A smaller study in 2019 did not find any significant increase in depressive disorders with COCP use in teenagers. I recommend having an open and honest discussion with your doctor of all the potential risks and benefits of the Pill before you reach a decision. You can be reassured that weight gain is not a side effect of the Pill. In my experience, seeing improvements in excess hair growth and clearing of skin on the Pill helps improve mood in many of my teenage patients. Your doctor should regularly ask you about your mood at your check up at six to 12 monthly intervals and before you pick up repeat prescriptions. Do remember to mention any symptoms that you may have noticed in recent weeks or months.

The Pill can be taken back-to-back, as there is no medical need for a monthly withdrawal bleed whilst on it, giving additional relief from painful or heavy periods, if that is an issue for you.

The Pill can be stopped at any time if you are unhappy with its effects. Having control and being involved in decision-making allows you to consider all options, which can improve your quality of life. Even small lifestyle changes alongside the Pill can help with PCOS symptoms. There are also other non-hormonal medications for acne and excess hair growth which may benefit you (see Chapters 16 and 17).

You may find patient resources and links to support groups helpful. They can encourage you to read more about your condition in your own time and speak to others in similar situations.

Case study outcome: Megan

Following our consultation, Megan had a few tests to confirm PCOS. We had a long discussion regarding the lifestyle changes that she would be willing to consider. I suggested adding one more fruit and one more vegetable to the ones she already liked and slowly building up to more. We discussed the importance of breakfast and not worrying about calorie counting. Links to support helpful groups (see page 382).

At Megan and her mum's request, I referred her to a private nutritionist for support and planning of her meals around foods she enjoyed. She loved dancing so I suggested she did 15 minutes of dancing a day in her room to music she enjoyed. The plan was to build on this. She did not wish to be referred to a therapist at this stage or to take the Pill and her mother agreed. I suggested they contact Megan's family doctor for a referral to a therapist via the NHS, if they changed their minds.

When we caught up three months later, Megan proudly told me she had not needed to miss school even for a single day. She had really started enjoying the dietary changes. She had had one period, had dropped a couple of sizes, and noticed her skin was clearer too. On review six months later, there was enough improvement for her to stay off the Pill as her periods were now coming every month.

I discharged Megan a year later, confident that she would maintain these changes and make even more as she went along, having seen the benefits first hand. She also understood that she could take the Pill for contraception without worrying about weight if she decided to go on it. Both Megan and her mother understood the importance of regular review with their own family doctor and to seek future specialist help if needed.

The PCOS Myth Buster

Myth: All teenagers have irregular periods.
The facts: This is not really true. Irregular menstrual cycles are acceptable only in the first year after menarche (the first period) as part of the transition into puberty. When irregular

menstrual cycles, such as missed or delayed periods, are present over three months in a row, the possibility of PCOS should be considered and medical advice sought (see Chapter 1).

PCOS POINTERS

- PCOS is thought to start in the teenage years.
- Menstrual irregularities and symptoms of androgen excess (acne and/or excess hair growth or evidence on blood tests) must both be present for diagnosis.
- An ultrasound scan is unreliable to diagnose PCOS in teenagers.
- Parents, caretakers and healthcare professionals should be sensitive in their handling of the situation.
- Screening questions should be asked regarding eating disorders, mood and sleep.
- Adopt an overall healthy way of eating rather than calorie counting or dieting, which can have a negative impact on mental and physical health.
- Lifestyle changes can help in both the short and the long term.
- Some teenagers will benefit from psychological therapy.
- The Pill can be useful in managing the symptoms of PCOS but you should be prescribed it only after a thorough discussion.

9

It's not fair
How PCOS affects people of colour

Why the ethnic and racial variations in those living with PCOS matter

This issue rarely gets enough attention. Most studies on PCOS have focused on white populations and the condition as currently understood is likely not representative of all. The prevalence of PCOS can vary widely depending on the populations studied and how hard we look for it. PCOS appears to affect South Asian, Black, Hispanic and Middle Eastern groups more than white groups. These groups also seem to be at a higher risk of excess weight, insulin resistance and many of the longer-term risks associated with PCOS for a number of reasons, including socioeconomic factors as well as historic and structural inequalities. If we fail to recognise these possible variations, many from these higher risk groups will miss out on the appropriate and timely treatment they need and deserve.

PCOS prevalence in racial subgroups

Evidence from a systematic review and meta-analysis in 2017[1] suggests that the highest prevalence of PCOS is seen in Black and Middle Eastern women (close to 20% had PCOS) followed by White European women, with the lowest prevalence (5.6%) among Chinese women.[2] The prevalence of PCOS in India ranged from 6% to 22.5% in studies, using different age groups and settings.[3]

Studies have confirmed the prevalence of PCOS in Mexican Americans to be at least twice as high as reported in other populations. They also appear to be more at risk of excess weight and insulin resistance.[4, 5] The prevalence of PCOS in Indigenous Australians in a small study was as high as 15% to 18%,[6, 7] while studies looking at European women from Spain and Greece found the prevalence to be much lower at 4-6%.[1, 8]

How symptoms vary in different groups

In the UK, women of South Asian origin with PCOS may have symptoms at a younger age and they may have more severe symptoms compared with white British women.[9, 10]

Symptoms of androgen excess, especially acne and excessive hair growth, may affect Hispanic women with PCOS more than women of Chinese Han origin with PCOS.[11] Excessive hair growth may be particularly troublesome for Middle Eastern, Hispanic and South Asian women living with PCOS.[12]

When compared with White women with PCOS, Black and Hispanic groups were more likely to be diagnosed with excess weight and Asian women were less likely; Asian and Hispanic women were more likely to have type 2 diabetes; and Black women were more likely to have higher body mass index (BMI) and raised blood pressure (hypertension).[13] However, I must stress that we shouldn't assume racial disparities in the symptoms of PCOS built on narratives that may not be true for you, as a specific individual. This may in turn put you at a disadvantage, irrespective of the colour of your skin.

Medical racism

Racism threatens and shortens lives, despite nearly 200 years of knowledge connecting racism to poor health outcomes.[13, 14] Health professionals will agree that disparities based on ethnicity are unacceptable. Most deny any conscious bias. However, we repeatedly see systemic biases that prevent Black and Indigenous people and people of colour accessing and receiving the care they urgently need. Inequalities based on ethnicity still permeate every aspect of healthcare, from conception to death. Most leading journals almost never publish scientific articles that name racism as a driver of poor health outcomes, with fewer than 1% including the word racism anywhere in the text.[15]

Maternal death rates were almost four times higher for women from Black ethnic backgrounds and almost two times higher for women from Asian ethnic backgrounds, compared with White women in the UK, in the 2021 MBRRACE-UK Confidential Enquiry report.[16] There was a similar finding in the 2019 report from the Oxford group, with Black women found to be five times more likely to die.[17] There has been a surprising lack of progress, with doctors and medical students of colour also often at the receiving end of discrimination.[18]

Black people are also less likely to be offered stronger pain relief, due to misconceptions dating back to slavery that Black people have higher pain tolerance.[19]

These inequalities were highlighted in the stark reality of the COVID-19 pandemic deaths, affecting many more from minority communities than others. These communities face significant health challenges, which include the effects of racism, discrimination, stress from daily micro and macro aggressions, poor access to green spaces, lack of access to appropriate housing and nutritious food, mental health stigma, and the effects of the criminal justice system. Chronic lifestyle diseases disproportionately affect minority groups.

Stereotyping in healthcare negatively impacts minority groups from accessing fertility treatment. The 'postcode lottery' (access to healthcare being dependent on where you live) and varying costs also have an impact. Women of colour are often seen as contributing to rapid population growth and having large families, which means individuals from these communities with fertility issues are sometimes unfairly dismissed.

In PCOS research too, interestingly there appears to be a racialised approach. Strong claims made by researchers about racial differences in 'male-pattern' hair growth in women with PCOS, as if they were established knowledge, can be dangerous, as highlighted in a recent 2020 paper on race and PCOS.[19]

If you suspect or know you have PCOS, try to find a family doctor you can trust and who understands your situation. Consider looking for local support groups which may help you with language translation and practical information.

PCOS in different ethnic groups

By using ethnic specific guidelines, screening for PCOS may need to be individualised for different racial or ethnic populations, as the same cut-off levels for insulin resistance tests and BMI used for the general population may result in missing the diagnosis of PCOS in many.[1]

I must stress that, irrespective of your ethnicity, if you notice symptoms that suggest that you may have PCOS, or if you notice a worsening of symptoms, you must seek medical guidance. This is because, regardless of your background, PCOS tends to be under-diagnosed and under-recognised, despite being the most common hormonal disorder to affect women. If you do not feel seen or heard, insist on seeing another health professional. There are many compassionate and non-judgemental doctors around.

The PCOS Myth Buster

Myth: Ethnic minorities are not really discriminated against in PCOS.
The facts: Unfortunately, this statement is not true, with both explicit and implicit bias existing amongst healthcare professionals and society against Black and Indigenous people and people of colour in all areas of health, including PCOS.

PCOS POINTERS

- Most studies on PCOS have focused on white populations.
- PCOS appears to affect Black and Indigenous people and people of colour more than White groups for complex reasons.
- Earlier screening for PCOS symptoms, especially for insulin resistance, should be offered for different groups.
- Medical racism exists and leads to poorer health outcomes.
- Insist on being heard and seek a second opinion if you feel dismissed.

Part Two

Making informed health choices

10

You are in the driving seat
Lifestyle Medicine

Case study: Nisha

Nisha, a 36-year-old lawyer by profession, had been diagnosed with PCOS 12 years earlier, following tests to investigate delayed periods. She had gone on the combined Pill (COCP) to manage her PCOS and for contraceptive purposes. For personal reasons, she had then decided to come off the Pill but her periods had not resumed. She was not worried initially but after a year of missing periods, Nisha came to see me in my clinic. She was not keen to return to taking the Pill.

I advised her to make lifestyle changes with a focus on nutrition and stress management. Within three months, her periods had returned and, after some initially longer cycles, she has had regular monthly periods for the last two years.

> When I see patient success stories like this, it makes all those long hours of training and years of hard work worthwhile.

The burden of chronic disease

Non-communicable chronic lifestyle diseases now make up seven of the world's top 10 causes of death, according to the World Health Organization's (WHO) 2019 Global Health Estimates. Heart disease is the number one killer worldwide, with dementia and diabetes both now in the top 10.[1] In the UK, heart disease kills twice as many women as breast cancer does.[2] Dementia is now worryingly the leading cause of death in women in the UK, accounting for 16.5% of all female deaths in 2018.[3] Western medicine is now dealing mainly with sick care rather than health care. Much of this death and disability appears to be avoidable, with similar statistics for all the high- and middle-income countries. Changes at policy level are even more important than those at an individual level.

This information is important for those with PCOS to know. Known longer-term risks of PCOS include womb cancer, metabolic syndrome, type 2 diabetes and possibly heart disease, especially for those with excess weight. Dementia risks also increase in the presence of excess weight.

More than just a job

The fulfilling career in Obstetrics and Gynaecology I chose over 35 years ago has never disappointed. It has been so gratifying to bring babies into the world, thrilling to save lives in acute emergencies and rewarding to perform complex surgical procedures to improve quality of life. From the start I loved what I did but, as the years went by, I became acutely aware that I was not preventing problems. I was seeing women after the disease process had already started. I felt as though I was firefighting a lot of the time and there had to be more to the puzzle. Surely, drugs and surgery could not be all that I had to offer my patients, even though that was what I had been taught in medical school?

A pill for all ills

When I trained to be a doctor, I did not receive any nutrition education, either in India or in the UK. To this day, most medical schools skim over nutrition as part of the curriculum. Doctors therefore tend to be confused about its role in preventing chronic lifestyle diseases; they typically offer pills and surgery rather than addressing diet and lifestyle factors to manage common conditions. Women's health is no exception. I too practised in this way for the first couple of decades of my medical career. Medications and surgery both still play very important roles in maintaining health for my patients when deployed correctly, but for long-term prevention and management of many health conditions, I feel differently.

In pursuit of the elixir of health, we often mistakenly think a pill will cure us of all ills. We hope that a health professional will have the answers. In reality, this isn't always true. In fact, there is a lot we can do for ourselves.

The missing pieces of the puzzle

Since 1986, I have treated thousands of patients. For decades, I have had the privilege of hearing about people's eating habits and lifestyles. It slowly dawned on me that the food we ate and the lifestyles we led were the missing pieces in the puzzle. These were the powerful tools I had been looking for to help my patients. I came to realise nutrition, along with other lifestyle interventions, goes hand in hand, complementing western medicine to promote health. These were the keys to good health. This is what we now know as Lifestyle Medicine.[4]

In 2012, I started to study in earnest and learn all about nutrition and lifestyle and their impact on health. There were thousands of scientific studies already out there. What I learnt was genuinely exciting. I could not wait to share my knowledge with my patients and with other health professionals, and have been delighted with the positive response.

Most of what other doctors and I see in our clinical practice is related to lifestyle, both in the community and in the hospital setting. This is not exclusive to women's health or the UK, but a worldwide phenomenon. It makes sense to use lifestyle to treat the very diseases it causes, starting with the food we put in our mouths. What we eat and how we live, the effects of sleep, stress, our environment, community and physical movement all have a huge impact on our mental and physical wellbeing, far greater than just our genes. These lifestyle factors also affect and modify how our genes are expressed, switching them on and off (see Chapter 2).

In 2014, I started to use a more holistic approach to help my patients, guiding them to choose the medical and surgical options most suited to them while also encouraging them to make a few lifestyle changes alongside this. I was inspired by what was possible and how receptive many of my patients were to the information, eager to transform their lives. Nisha is just one of the many patients who have made dramatic improvements to their lives. For those still needing medications or surgery, many have seen significant positive benefits to other aspects of their health by making small changes.

Prevention is the key to health

According to the WHO, up to 80% of cases of coronary heart disease, 90% of type 2 diabetes cases, and one-third of cancers could be avoided by adopting a healthier diet, increasing physical activity and stopping smoking. This is not new information and has been around for decades, yet western medicine has failed to acknowledge the very real impact of nutrition and lifestyle factors in both causing illness and maintaining good health.

Our lack of understanding of the causative link between food and chronic lifestyle diseases is costing lives. The Global Burden of Disease study, published in the leading journal *The Lancet*, is the most comprehensive worldwide observational epidemiological (population-based) study to date. The study analysed trends in consumption of 15 dietary factors from 1990 to 2017 in 195 countries and concluded more deaths and disabilities were caused by unhealthy diets, with too low intake of foods such as whole grains, fruit, vegetables, nuts and seeds, than by any other factors.[5] Cardiovascular disease was the leading cause of diet-related deaths and disability, with food-related risk factors, including excess weight and a diet high in saturated fat, playing a significant role.

People in almost every region of the world could benefit from urgently rebalancing their diets. In the UK, over half of the standard diet now consists of ultra-processed foods, and less than a third (only 28%) of adults were eating the recommended five portions of fruit and vegetables per day in 2018, with eight in 10 children not reaching their daily target.[6]

Lifestyle Medicine

Lifestyle Medicine is old in its principles, but a fairly new discipline of medicine, which means many doctors haven't heard of it either. It is defined as the use of evidence-based lifestyle interventions for the prevention and treatment of lifestyle-related chronic disease. In simple words, doctors should be recommending the use of lifestyle measures where possible to alleviate the chronic diseases caused by lifestyle and reduce the use of medications and surgical procedures, which are often accompanied by unwanted side effects.

The American College of Lifestyle Medicine (ACLM), established in 2004, came out with their dietary position statement in September 2018.[7] Lifestyle Medicine has been growing since then and now healthcare professionals have formed societies all over the world, embracing the power of lifestyle in treating people. The British Society of Lifestyle Medicine and Plant-Based Health Professionals are two organisations raising awareness among both healthcare professionals and the general public.

Lifestyle Medicine complements conventional western medicine. Both disciplines are based on science and evidence-based medicine. A key difference is that in Lifestyle Medicine, the patient is in the driving seat while in western medicine, it is your doctor who does the driving and decides management. Self-care and self-management are fundamental in Lifestyle Medicine, with your doctor working alongside you as a guide rather than deciding for you.

I advocate for lifestyle changes to be considered as the first choice in preventing many of these chronic illnesses that come with huge costs to the person, to their loved ones and to wider society. PCOS, with its similarities to type 2 diabetes, another lifestyle-related chronic condition, should also be considered a metabolic condition that can be largely managed through lifestyle and often prevented through early intervention.

Women's health benefits from Lifestyle Medicine too

People often make the mistake of assuming that the role of Lifestyle Medicine is mainly to prevent heart disease and type 2 diabetes, deadly diseases that also affect women. However, specific women's health issues are also adversely affected by lifestyle factors. Conditions such as PCOS, endometriosis, painful periods, depression, acne, weight management, autoimmune conditions and reproductive organ cancers can all benefit from dietary and lifestyle modifications just as much as heart disease, lifestyle cancers and type 2 diabetes.[7, 8] People of all ages and at every life stage, including puberty, pregnancy and menopause, can benefit from making dietary and lifestyle changes. In fact, most aspects of health benefit hugely from Lifestyle Medicine.

The six pillars of Lifestyle Medicine in PCOS

There are six main principles (known as 'pillars') in Lifestyle Medicine that can help benefit anyone looking to stay healthy or wishing to prevent or manage their health condition. These are nutrition, activity, sleep, stress reduction, avoidance of risky substances, and positive social relationships. I will describe how these six pillars of lifestyle can help you manage PCOS in detail in the next chapter, The domino effect.

Case study outcome: Nisha

When Nisha first came to see me, all she wanted was to have her periods and her energy back. I took a detailed medical history and ran tests to ensure there was no other reason for her missing periods. I confirmed it was PCOS that was responsible for her symptoms. I sat down with her to discuss both medical and lifestyle options but she was absolutely clear that she did not want to try any other form of pharmacological treatment, at least for another few months.

She had been delaying prioritising her health due to her busy work and social schedules. She admitted to being chronically stressed. She listened intently as I explained the benefits of lifestyle modifications and was eager to go the whole way and follow my recommendations.

Nisha continues to do well. She is managing her PCOS through a healthy lifestyle, has regular periods and remains happy with her improved energy levels.

I encourage my patients to be fully informed and engaged in their own treatment. Being in the driving seat allows people to decide for themselves how far they want to commit. I want to be their guide, not their driver. I wish the same for you. After all, just like Nisha and all my other patients, you know your body best.

The PCOS Myth Buster

Myth: Lifestyle Medicine is the same as alternative medicine.
The facts: Lifestyle Medicine is not alternative medicine, functional medicine, integrative medicine, homeopathy or acupuncture. It may work alongside and use some of their scientific principles if appropriate, but it is not considered to be any of these. Lifestyle Medicine also steers clear of most supplements and unproven theories. This is medicine as it was truly designed to be, free of negative side effects and always based on science. I explore these lifestyle changes in detail in the next chapter.

PCOS POINTERS

- Most deaths in the UK are caused by chronic lifestyle-related diseases, including heart disease, certain cancers and type 2 diabetes.
- PCOS is a condition that benefits from lifestyle changes.
- Lifestyle Medicine complements western medicine.
- Lifestyle changes have positive benefits for most aspects of women's health.
- There are six pillars of Lifestyle Medicine – nutrition, activity, sleep, stress management, avoidance of risky substances, and positive social relationships.

11

The domino effect
The six pillars of lifestyle in PCOS

People benefit from lifestyle interventions, even when conventional medical approaches are needed for particular conditions. Many of my patients with PCOS tell me regularly how introducing a few simple and small achievable changes to their lifestyle has helped them to successfully manage their PCOS. Not everyone needs, or is able, to make all the lifestyle changes I discuss below to see benefits in their health.

Addressing lifestyle in PCOS

PCOS is a lifestyle-related condition where metabolic and environmental factors interact with genetics to create the perfect storm of hormonal imbalance. The condition therefore lends itself to being very successfully managed with lifestyle changes.

International and national guidelines for PCOS agree that health professionals should offer dietary and lifestyle advice along with behavioural strategies as the first line of management for those diagnosed with PCOS, whether or not conventional medicine is offered as well.[1, 2, 3, 4] Experts say lifestyle advice should be recommended not only for those with PCOS who would benefit from weight reduction to improve insulin resistance but also for all living with the condition to achieve and/or maintain a healthy weight in order to optimise hormonal outcomes and general health and improve their quality of life.[3] Even so, confusion reigns in both the medical community and the general population, with remarkably few patients receiving any detailed or meaningful lifestyle guidance from qualified health professionals when diagnosed with PCOS.

Lifestyle interventions help with managing PCOS

PCOS is characterised by insulin resistance, excess body weight and androgen excess, often as a result of a background of chronic low-grade inflammation and oxidative stress. Oxidative stress is the result of an imbalance between the production of free radicals (reactive oxygen species) and the body's antioxidant defence system. This in turn causes damage to tissues at the molecular and cellular level, with people with PCOS showing many of the signs and symptoms we discussed in Chapter 3. These are all factors that are heavily influenced positively or negatively by dietary and lifestyle choices. Evidence suggests that lifestyle interventions, such as diet, exercise and behavioural interventions, can improve the key underlying metabolic issues implicated in PCOS – namely, insulin resistance and androgen excess – with a visible improvement in both physical signs and symptoms as well as blood test results.[2, 3, 4] An improvement in quality of life and emotional wellbeing outcomes was also noted.[3] There may be benefits for reproductive health as well.[5]

A 'healthy lifestyle' is also more effective for losing weight than anti-obesity medications, as shown in studies, and can offer benefits even when weight loss is not needed in those living with PCOS.[3, 4]

Defining a 'healthy lifestyle'

Despite this clear guidance from all major medical guidelines, women with PCOS around the world report that excess weight causes significant distress yet there is still inadequate information and support around lifestyle change.[3, 6] This has been my experience too, with patients usually being told to follow a 'healthy lifestyle' with little or no direction prior to them coming to me. Everyone has their own idea of what a 'healthy lifestyle' is and what 'moderation' stands for, which means most people are genuinely confused as to what that lifestyle advice should look like.

Where there is confusion, misinformation usually thrives. Non-evidence-based unscientific fads and restrictive diets as well as expensive supplements are peddled by individuals and companies as guarantees for weight loss and improving PCOS. This billion-dollar industry is looking to make a quick buck and once the miracle cure has been sold to the vulnerable consumer, those consumers are left to fend for themselves after realising there is no shortcut to health.

It is important to understand how and why making lifestyle changes can help you achieve better control of your PCOS and opti-mise your overall health. It is also important to highlight that the lifestyle that manages the condition of PCOS successfully is also the same lifestyle that helps prevent many other serious conditions. Lifestyle interventions have been shown to halt the progression of many chronic lifestyle diseases, such as type 2 diabetes, heart dis-ease, dementia and certain cancers such as breast, bowel, womb and prostate. They can reduce the risk of dying, and, if adopted early enough, help prevent many of these life-threatening conditions.[7, 8, 9]

The six pillars of lifestyle

The six pillars of lifestyle behave like dominos. When one falls, the rest tend to follow.

By nurturing each of the six pillars (see Box below), you will feel equipped to manage your PCOS better, in both the short term and the longer term. The positive changes in your lifestyle will help you live PCOS free.

THE SIX PILLARS OF LIFESTYLE

1. **NUTRITION:** predominantly whole food plant-based
2. **ACTIVITY:** regular physical movement
3. **SLEEP:** restorative sleep
4. **STRESS MANAGEMENT:** identify triggers and manage stress
5. **AVOIDANCE** of risky substances such as alcohol and tobacco
6. **SOCIAL RELATIONSHIPS:** positive social connections.

Pillar One: NUTRITION – Predominantly whole food plant-based (WFPB)

A plant-predominant diet that focuses on consuming whole or minimally processed plant foods most of the time has been shown in numerous studies to help prevent, treat and, in some cases, reverse chronic lifestyle diseases.[8, 10, 11] Simply put, whole plant foods are foods that have been refined or processed as little as possible and are eaten in their natural state, such as fresh fruit. Ultra-processed foods are made mostly from substances (including starches, added sugars, fats and hydrogenated fats) extracted from foods, and end up bearing little resemblance to the original food. Think crisps/chips, sausages and industrialised bread. One in four deaths globally are now attributed to a poor diet low in fruit, vegetables, nuts, seeds and whole grains and high in sodium from ultra-processed foods.[10, 11] Fruit and vegetable intake remains 50% below the recommended level of five servings per day that is considered healthy, and legume and nut intakes are each more than two thirds below the recommended two servings per day.[11a]

A predominantly whole food plant-based diet means enjoying an abundance of colourful vegetables, fruit, legumes (beans, peas, soya and lentils), whole grains, nuts, seeds, herbs and spices, with water as the drink of choice to optimise good health. These vibrant plant foods are all full of hormone-regulating fibre, health-promoting micronutrients and inflammation-busting antioxidants. Eating this way most of the time is both joyful and free of calorie counting. Rather than feeling restricted, you can discover many delicious world cuisines which celebrate plants, as you will find in our recipes.

As nutrition is probably the most important of all lifestyle pillars for regaining hormonal health, we have an entire chapter (Chapter 12) on how plant-based nutrition can help you manage your PCOS effectively as well as Part 4 packed with practical advice. The rest of this chapter will focus on the other five pillars of lifestyle, each one playing a critical part in the successful management of your PCOS.

Pillar Two: ACTIVITY – Regular physical movement

Most wealthy societies have become sedentary over the last hundred years or so. This is now becoming increasingly common around the world, even in low- and middle-income countries. Modern technologies and the way we work and relax mean that many of us spend significant parts of our waking hours in front of a screen. However, we need to find ways to keep moving to remain healthy.

This means we need to be doing physical activity (any bodily movement produced by skeletal muscles that requires energy expenditure) and structured exercise (any activity requiring physical effort, carried out to sustain or improve health and fitness). Sedentary behaviours (activities during waking hours in a seated or reclined position with energy expenditure less than 1.5 times resting metabolic rate) have been shown to have adverse health impacts. Any physical activity is better than none. Exercising for as little as 15 minutes a day has been shown to reduce mortality.[12]

Exercise has several proven and established benefits for the mind and body. It helps to:

- Improve mood and lower stress levels.
- Reduce the severity and duration of period pain.
- Improve sleep.
- Improve muscle tone and bone strength.
- Maintain a healthy weight.
- Reduce the risk of many chronic and deadly lifestyle-related illnesses.

Lack of exercise puts one in four people at risk of heart disease, type 2 diabetes and some cancers, according to figures published by the World Health Organization (WHO) in 2018.[13]

Aerobic exercise

Only 63.3% of people in England aged 16 and over are 'physically active', defined as engaging in at least 150 minutes of moderate-intensity physical activity a week (30 minutes, five days a week).[14] Moderate aerobic activity means any activity that uses large muscle groups and improves blood flow to the muscles, lungs and heart. Examples include brisk walking, dancing and pushing a lawnmower. Worryingly, close to 40% of women are not meeting the guidelines and of all groups and genders, British women of Southeast Asian heritage are the least likely to exercise.[14]

Exercise helps manage PCOS

Exercise offers several health benefits for women with PCOS, but most of these women do not receive advice on the specifics of the type and intensity of exercise they should be doing and the interaction between diet and exercise.[15] This is also partly due to limited research in PCOS. As with most women's health issues, there is not a lot of high-quality evidence when it comes to determining the exact type and effect of exercise on major health outcomes in PCOS. A systematic review and meta-analysis of randomised controlled trials in 2020 showed with moderate certainty that aerobic exercise alone is beneficial for reducing body mass index (BMI) in women with PCOS.[16] Formal exercise, both aerobic and muscle-strengthening, as well as physical activity, were found to improve body composition and make tissues more sensitive to insulin, thereby improving insulin resistance and blood sugar control, as well as cardio-metabolic function.[15, 16, 17, 18] Similarly, in smaller studies, both mental health and reproductive outcomes seemed to improve in those with PCOS.[3] All these effects seem to be independent of significant weight loss. Combining exercise with diet changes seemed to have added benefits.

Interestingly, women with PCOS often show greater muscle strength, irrespective of body composition, compared with those without the condition. PCOS is the most common cause of menstrual disorders among Olympic sportswomen.[10]

More good-quality research is needed to understand how best to guide women with PCOS to achieve maximum benefit from exercise[16] but it is clear from current evidence that being sedentary is detrimental. Physical activity, no matter the type of exercise, is beneficial in PCOS.

Physical activity recommendations

Remember to consult your doctor if you have any concerns about exercising, a serious medical condition or are on medications before you undertake exercise that you are not already used to. This is to decrease your risk of a sudden medical emergency.

Initially do exercises that you are used to and listen to your body, so you know how much you can push yourself. Make small increases to get into the habit of moving naturally throughout the day, whether it is by walking, dancing, gardening, washing dishes, cleaning or investing in a standing desk. If you have a sedentary job, taking a break every 20 minutes or so to stretch or do a few simple exercises at your desk can be helpful.

Helping yourself

I suggest building up over time to an hour of moderate-intensity exercise per day, five days of the week, along with a couple of sessions of muscle-strengthening exercises. UK national guidelines tell us to aim for at least 150 minutes of moderate-intensity exercise, which is half an hour a day, five days a week. However, studies have shown that 300 minutes of moderate or 150 minutes of intense exercise per week is ideal, especially if you have a medical condition such as type 2 diabetes or high blood pressure.[19, 10] This is applicable to PCOS as it is a chronic condition with similarities to type 2 diabetes, as we have seen (Chapter 10). In addition, 30 minutes of resistance exercise twice a week, working all muscle groups, is highly recommended to make our cells sensitive to insulin again and also to prevent muscle wasting (sarcopenia) as we get older. Balance training as well as aerobic and muscle-strengthening activities can help prevent falls and hip fractures later in life.

For teenagers, at least 60 minutes of moderate- to vigorous-intensity physical activity every day is recommended, including exercise strengthening muscle and bone at least three times weekly. I recommend this for teenagers with adolescent PCOS.

Choosing the type of exercise

The exercise you enjoy is the one that is best for you and the one you can do consistently. Regular sustained exercise, such as brisk walking, running, cycling, swimming, yoga and Pilates have been shown to help with overall health, which will benefit PCOS. Aerobic exercise can improve psychological health and quality of life by both improving mood and reducing insomnia along with cardio-metabolic benefits. Exercises that force one's body to work against gravity are known as weight-bearing exercises. Weight-bearing exercises help with improving body composition and insulin resistance. Aim to perform the activity in at least 10-minute bouts or around 1000 steps. Ideally, the exercise should be spread out throughout the week but if you want to be a weekend warrior, that is acceptable too. Try out the different types of exercise to find what you prefer.[19, 20]

The clear message from all studies is that exercise can help you when you have PCOS. The best exercise is the one you will do regularly, especially if you enjoy it.

Pillar Three: SLEEP – restorative sleep

Insomnia is thought to affect about a third of people in western countries at least once a week, with almost twice as many women compared to men affected, and results in impaired daytime functioning.[21] It is defined as difficulty in getting to sleep, difficulty in maintaining sleep, early wakening, or non-restorative sleep despite enough opportunities for sleep. Non-restorative sleep is defined as the experience that sleep has not been sufficiently refreshing or restorative.

Effects of sleep deprivation

Sleep seems to be one aspect in our lives that many compromise on quite readily in modern life. Disturbed sleep and insomnia affect teenagers and young people too and are particularly high in adolescent girls with anxiety-related symptoms.[22] The effects of chronic sleep deprivation creep up on us over time. People who consistently sleep less than five hours per night should be regarded as a population at higher risk for cardiovascular events and death.[23] Blood sugar, blood pressure and weight control become problems with chronic sleep deprivation, as shown in studies comparing nurses who do only night shifts with those who work in the day, increasing the risk of diabetes, heart attacks and excess weight.[24] Night-shift work also appears to be a risk factor for breast cancer.[25]

The importance of sleep

Seven to nine hours of restful sleep allows for DNA and cell repair, as well as reduction in stress hormones such as cortisol.[23] Not surprisingly, sleep also improves mood. Good quality sleep is invaluable for unlearning fearful memories and for memory building.[26] Too little or too much sleep can both affect health. Too much sleep may also increase the risk of chronic lifestyle diseases. Those with raised BMI, PCOS and/or mental health issues seem to be at higher risk of oversleeping.[27] The exact cause is not well understood.

PCOS and sleep

Sleep is critical for hormonal health along with all the other benefits mentioned above, and sleep disturbances are common in PCOS (see Chapter 21). Women, with or without PCOS, tend to suffer from sleep disturbances more than men, which may be in part due to the fluctuations in oestrogen and progesterone (as well as cortisol) that often occur throughout the menstrual cycle, in pregnancy and in women before and during menopause. A disturbed sleep pattern can make premenstrual (PMS) symptoms worse.[28] Period pain can also affect sleep quality during periods.

Insomnia and sleep apnoea, which is when breathing stops and starts during sleep, are under-reported in many living with PCOS. Disturbed sleep patterns in PCOS may lead to increased cortisol levels, which in turn increase stress levels, and poor sleep has been found to worsen anxiety and depression, which are often seen in PCOS. Disturbed nights lead to further hormonal disruption, fluctuations in blood sugar control and androgen excess, with worsening symptoms that lead to irritability, lack of concentration, feeling tired during the day and ultimately chronic sleep deprivation.

Oversleeping and excessive daytime sleepiness can be an issue in PCOS too. This relentless cycle should be addressed early to avoid worsening of symptoms.

Helping yourself

If you think you are sleep-deprived or are not feeling refreshed after spending seven to nine hours in bed, or if you are constantly tired during the day, try and make the following changes. If you see little improvement, then seek the advice of your doctor.

- Regular exercise such as yoga, walking, swimming or going to the gym can all help with a good night's sleep, with intense workouts ideally earlier in the day. Spending time in nature can be especially relaxing.

- A short nap of less than 30 minutes, ideally no longer than 60 minutes, early in the day may be beneficial for some of you.

- Both alcohol and caffeine can act as stimulants and can disturb sleep. They can also increase urinary frequency, creating the need to get up to pass urine more often, especially at night. Instead, consider a cup of relaxing caffeine-free herbal tea a couple of hours before bedtime and drink your coffee before midday if you cannot go without it.

- Eating your main meal early, ideally before 7:00 pm, in tune with the circadian rhythm, or at least a couple of hours before going to bed, helps with restful sleep by avoiding reflux and indigestion. A complex carbohydrate starch-based meal, such as beans with sweet potatoes, is ideal as it keeps you fuller for longer.[29] A Mediterranean-style diet, typically rich in plant foods, is associated with adequate sleep duration and fewer insomnia symptoms.[30]

- Consider unwinding with a pleasant book or soothing music to relax your mind, or take a bath.

- Mindfulness and meditation techniques desensitise the amygdala, the part of your brain that initiates stress and anxiety. They can reduce your stress levels and improve sleep quality.

- It helps to turn the central heating down and layer clothes to avoid overheating, which can result in a restless night.

- You may find you sleep better in a completely darkened room, using blackout curtains or an eye shield. Bright lights, television and smartphones can all suppress melatonin, a hormone produced in the brain, the levels of which need to rise in the evening to enable us to fall asleep. Be diligent about removing all electronic devices from the bedroom that emit light that suppresses melatonin. An old-fashioned alarm clock might be a good option.

- Some people will benefit from psychological approaches, of which cognitive behavioural therapy for chronic insomnia (CBT-I) appears to be the most effective treatment, with improvement in 70% of cases. You should be able to request a referral after discussion with your doctor.

- In some situations, especially as a short-term solution, your doctor may prescribe you sleeping pills after checking your other medications if you are struggling to sleep. These pills may come with side effects, such as daytime sedation, or alter your pattern of sleep. They have not been found to be superior to CBT and may even cause rebound insomnia when you stop them. The effects of CBT for insomnia also appear to be much longer lasting; a study has shown they continue for as long as five years after you stop the therapy.[31]

Pillar Four: STRESS MANAGEMENT – Identify triggers and manage stress

In our hectic modern-day lives, stress is an invisible factor in most health conditions, with 81% of women in the UK admitting to regularly feeling overwhelmed.[32] Stress is the body's reaction to feeling threatened or under pressure and is fuelled by hormones such as cortisol and adrenaline. Some stress is good and can be motivating in certain situations, helping us achieve goals we may set ourselves, be it to host a dinner party, give a presentation or complete a workout class.

However, too much stress can affect our mood, our body and our relationships and becomes harmful when the level of stress feels out of our control. Stress can make us feel anxious and irritable, affecting our self-esteem. Chronic stress can lower mood, disturb sleep, lead to poor dietary choices and to the avoidance of physical activity. It makes us less likely to connect with others, and work and relationships are also likely to suffer. Over time, it becomes a vicious cycle, and our mental and physical health starts to suffer, as they are closely linked together.

Health impact of social media

The ever-increasing use of social media is a double-edged sword, with systematic reviews suggesting a correlation between addiction, activity and time spent on social networking sites and anxiety, depression, self-harm and psychological distress in adolescents and young people.[33, 34] Some reviews have suggested positive benefits associated with social media use and depression. Whether the overall effect of social media is beneficial or harmful depends on many factors, not least the quality of the online environment that you surround yourself with.

PCOS and stress

Those living with PCOS have higher levels of anxiety than the general population, which cannot be attributed solely to physical symptoms such as excess weight, acne or increased face and body hair growth, or subfertility, although these are often genuine contributors to stress levels and mood disorders in those living with PCOS (see Chapter 19).

There are certain situations in which women may notice their anxiety levels to be particularly high. Times such as just before your periods, during pregnancy and around menopause can increase anxiety levels significantly. If you have PCOS, a condition associated with anxiety and depression, stress can make it even harder to deal with other health conditions such as premenstrual syndrome, subfertility and cancers.[35]

Stress is believed to be an important component of PCOS and seems to precede many long-term health problems, triggering inflammation and increasing your risk of type 2 diabetes, excess weight gain and heart disease.[36] Stress includes inflammatory and oxidative stress as described earlier.

The higher prevalence of altered cortisol levels and other stress-associated factors compared with age-matched controls (people of the same age who do not have PCOS) may have a critical role to play in the altered body composition and excess weight seen in many living with PCOS.[37, 38]

Helping yourself

Most of us find we are better at dealing with acute (short-lived) stress but when it becomes chronic, it starts to wear us down. It helps to try and figure out if your stress is acute or chronic. It may be that it is a family member who needs your attention because they are sick, or it may be your relationship, work-related stress and deadlines, or even bullying and harassment. Chronic stress is a prolonged and constant feeling of stress that can negatively affect your health if it goes untreated. By identifying and acknowledging stress triggers, you may feel better equipped to deal with the situation.

Regular exercise

You may find there are some physical measures that can help manage your stress and anxiety levels. Initially you may find it hard to motivate yourself so try doing a fitness class or walk with a loved one.

Regular exercise improves the feel-good factor and can help reduce anxiety levels. Walking or working out, especially in natural light, can help increase endorphins, also known as the happy hormones. Spending time outdoors in nature has been found to ease stress. Sunlight seems to be beneficial for seasonal affective disorder (SAD), a type of depression that comes and goes in a seasonal pattern, usually during the winter.

Stress management techniques

Gratitude practices and thinking of a few positive areas that are going well in your life can help relieve stress levels. Yoga, meditation or simple mindfulness and breathing techniques can calm the mind and reduce anxiety levels.

Writing your fears or concerns in a diary or journal may help you to see the situation more clearly. Talking about your fears with a trusted friend or family member or qualified therapist can help hugely with improving mental health.

Spending time in nature reduces stress. Studies have found that the Japanese practice of *shinrin-yoku*, translated as 'forest bathing', can lower blood pressure and improve immune function and mental health. Forest bathing involves immersing oneself in nature by mindfully using all five senses.[39, 40]

With regard to social media, follow accounts that inspire you, make you smile or feel good about life rather than accounts that arouse negative feelings about how you view yourself in comparison with others or accounts that promote toxic diet culture. These can be detrimental to the healing process and behavioural change that are critical for you to be in control of your PCOS. If you are sensitive, try to limit your consumption of news media. Establishing clear boundaries with work, social media and those around us, helps safeguard our time and energy.

Food and mood

Unhealthy dietary patterns with high consumption of refined grains, sweets, red and processed meat and high-fat dairy products (such as butter) have been consistently associated with lower scores of health-related quality of life, including mood, compared with plant-predominant diets with low intakes of animal foods.[41, 42] Depression can be helped by cutting out ultra-processed foods as they often contain various compounds that can affect mood, such as nitrites in processed meats.[43, 44] Instead, add more colourful fruit and vegetables into your daily diet as the intake of these anti-inflammatory foods reduces the very hormones that increase our stress levels.

Finally, if none of these suggestions appeals to you or provides relief, I would suggest seeking medical advice from a sympathetic health professional, as therapy can really help. Some of you may benefit from taking medications. You can still continue with lifestyle modifications alongside this.

Pillar Five: AVOIDANCE of risky substances

There are no health benefits from drinking alcohol, whatever claims you may hear. Alcohol misuse is the biggest risk factor for death, ill-health, and disability among 15 to 49-year-olds in the UK. Alcohol is a causal factor in more than 60 medical conditions, including high blood pressure, depression, liver disease and seven types of cancer, including breast cancer, with the WHO attributing more than 200 disease and injury conditions to alcohol.[45, 46]

Cigarette smoking and alcohol are both Class 1 carcinogens, which means that they are known to cause cancer.[47] Tobacco use is still unfortunately the leading preventable cause of cancer and cancer deaths, being implicated in as many as 14 different types of cancer, including cancer of the cervix and ovary, with the toxic chemicals in cigarettes causing DNA and cell damage.[48] Smoking causes other diseases too, such as heart disease and various lung diseases.

Risky substances and PCOS

There is limited clinical human research on the effects of smoking, alcohol intake and addictive drugs on PCOS. However, we do know that smoking significantly worsens the already increased risk of metabolic syndrome and insulin resistance in those with PCOS compared with non-smokers and the effect appears to be independent of changes in androgen levels. Smokers with PCOS also have higher triglyceride levels than non-smokers,[49] which in turn increases the risks of heart disease and stroke.

Mental health effects

Alcohol and smoking can have negative health effects, especially on mood and sleep, making already existing symptoms worse. The chemical changes in your brain induced by alcohol can mean more negative feelings start to take over and a loss of inhibition under the influence of alcohol may result in risk-taking behaviour or over-indulging, with feelings of guilt later.

Fertility

Overall, clinical studies suggest that smoking is associated with reduced fertility and passive smoking is also likely to reduce your chances of conceiving.[50] There is scant information on the effect of addictive drugs, due to use of more than one drug at the same time, but these should also be avoided.[50, 51]

Studies have not been able to confirm the role of alcohol and even stimulants such as caffeine in impairing ovulation to the point of decreasing fertility. However, alcohol does appear to increase oestrogen and decrease progesterone levels in pre-menopausal women, which in turn can affect fertility.[52]

There does seem to be an association between soft drinks and ovulatory subfertility but this does not appear to be attributable to their caffeine or sugar content.[53] Further research is urgently warranted in this area, specifically in those with PCOS, given that the alcohol, soft-drink and tobacco industries are known to target young people.

Breast cancer

In the UK, one in seven women will receive a diagnosis of breast cancer in their lifetime.[54] Research consistently shows that drinking any form of alcohol increases a woman's risk of breast cancer. Breast cancer risk appears to be increased by the build-up of acetaldehyde, a toxic substance which is produced as alcohol is broken down, damaging the cellular DNA.[55] Alcohol can also increase levels of oestrogen and other hormones associated with hormone-receptor-positive breast cancer. As PCOS is associated with higher-than-normal levels of oestrogen, especially in those carrying excess weight, it would be advisable to avoid alcohol that can further raise levels of oestrogen.

Compared with women who do not drink at all, women who have three alcoholic drinks per week have a 15% higher risk of breast cancer.[48] Experts estimate that the risk of breast cancer goes up another 10% for each additional drink women regularly have each day. Adolescents who consume alcohol are also at increased future risk.

When it comes to other aspects of women's health, excess weight gain and worse menopausal symptoms, such as hot flushes, are just some of the negative consequences of consuming alcohol. Consumption of alcohol, especially beer, appears to be associated with an increased risk of developing fibroids.[56]

No level of alcohol can be considered safe in pregnancy so abstinence is the safest option, particularly for women trying to conceive or those in the first three months of pregnancy as recommended by experts.[57]

Helping yourself

There are no safe limits for these risky substances and my medical advice is to avoid them as much as possible, especially if you are trying to conceive or are pregnant. If you choose not to drink, you do not need to explain yourself to others. It is never too late to stop and the body will in time heal itself. In the UK, therapy and support to help you quit are available on the NHS through your doctor.

Set yourself small goals using the SMART objectives – Specific, Measurable, Achievable, Realistic and Time-Bound – so you can make progress rather than getting overwhelmed. For example, start by setting specific alcohol-free days or a set period of abstinence. Smart swaps, such as swapping a cigarette for a telephone call with a friend, a warm bath or even sugar-free chewing gum, or an alcoholic drink for sparkling water, are just a few suggestions.

Safer sex

Practising safer sex by using condoms, attending regular cervical screening appointments and having the HPV vaccine as recommended by your national programme, all help in reducing sexually transmitted infections and lowering the risk of genital warts, cervical cancer and subfertility. The use of alcohol and mood-enhancing drugs increase the likelihood of taking unnecessary risks. You must insist on a condom or dental dams in new relationships to avoid unwanted infections. I advise both you and your partner(s) to get tested for sexually transmitted infections before becoming intimate.

Pillar Six: SOCIAL RELATIONSHIPS – Positive social connections

Studies have shown that those in positive relationships tend to have more rewarding and less stressful lives and enjoy better health. Loneliness can and does affect anyone and at any age. People can be isolated, as in physically alone, yet not feel lonely. People can be surrounded by other people, yet still feel lonely.[58] Loneliness is as prevalent as excess weight and has a similar impact to smoking 15 cigarettes a day, shortening lifespan by as much as eight years.[59, 60] Loneliness is a source of chronic stress and is associated with increased risk of heart disease, high blood pressure and type 2 diabetes.[61]

According to Age UK, more than two million people in England over the age of 75 live alone, and more than one million older people say they go for over a month without speaking to a friend, neighbour or family member.[58] The COVID-19 pandemic and enforced social isolation have had a severe impact on mood and anxiety in all age groups.

PCOS, loneliness and social isolation

Body image is complex and is defined as the way a person may feel, think about and view their body, including their appearance.[3] Sociocultural factors all influence body image in those living with PCOS. These include negative perceptions of one's body, feeling judged about body size, feeling conscious of androgen excess symptoms such as acne, excessive facial or body hair, scalp hair loss, and lack of regular periods with a feeling of loss of feminine identity as a result.[62] This can create an acute sense of loneliness and low self-esteem leading to avoidance of social situations and increasing isolation in PCOS. This loneliness may lead to disrupted relationships, sexual dysfunction and increasing isolation, worsening symptoms of anxiety, depression and low mood. Studies have suggested that women with PCOS have a lower quality of life compared with women without PCOS.[3]

Helping yourself

I encourage you to actively start building a meaningful social network of friends who genuinely matter to you and care about you.

Valuing friendships is generally associated with better health, well-being, and happiness.[63] Reach out to friends or family members who make you feel positive about yourself.

Whether it is by helping an elderly neighbour, making a meal for someone in need or doing community work, those who contribute positively to society seem to live happier and healthier lives. Maybe this is something you can try out to see if it helps you feel better. There are benefits to ourselves and others if we try and adopt these positive behaviours.

Finding areas of interest and activities that you like, and connecting with groups, preferably face-to-face, can bring joy. These could be book clubs, running, dance or theatre groups, volunteering or learning a new skill or language. Carefully chosen support groups where you can share your mutual concerns may also help combat loneliness and isolation.

The PCOS Myth Buster

Myth: Lifestyle cannot be that important – otherwise doctors would tell us much more about it and less about pills.
The facts: Most doctors do know lifestyle is important but as we do not learn about it in detail in medical school, we are often at a loss to help our patients. This knowledge is improving but you do not have to wait for medical knowledge to catch up. When you start to improve one aspect of your life, you will almost always see benefits in other areas. You will find that when you choose foods that are nourishing and filling, you will have more energy to take that walk in the park with a friend, laughing and connecting, thereby lowering your stress levels. You will likely sleep better at night, helping to regulate your hormones, and a good night's sleep in turn will help you make

healthier food and drink choices. Science suggests that the way we eat and how we live have a great impact on our mental and physical wellbeing. The same is true even if you do not have PCOS.

Figure 5: *The six pillars of lifestyle*

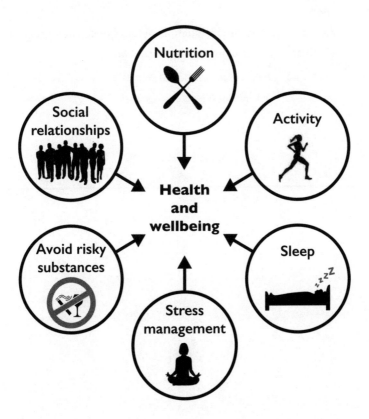

PCOS POINTERS

- Eat mostly whole plant foods, avoiding ultra-processed foods.
- Include physical movement every day.
- Aim for regular restorative sleep of seven to nine hours every night.
- Identify your stress triggers and find ways to manage them.
- Avoid risky substances such as alcohol and smoking.
- Build social connections when you can.

12

Full of beans
The benefits of plant-based nutrition for PCOS

My patients often ask me how closely they need to follow my advice regarding the dietary and lifestyle changes to help manage and treat their condition. Like them, you may wonder if you need to go all the way. My advice is to bring in lifestyle changes to the best of your ability. Do not be too hard on yourself; any changes in a positive direction would be an improvement.

Progress, not perfection

It really depends on your starting point, your age, what medical conditions you have, your family history, your risk factors and, above all, what changes you are prepared or able to make. Any change is better than no change, whether it is with the food you eat or with exercise. The more positive changes you make, the more benefits you will see. Don't give up as it may take more than two months – 66 days according to a study published in the *European Journal of Social Psychology* – for a new habit to become automatic.[1] Some people are ready to make the leap straightaway while many of my patients need a three-to-six-month transition period to a healthier way of eating, especially after a lifetime of eating a standard western diet. Some may never make the full transition and may not even wish to.

Habits tend to improve with persistence, so it is better to build up over time rather than have unrealistic expectations, which usually lead to disappointment and frustration. That is why we have a 21-day programme (page 315) that can help you break some of those habits and get you started on your journey to *Living PCOS Free*.

Weight loss as a goal

When it comes to weight loss, experts say there is no good evidence that one type of diet is superior to another for women with PCOS. Most diets work in the short term when it comes to losing weight as they all work on the principle of calorie restriction. Keeping weight off in the long term is much more challenging and, after an initial weight loss and plateau, weight regain is typical.[2] In a meta-analysis of 29 long-term weight-loss studies, more than half of the weight that was lost had been regained within two years, and by five years more than 80% of the weight lost had been regained.[2, 3] Cycles of yo-yo dieting, also known as 'weight cycling', can also lead to increased weight gain in the longer term. Weight oscillations cause hormonal fluctuations which affect sleep cycles.[4] Low-calorie dieting increases levels of stress and of the stress hormone cortisol, which are higher in women with PCOS.[5]

So, if the only goal is to lose weight in PCOS, then any diet can work, at least in the short term, with improvement in some of the symptoms of PCOS. However, virtually every diet appears to be destined to fail in the longer term if it doesn't become part of a healthy, sustainable lifestyle with realistic goals and a positive mindset. Most people, particularly women, have been on a number of diets and after an initial weight loss, as the scientific evidence shows, they mostly put all the weight back on, leaving them frustrated and willing to try yet another expensive and unhealthy fad programme. They are also more likely to be more vulnerable to eating disorders within this cycle of dieting.

The optimal diet for PCOS

The goal should be to permanently improve the symptoms of PCOS in a healthful, sustainable way. Weight loss, if desired, may be a pleasant side effect, with the aim of keeping the weight off and maintaining a healthy weight in the long term. While we can't say one specific diet is best for human health, what we can say, based on best available current scientific evidence, is that eating mostly plants, especially in their whole or minimally processed forms, alongside other positive behaviour changes is without doubt the healthiest option.

Eating plants for PCOS

A whole food plant-based (WFPB) diet that emphasises fruit and vegetables, legumes and whole grains, and includes nuts and seeds is recommended for optimal human health and disease prevention and management. It eliminates or minimises animal foods, such as red and white meat, poultry, eggs, fish and dairy, as well as ultra-processed foods that include added sugars and oils. PCOS is no different and responds extremely well to adopting this way of eating.

A dietary pattern like this also includes herbs, spices, mushrooms and starchy vegetables, such as sweet potatoes, potatoes in their skins, yams and squashes. I would like to clarify that the whole grains should ideally be intact (e.g. oat groats) or minimally processed (steel cut oats) and, by 'legumes', we mean beans, soya, peas and lentils.

The vast majority of the human population eats a meagre 200 of the 300,000 edible plant species, with half our plant-sourced protein and calories coming from just three: maize, rice and wheat. It is time to start enjoying the abundance found in nature.

The evidence for plant-based eating

There are population studies, especially from the five Blue Zones around the world, which are places where people consistently live to over 100 years old in good health: Okinawa, Japan; Sardinia, Italy; Nicoya, Costa Rica; Ikaria, Greece; and Loma Linda, California. The diets of these long-living populations are typically 85-95% plant-based and, in the case of Loma Linda, exclusively plant-based. These regions are proof in action that eating more fruit, vegetables, whole grains and beans while reducing or avoiding ultra-processed foods and animal foods is healthful for all people at all ages and stages in their lives for disease prevention and disease management.

A healthy plant-based diet reduces the risk of type 2 diabetes by at least 50%, coronary heart disease by 25% and certain cancers by around 15%. These diseases affect all genders.[15, 16, 17, 18, 19] This way of eating could benefit health in countless ways, including lowering the odds of moderate-to-severe COVID-19.[20] Many people find motivation in the ethical and environmental reasons to go plant-based too (see Chapter 34).

The research on type 2 diabetes

PCOS has remarkable similarities to type 2 diabetes. One of the biggest contributors to serious illness and death (heart disease, dementia, blindness, kidney failure, for example), type 2 diabetes is now a common condition all over the world. Insulin resistance and impaired blood sugar control are common to both type 2 diabetes and PCOS.

Informed by the latest research around type 2 diabetes management, the American College of Lifestyle Medicine (ACLM) put out a position statement in June 2020, stating clearly that sufficiently intensive lifestyle modifications can produce significant clinical improvements in patients with type 2 diabetes. The optimal treatment to bring about remission of diabetes includes a whole food, plant-based dietary pattern coupled with moderate exercise. The success was similar to weight loss (bariatric) surgery but with significantly fewer side effects. This is ground-breaking evidence and if implemented properly at policy level could help save millions of lives around the world.

Not all carbs are the same

Carbohydrates are one of the three macronutrients (protein and fat being the other two) found in our food. Carbohydrates have been much maligned in recent years but they are a broad category.

When we use the word 'carbohydrate', we must distinguish between the type and quality of a carbohydrate based on its degree of processing. Fibre-rich unprocessed or minimally processed carbohydrates in a dietary pattern based around fruit, vegetables, whole grains and legumes are wholly different from fibre-deficient, ultraprocessed carbohydrates found in large proportions in a typical western diet, such as cakes, biscuits, refined sugar, white rice, white bread and other ultra-processed foods.

Low-carbohydrate animal-based diets can harm you

The term 'low-carbohydrate diet' is usually used for any of the following low–carb, high-animal-fat or low-carb high-animal-protein diets, such as keto, paleo, Atkins and various combinations of these diets that all result in carbohydrates, including healthy complex carbohydrates, being kept to a minimum (from <12% to <40% of total calorie intake). There are relatively few people who do low-carbohydrate diets based mainly on plant-based protein and fat sources, such as the Eco-Atkins diet.[8a]

In a large 2018 study, low-carbohydrate diets which had high animal-derived protein and fat from sources such as lamb, beef, pork and chicken were consistently associated with higher mortality.[9] Those favouring plant-derived protein and fat intake from sources such as vegetables, nuts, peanut butter and whole-grain breads were associated with lower mortality. This suggests that the type and source of food make a big difference in the association between carbohydrate intake and mortality. Both extremely high and low percentages of carbohydrate in diets have been associated with increased mortality. A carbohydrate intake of around 50–55% of one's diet has been observed to be optimal, with the lowest risk of death.[9] A diet high in animal foods is thought to stimulate inflammatory pathways, biological ageing and oxidative stress.[8, 22]

The main types of fat in our diet should be unsaturated fats from plant sources rather than animal fat, just as the main sources of protein in our diets should be plant-derived. A whole food plant-based diet is high in fibre and usually low in fats, especially the processed ones that leap into the bloodstream causing adverse physiological effects (insulin resistance, vascular dysfunction, etc), unlike the fats in whole walnuts, seeds and avocados. This delicious way of eating should be celebrated by all of us, including those living with PCOS.

Low-carb vs plant-based diets in PCOS

Although low-carbohydrate diets have become popular for women with PCOS, this is based upon the assumption that less carbohydrate leads to less abnormally high levels of insulin in your body and therefore less insulin resistance. Scientific evidence tells a different story. For example, in a small 12-week study of 28 women with PCOS wanting to lose excess weight, a high-protein/low-carbohydrate diet (30% protein, 40% carbohydrate, 30% fat) and a low-protein/high-carbohydrate diet (15% protein, 55% carbohydrate, 30% fat) were equally effective for weight loss, improvements in menstrual cycles, insulin resistance, abnormal lipid levels and abdominal fat. However, we know that in the longer term, low-carbohydrate diets increase the risk of the chronic diseases that people with PCOS are predisposed to, such as type 2 diabetes.

In a randomised controlled trial in 2015, 48 women with PCOS and excess weight were randomly assigned for eight weeks either to a control group or to adopt the well-known DASH (Dietary Approaches to Stop Hypertension) diet which focuses on increasing fruit, vegetables, wholegrains and low-fat dairy[28] while reducing saturated fats, cholesterol, refined grains and sweets. The diet of the control group included foods they normally ate, and both diets had the same distribution of the macronutrients (52% carbohydrates, 18% proteins and 30% total fats). Those on the DASH diet saw an improvement in insulin resistance, inflammatory markers and reduction in belly fat compared with controls.[29]

A systematic review in 2019 found lifestyle interventions (diet, exercise and behaviour) could improve the markers of androgen excess and body weight. Most of the available studies included in this review were of low quality and at risk of bias; research with large-scale, well-designed studies of dietary patterns is urgently needed in PCOS specifically.

Based on available evidence looking at other chronic diseases, especially type 2 diabetes, it would be sensible to opt for a whole food plant-based diet, especially if keeping weight off is the goal[12, 31] while seeing symptom improvement in PCOS.[32, 33] If one does wish to do a low-carb diet, then it would be wise to choose plant-derived sources of protein and fat rather than animal-based sources, for reasons explained previously.

Eating a plant-based diet is a good idea for PCOS

A plant-based way of eating helps reduce many of the symptoms of PCOS through several mechanisms. PCOS is characterised by low-grade inflammation as evidenced by raised levels of inflammatory markers such as IL-6, homocysteine and C-reactive protein. Eating whole plant foods helps to reduce this chronic inflammation that is harmful to our body in the longer term, especially damaging to our blood vessels and ovaries. For lowering inflammation, colourful, antioxidant-rich foods are particularly helpful. These include berries, pineapple, dark green leafy vegetables, nuts and seeds such as walnuts, flaxseeds, beans, lentils and herbs and spices such as turmeric and cinnamon.

This way of eating also works extremely well by reducing insulin levels and improving insulin resistance, the main driver for the symptoms of PCOS (see Chapter 5).

Eating more plants which are nutrient-dense yet calorie-light helps with weight loss. By minimising or excluding animal foods, circulating levels of excess oestrogen drop; this improves androgen-excess symptoms of PCOS and helps to address menstrual irregularities. Levels of SHBG (sex hormone binding globulin) increase, which helps bind excess circulating testosterone, improving PCOS symptoms also.

Replacing protein-rich animal products (e.g. meat, poultry and fish) with protein-rich soya foods (e.g. tofu, tempeh, edamame and soya milk) can also help with both weight loss and lowering insulin resistance.

Soya, as well as fruit such as apples, cacao and watermelon, can improve sexual function by increasing vaginal blood flow, lubrication and vaginal collagen content while reducing discomfort during sex. This may be because they enhance nitric oxide (NO) activity that dilates blood vessels. Other fruit also probably have the same effect. This may be relevant as women with PCOS approach meno-pause, when typically, these vaginal symptoms are more noticeable.

A plant-based diet brings many of its benefits through its unique property of containing high amounts of health-promoting fibre and phytonutrients that improve gut health and the gut microbiome.

Remember only plants contain fibre

There is strong scientific evidence that fibre is good for our health. Fibre is not actually a single nutrient but a collective group of car-bohydrates or carbohydrate-containing foods. A higher intake of dietary fibre has been associated with a reduced risk of death.[38] Fibre intake seems to be inversely associated with PCOS, suggesting higher intake of fibre (plants) lowers the risk of PCOS. Conversely, a low-fibre intake and high intake of refined foods is significantly associated with PCOS.[39] High intake of a variety of plant foods con-taining soluble and insoluble fibre (see Chapter 24) is associated with less chronic inflammation as measured by certain inflamma-tory markers, such as IL-6 and TNF-alpha.[40]

A constipated nation

In the UK, most people do not get enough fibre, with the aver-age intake being 17.8 g per day for women and 22.4 g per day for men.[41] The recommended average intake for adults is 30 g per day as per the advice of the British Dietetic Association[42] and we have evolved eating a diverse range of plants that regularly contributed up to and often more than 100 g of fibre per day over millions of years.[43] Eating whole plants allows you to hit your target for fibre rather easily as only plant foods contain fibre. There is minimal fibre in ultra-processed foods and zero fibre in animal foods. People are always surprised to hear that animal foods have no fibre. That's right, unfortunately none at all.

One result of this is that constipation is a real problem for many in the UK as most eat a standard diet made up of at least 50% highly processed foods.[44] Taking laxatives or fibre supplements misses the point and stops working after a while. As Dr Denis Burkitt, a British doctor who worked for years in Africa, famously observed, 'Societies that eat unrefined foods produce large stools and build small hospitals; societies that eat fibre-depleted foods produce small stools and build large hospitals.'[45]

Feeding our healthy gut bacteria in PCOS

A fibre-rich plant-based way of eating helps promote a healthy gut microbiome in PCOS. Scientists now believe that the trillions of beneficial bacteria and other helpful micro-organisms that we harbour in our gut feast on these fibre-rich plant foods, producing short chain fatty acids (SCFA) that are critical not just to our general health (gut, heart, brain health, for example) but also to our hormonal health. These good bacteria keep the bad bugs, such as *E. coli* and *Salmonella* and thrush-causing *Candida* in check, all of which can negatively impact women's health. The significant lack of fibre in a typical western diet means that the healthy colonies of bacteria, such as *Firmicutes* do not flourish. Instead, the gut harbours an environment that allows inflammatory colonies of microbes, such as *Bacteroides, Bilophila wadsworthia, Clostridium* and entero-invasive *E. coli* to run riot, releasing endotoxins such as amines, sulphides and secondary bile salts amongst other harmful substances that damage the delicate gut lining over time and promote ill health.

When examined, stool from those with PCOS had lower bacterial diversity and there were higher numbers of bacterial colonies such as *Prevotella* that promoted androgen excess and insulin resistance as well as worsening lipid levels. Correcting this gut 'dysbiosis' (unbalanced flora) was found to help improve symptoms of PCOS. Our gut is very forgiving and making dietary changes to include more nourishing whole plant foods allows the healthy bacterial colonies to return.

The oestrobolome

The oestrobolome is the collection of microbes in our gut that is one of the principal regulators of circulating oestrogens in our body, as they can break down (metabolise) oestrogen.[37] Much of this unwanted excess oestrogen gets excreted from your gut in your poo, bound to the fibre from the plants you eat. This trapping by the fibre in the food we eat prevents the excess hormones from re-entering the blood circulation via the liver, by a mechanism called the enterohepatic circulation. Those on plant-based diets tend to excrete two to three times more of the unwanted oestrogen.[47] This is exciting as we know PCOS and other women's health conditions, such as endometriosis, fibroids, adenomyosis and certain cancers such as breast and womb cancers, are associated with higher levels of excess oestrogen, produced both from excess body fat and also found in animal foods.[48]

A group of researchers led by B Zhang have studied the gut microbiome as a potential target for treatment of PCOS.[46] Their findings identified gut dysbiosis in PCOS, suggesting that it may be possible to intervene in PCOS by targeting the gut bacteria, replacing harmful colonies with health-promoting gut-friendly bacteria.

Foods to crowd out in PCOS

By focusing on foods to bring into your diet, you will naturally move away from, or 'crowd out', less beneficial foods. In general, the closer a food is to its whole form, the better it is for you. That is why it is best to avoid highly refined foods such as sugar or white bread and emphasise fibre-rich whole-plant foods.

The reason doctors ask you to stay away from ultra-processed foods is because these biscuits, cakes, sugar-sweetened beverages and takeaways tend to be high in unhealthy fats such as hydrogenated oils or tropical oils rich in saturated fat. They also contain added chemicals, salt and sugars, promoting inflammation, a major trigger for most chronic diseases. Saturated fats are consistently associated with elevated blood cholesterol levels. Increasing fibre and reducing unhealthy fats was associated with metabolic improvement in those with PCOS and excess weight in a randomised controlled trial.[49]

The same goes for many oils, with some exceptions (see Chapter 25), and shop-bought fruit juices as these too are highly processed, a dense source of calories and lack the fibre the body needs to thrive. Consuming these in large amounts regularly deprives us of the wonderful array of micronutrients that whole plant foods contain that are so good for our health.

Animal-derived products

You should try to eliminate or limit animal-derived foods, especially red meat and processed meats.[8] The latter have high levels of saturated fat and unwanted excess protein while being devoid of any fibre. Animal-derived foods also promote oxidative stress and inflammation in our bodies through the various inflammatory compounds that are naturally present in them, such as carnitine and Neu5Gc, as well as carrying harmful bacterial endotoxins, antibiotics, plastic and persistent organic pollutants.[19, 50, 51] The higher levels of growth hormones, insulin-like growth factors, sex hormones, added chemicals, pesticides and antibiotics found in these animal foods worsen the inflammation associated with PCOS. An increased intake of saturated fat may worsen the cardiovascular risk profile in PCOS.[52]

The role of advanced glycation end products (AGEs) in PCOS

AGEs are highly reactive compounds which form inside the body when sugars attach to protein molecules (glycotoxins) and are thought to accelerate the ageing process. A small amount of AGEs are produced internally as natural waste products of metabolism, but the other source is from our diet, especially from food cooked at high temperatures.

AGEs crosslink proteins together, causing tissue stiffness, oxidative stress, insulin resistance, cellular damage and inflammation. Women with PCOS tend to have higher levels of circulating AGEs in their bloodstream[53] as well as higher levels of AGEs and AGE receptors in their ovaries.[40, 54] As a result, the ovaries seem to be particularly sensitive to the negative effects of AGEs. High AGE levels are seen in those with PCOS and excess weight as well as in lean PCOS.[55]

Diet and AGEs

The biggest dietary sources of AGEs which worsen PCOS symptoms are foods high in animal protein and animal fat, including beef, pork, chicken, cheese, butter, cream cheese and ultra-processed snacks and breakfast cereals.[56] Diets low in AGEs include whole grains, legumes, vegetables and fruit, which all help reduce inflammation and improve insulin resistance.[40]

Increasing intake of foods that help pull AGEs out of the body, like brown rice and mushrooms, can help in PCOS, as well as eating anti-inflammatory antioxidant-rich foods, such as berries, greens, herbs and spices, like turmeric and cinnamon. Try to include more raw foods in your diet (fruit, vegetables) and raw nuts and raw nut butters, as the latter may have 30 times fewer AGEs compared with roasted nuts.

You can also reduce your dietary AGE intake by changing the method of cooking from high-temperature dry-cooking ways of preparing foods (barbecuing, grilling, frying) to low-heat, higher-humidity (stewing, steaming and boiling) methods.

The right time to start

Adopting an anti-inflammatory whole-food plant-based way of eating early in life helps with both short-term and long-term health but it is never too late to start, as benefits can often be seen within weeks and months.

The PCOS Myth Buster

Myth: I can't get enough nutrients on a plant-based diet.
The facts: This statement could not be further from the truth. Just by eating a variety of mostly whole plant foods, you can get enough calories, more than enough protein, fat and carbohydrates and, in addition, countless phytochemicals, micronutrients and cancer-fighting antioxidants not really found elsewhere in our food. All these foods can be culturally adapted and there is no need to feel you are missing out. We discuss how you can smoothly make this transition in Chapter 24 on transitioning to a plant-based diet and Chapter 27 on the key supplements for PCOS.

PCOS POINTERS

- A whole food plant-based (WFPB) diet is beneficial for PCOS as it:
  - Reduces inflammation and oxidative stress.
  - Improves insulin resistance.
  - Promotes weight loss and weight maintenance.
  - Lowers excess oestrogen levels.
  - Promotes healthy gut bacteria.
- Focus on fruit, vegetables, legumes, whole grains, nuts and seeds.
- Limit animal foods.
- Avoid or minimise ultra-processed foods.
- Low-carbohydrate high-animal-protein or high-animal-fat diets are consistently associated with worse health outcomes, especially long-term increased death rates.

13

You cannot meditate away a broken leg
Lifestyle Medicine complements conventional medicine

Case history: Alison

At 29, Alison enjoyed her job as a personal trainer, did not smoke, hardly drank alcohol and loved her fruit and vegetables. She had decided against taking the Pill when she had been diagnosed with PCOS two years earlier, preferring to try a more holistic approach. She did not want to consider starting a family for a few more years and needed effective contraception. Her heavy periods, fatigue and cystic acne had been starting to get her down over the last couple of years and she remarked that she felt like a failure.

Alison had been advised by her GP that the Pill was probably going to give her the much-needed relief from her irregular and heavy periods, help with her acne while

---

offering her highly effective contraception. Alison felt she was letting herself down by agreeing to take the Pill as she had been set on holistic methods.

She had come to see me for a second opinion. After appropriate tests and a discussion of all the lifestyle pillars and medical options, the Pill was certainly the most suitable of all her options to give her the relief from her symptoms of PCOS and the contraception she desired.

Lifestyle medicine complements conventional medicine

If you have a major fracture, you cannot heal it through meditation, as much as that may help you to cope with the pain. You will almost always need surgery and medications. If a cancerous growth is discovered which is suitable for surgery, you should be encouraged to have it removed. I have seen too many patients in the course of my career who have gone off to try natural methods, sadly to return to die in hospital a little while later, after the cancer had spread everywhere. It is not just patients with cancer who are sometimes misguided and confused by conflicting information put out there. I have seen patients with large fibroids (non-cancerous growths that develop in or around the womb) with severe anaemia from resulting heavy periods try natural methods, only to end up needing emergency surgery or blood transfusions.

Following a healthy lifestyle is invaluable and can help significantly in the prevention and management of many chronic lifestyle diseases, including several women's health conditions, but it cannot necessarily replace conventional medicine, especially when there is evidence of established disease. Lifestyle medicine does not replace conventional medicine and nor does conventional medicine replace lifestyle medicine. Both are invaluable for good health, when used appropriately.

Pick a side

Some think you must either be on the side of conventional medicine or against it. It does not have to be this way. The use of penicillin, discovered by Dr Alexander Fleming in 1942, has over time saved millions of people from life-threatening infections.[1] Another example is the simple act of hand washing, introduced by Dr Semmelweis a century earlier, in 1840, which dramatically reduced the incidence of deadly puerperal sepsis (postpartum sepsis or childbed fever) on the obstetric wards of a Viennese hospital.[2] Both have a place in modern medicine in saving lives. One is treatment, the other is prevention. One does not replace the other. With the COVID-19 pandemic of 2020,[3] hand washing, wearing a mask and social distancing proved to be preventative measures to stop the spread of infection. An effective vaccine, however, has allowed people to get back to some degree of normality.

When it comes to treating life-threatening infections, cancer or mending broken bones, modern medicine must be the first choice.

The combined oral contraceptive pill (COCP)

If you do not wish to get pregnant, then hormonal contraception, especially the combined oral contraceptive Pill (COCP or the Pill) is a highly suitable option in PCOS, after your doctor checks you have no absolute contraindications – for example, a history of blood clots or migraines with aura or breast cancer. The COCP contains a combination of the hormones, a combination of an oestrogen (usually ethinylestradiol) and a progestogen (specifically a progestin). Natural methods of contraception have a much higher failure rate and are not necessarily reliable, especially for women with PCOS with irregular periods.

There are many non-contraceptive benefits of the Pill, which can significantly improve quality of life by providing relief from many of the symptoms of PCOS as well as from heavy or painful periods and from the effects of iron-deficiency anaemia.[4] Taking the Pill for four to five years is protective against cancer and the longer someone takes the combined Pill, the lower the risk of ovarian, colorectal and womb cancers, with the protection often lasting for years after stopping the Pill.[5, 6] This is in contrast to the very small increase in risk in breast cancer when the Pill is taken for longer than 12 years, with the risk returning back to the background risk on stopping.[6] The small risk of side effects, such as mood changes in some, especially teenagers, should be discussed but should not be a deterrent if it is the most appropriate option after a thorough discussion with your doctor (see Chapter 8).

The Pill is especially useful to manage missed or delayed periods and can be used to have a scheduled and more controlled bleed. The Pill prevents a build-up of womb lining when used to treat missed periods of PCOS, which can result in overgrowth of womb lining cells (endometrial hyperplasia, a risk factor for womb cancer, see Chapter 23) or prolonged bouts of heavy bleeding. The Pill may be taken back-to-back with a break every few months as desired, as there is no medical reason to have a monthly withdrawal bleed. This is contrary to popular belief but many women do prefer to take it back-to-back, and in this situation, there is no lining build up as the womb lining is suppressed with the hormones you are taking.

Before you start taking the Pill or any hormonal contraception (progesterone only pill, injection, implant or coil, for example), whether it is for managing PCOS symptoms or for contraception, you should have a detailed discussion with your doctor both about hormonal contraception and about possible alternative options, including the side effects and benefits of the different treatment options. Any decision to take any form of medication, including the Pill, should be with your informed consent. You should know that if it does not agree with you, with medical guidance, you can come off your medication while considering other options.

Case study outcome: Alison

I explained to Alison that her healthy lifestyle had really helped her PCOS as well as her general health and would continue to do so. She agreed that this was indeed the case. She did not want to reconsider other forms of hormonal contraception or other specific medications for her acne management, having tried them before. The copper coil was inappropriate for her given her heavy periods as it could make them worse. The Pill was the most likely option to offer her both symptom relief for her PCOS-related cystic acne as well as highly effective contraception. It was really not a case of choosing holistic methods over medication or vice versa, and it was my job as a healthcare professional to help her see the benefits of both. I also reassured Alison that she could have a trial of the medication for six months and, if she saw no benefit, if it did not suit her or if her circumstances changed, she could always reconsider.

Alison found the Pill did suit her and was happy to stay on it while remaining mindful of all the lifestyle measures that had helped her PCOS so far.

The PCOS Myth Buster

Myth: I have heard I should avoid the Pill due to the increased risk of clots as I have PCOS.

The facts: Combined oestrogen-progesterone oral contraceptives (COCPs) are the most useful of all medical treatments in PCOS, especially when it comes to managing androgen excess and menstrual disorders as well as providing contraception. Currently available information does not support PCOS being an additional risk factor for blood clots (venous thromboembolism). The Pill is safe and effective, although it slightly increases the risk of blood clots in the legs or lungs. This is a rare complication in young, healthy women who do not smoke, but it is more of a concern in women who are medically obese, if one has a genetic blood clotting factor or disorder, and in older women.[7] After thorough assessment of risk factors and proper counselling, as in the case of anyone being offered the Pill, there is no need to be denied the Pill if you have PCOS, if this is the most suitable option for you.

PCOS POINTERS

- Take time to understand your condition where possible, so you can reach an informed decision.
- Ask healthcare professionals to discuss all suitable options that can help manage your condition.
- Lifestyle medicine and conventional medicine complement each other; it is not one or the other.
- Ask to be referred to a professional who can help you if your current healthcare professional cannot.
- Do not reject lifesaving or life-enhancing vaccines, medicines and surgery without due consideration of the benefits and risks.
- PCOS does not put you at a higher risk of blood clots when compared with people without PCOS.
- The Pill is safe and is the most useful of all medical treatments in PCOS.

Part Three

Managing PCOS

The use of lifestyle approaches and nutrition to manage the condition of PCOS

Section 3.1: Symptoms of anovulation in PCOS: Periods, fertility

14

When your periods go missing
Periods in PCOS

Case study: Keisha

Keisha, a 25-year-old office worker, had not seen her period
for four months. When they finally started, she was initially
relieved but it soon felt as if the floodgates had opened. She
had not stopped bleeding for the last four weeks. Every time
she felt they were stopping, she started passing clots again.

She had been diagnosed with possible PCOS a few years
before and had been offered the Pill as treatment for her
irregular periods. It had helped her through university.
Since coming off the Pill a couple of years before seeing me,
her periods had once again become unpredictable, coming
every six to eight weeks and were noticeably heavier but she
had never gone this long before without a period.

Periods in PCOS

In Chapter 1, I explained how the menstrual cycle results from a complex feedback loop involving the brain, ovaries and uterus. Irregular menstrual cycles are the most common and best known of all symptoms of PCOS. This usually presents as infrequent periods, either missed or delayed in timing.

Other period problems which may also occur in PCOS include heavy or prolonged periods, bleeding between periods and painful periods. There are other possible causes for these menstrual problems, such as endometrial polyps, fibroids, endometriosis and pelvic inflammatory disease. These are usually unrelated to PCOS but may co-exist with the condition. A detailed medical history and clinical examination along with simple blood tests and a pelvic ultrasound scan will usually point to the right diagnosis, so correct treatment can be offered. This chapter focuses on PCOS as a cause of period problems.

Tracking the menstrual cycle

I recommend that all people with uteruses track their cycle from their first ever period until they completely stop at menopause (defined as no periods for more than 12 months). Tracking is not only for those who are trying to conceive. You can use a simple calendar to mark the days or one of the reliable apps on your smartphone. This way, you will know if there are major variations in your cycle or if you have bleeding when you shouldn't.

The length of the normal menstrual cycle is usually 24-35 days and is calculated as the number of days from the first day of the start of your period to the day before the start of your next period. Most cycle lengths are fairly consistent and vary by just a few days in general for an individual. For example, if your cycle is 32 days, a normal cycle may be 30-32-33-31 days and not usually 35-24-34-25 days.

The duration of your period is the number of days you bleed and typically lasts between two and seven days. Remember to include spotting or brown loss in your calculations, both for your cycle length and for the duration of your period.

When to be concerned about periods

Each individual will usually have their own cycle pattern, which also varies as a result of many factors including age, hormonal contraception and pregnancy. If the gap between your periods keeps changing significantly and this change lasts for more than three cycles in a row, you should see a doctor. If you are concerned about the nature, timing or amount of bleeding, if you notice bleeding after sex or if you are having prolonged bleeding – i.e., your period is lasting much longer than a week – it is best not to ignore these symptoms and to get checked out sooner rather than later.

Missing periods

If you miss your periods more than three months in a row and there is no obvious explanation, such as hormonal contraception, pregnancy or lactation, you should seek medical advice. The finely tuned hormones that regulate the menstrual cycle are also influenced by our environment, both internal and external. Stress can affect the length of your cycle. Even moving to a new place, starting university, travel, a new job, a breakup or grief can affect your periods and your cycle length.

Functional hypothalamic amenorrhea (HA)

Functional HA (amenorrhoea means 'without menstruation') suggests there is no known underlying medical cause or medication stopping periods. The signalling to the brain that regulates the menstrual cycle is altered, with low levels of hormones including oestrogen, leading to periods stopping. This may be from one or a combination of:

- weight loss from eating too few calories to meet your needs
- an eating disorder
- low body fat as seen in some athletes
- excessive exercise (often more than 2-3 hours a day).

HA can affect people of all sizes, including those with PCOS. It is important to seek medical advice early to investigate and manage this condition as long-term complications include bone loss in as little as six months of period loss,[1] skin and hair changes and infertility. The condition can often be reversed with a multidisciplinary approach such as cognitive behavioural therapy (CBT) alongside lifestyle changes with a focus on nutrition and stress management.

Don't ignore missed or infrequent periods

Acute or chronic illness, sudden and rapid weight gain, thyroid problems, cancer treatment and substance misuse are some of the other situations that can also cause missed periods. Whatever the underlying cause of your missed cycles, it is best never to ignore this symptom, as periods are such an important indicator of general health. In fact, doctors are recommending periods be considered the fifth 'vital sign' and as important as the four other vital signs (see Chapter 1).

If you are having fewer than six to eight periods per year, this is known as oligomenorrhea, the medical term for infrequent menstrual cycles. The term amenorrhea refers to no periods for three months or more. You should ask your doctor to check you for PCOS or any other underlying cause in this situation.

Period problems in PCOS often start in the teenage years

As ovulation is not yet fully established in young menstruating people, it is common to have variable periods for a year from when you first start (menarche). However, the condition of PCOS does seem to start around puberty (see Chapter 6).

The cause of irregular periods in PCOS

The hormonal surges from the brain as well as the oestrogen and progesterone levels in the ovary all depend on the release of an egg from the ovary (ovulation). The multiple immature follicles seen within the ovaries of those with PCOS do not get selected for at least one follicle to grow to the size needed to trigger ovulation.[2] Missed or delayed periods result from this anovulation (when an egg doesn't release from the ovary during the menstrual cycle). Ovulatory dysfunction, when eggs are not released regularly, is often seen in PCOS due to the androgen excess or oestrogen excess (see Chapters 4 and 6).

Some women with PCOS can have ovulatory dysfunction even in the presence of regular periods. There are blood tests to check for ovulation if needed, such as if subfertility is suspected.[3]

Heavy or prolonged periods in PCOS

When ovulation does not occur or happens infrequently, periods are missed or delayed and the endometrial lining of the womb becomes thicker than normal and builds up over time. Eventually, when the endometrial lining does shed, it does so rather patchily, resulting in heavy and often prolonged bleeding. The lining does not grow or shed evenly as it does in an ovulatory menstrual cycle. People with PCOS who have missed periods for several months are at higher risk of endometrial hyperplasia (overgrowth of the womb lining), which in turn can increase the risk of womb cancer.

There are other causes for heavy or prolonged periods and some of these, such as endometrial polyps, fibroids, endometriosis and adenomyosis, may also be seen in women with PCOS. These are oestrogen-dependent conditions, so occur in the reproductive age group (15- 49 years) and often go hand in hand with each other.

Defining heavy periods

The average blood loss in a normal period is about 30 ml, or five teaspoons. Menstrual flow consists of some blood mostly mixed with cells from the womb lining, vaginal secretions and cervical mucus and is not all blood. This why it appears to be more than five teaspoons. If the menstrual blood loss is more than 80 ml or five *tablespoons*, then this is called heavy menstrual bleeding (HMB) in medical terms. We never really measure blood loss except in a research situation as there are many limitations to measuring this accurately.[4] If you think your period is heavy, then it is. Your perception is the most important. Doctors agree that if a woman says her periods are heavy, then they are. The National Institute for Health and Care Excellence (NICE) in the United Kingdom defines HMB as excessive menstrual blood loss that interferes with a woman's physical, emotional, social and material quality of life. Up to half of people who menstruate can experience heavy periods.

You may notice this as flooding where you experience gushes of blood, large clots bigger than your thumbnail (10 pence coin), leaking through your menstrual product or needing to wear double protection (for example pad and period panties, pad and tampon).

Periods are considered heavy if:

- They interfere with your quality of life.
- They stop you from going to work.
- You cannot do your normal activities.
- You are passing large clots (2.5 cm/10 p coin).
- You have flooding or leaking through.
- You need to change every couple of hours.
- You need to use double protection.
- They last much longer than a week.

Painful periods

Painful periods can affect women at all ages during their reproductive life, whether you have PCOS or not. A large survey of 32,000 women in the Netherlands published in 2019 revealed that menstrual symptoms, including pain, heavy bleeding and low mood, may be linked to nearly nine days of lost productivity per woman every year.[5] That's nearly two weeks' worth of working days. More importantly, a staggering eight out of 10 women reported working while feeling unwell. Periods usually tend to become less painful as one gets older and after childbirth, but not always.

The cause of painful periods

The main reason for period pain is the release of pain-producing chemicals, called prostaglandins, as the uterine lining sheds. Any cramps felt are due to the uterine muscle contracting in response to these pain chemicals which act to reduce the blood supply and oxygen to the uterus. You may also notice nausea, vomiting, headache, dizziness and an upset tummy. Painful periods that do not have an underlying cause are known by the medical term 'primary dysmen-orrhoea'. The pain usually begins as your period starts or just before, and fades in a couple of days. Having a particularly heavy flow with clots may also make periods more painful as the clots make their way into the vagina, stretching the neck of the womb (cervix).

Some people with PCOS seem to suffer more from period pain than those who do not have the condition, according to a study of young Korean women published in 2019. The reasons for this are not entirely clear and much more research is needed in this area.[6]

Sometimes, there is an underlying cause for your painful periods. If so, it is called secondary dysmenorrhoea. Conditions such as endometriosis, adenomyosis, fibroids and pelvic inflammatory disease may be present alongside PCOS. You should see your doctor if you have new or recent pain during your periods or in the lead-up to your monthly period.

Endometriosis, a condition that can cause painful periods in as many as 10% of people who menstruate may be seen more often in those with PCOS, especially when subfertility is also a factor as endometriosis can make it harder to conceive.[7]

Recommended tests for detecting menstrual disorders

As discussed in Chapter 3, a thorough medical history and examination and tests as appropriate will not only help with the diagnosis of PCOS but will also give your doctor information regarding other associated conditions. What you tell your doctor about the timing, length and flow of your periods is really helpful to arrive at an accurate diagnosis of PCOS. A pelvic ultrasound scan can be helpful as it gives more information about your womb and ovaries, pointing to the possible causes of painful or heavy periods discussed above.

A full blood count with haemoglobin and ferritin levels to check your iron stores is a quick and easy way of testing for iron-deficiency anaemia. More detailed blood tests and specialised scans may be recommended by your doctor, depending on the situation.

Helping yourself

Track your cycle

With the help of a free app on your smartphone or a good old-fashioned diary, start tracking your periods as it is helpful to know your menstrual pattern, recording any changes.

Seek medical help

It's really important to seek qualified medical help early if you suspect you have heavy periods or PCOS-related menstrual problems.

Lifestyle advice

Most people who have irregular menstrual cycles in PCOS have an excess of androgens from insulin resistance or excess body weight. Addressing this through lifestyle and dietary modifications and medications as appropriate is key (Chapters 11 and 12). We will look at how nutrition can specifically help with painful and heavy periods here.

Eat more whole plant foods

Eating a whole food plant-based diet can help make periods both less painful and lighter.[8] This exact mechanism is unclear, but the anti-inflammatory nature of plant foods (think fruit, vegetables, beans, herbs, spices and whole grains) has positive effects on the pathways in periods. This includes arachidonic acid and prostaglandin synthesis, which in turn is intimately related to the flow and pain associated with periods.

As our body fat is a storehouse of hormones, losing excess fat helps not just to bring periods back but often normalises menstrual blood flow and helps with improving reproductive function.[9, 10] Plants tend to be much lower in calories but occupy more space in our stomachs when compared with similar weights of animal-derived foods or ultra-processed foods. As a result, when we eat a plant-predominant diet, we feel fuller despite consuming fewer calories and this helps with losing weight without having to reduce the amount of food one eats.

Enjoy a variety of iron-rich plant foods daily

Some of these foods can help keep your iron levels up:

- Green leafy vegetables (such as kale, broccoli and bok choy)
- Pulses and legumes (beans, lentils, peas, tofu)
- Nuts and seeds
- Dried fruit (such as dried apricots, dates and raisins)
- Blackstrap molasses.

We advise women to pair these sources with vitamin C-rich foods, such as kiwis, oranges, lemons, bell peppers and strawberries, to increase iron absorption. Soaking, germinating and fermenting grains and legumes improves the bioavailability of micronutrients, including non-haem iron, the type of iron found in plant foods. In other words, it means there is more active iron available for use by our body.

Avoiding cocoa, coffee, red wine and tea, especially black tea and green tea (all these contain polyphenols such as tannins) at mealtimes or within an hour of a meal is advised as these foods hinder iron absorption.

Whole grain cereals containing phytates may make it harder to absorb iron so combine these with vibrant carotenoid-containing vegetables, such as bell peppers, carrots, squash and asparagus, to reduce this effect; a simple reminder is to 'eat the rainbow'.

Iron-deficiency anaemia with lower iron stores is a common problem in menstruating women, irrespective of diet, although those on a plant-based diet may have lower levels than those on an omnivore diet.[11] It is important to take particular care to include iron-rich foods on a plant-based diet and to have blood tests for iron levels (haemoglobin and ferritin), initially as a baseline and more regularly if there have been any concerns. Low plasma zinc levels can lead to iron-deficiency anemia. Add in zinc-rich plant foods such as peas, corn, nuts, carrots, whole grains, wheat germ, cabbage, radish, watercress, soya beans and other legumes. It is important to include iron-rich foods, especially for menstruating people as the requirement is higher at 14.8 mg (NHS UK), or 18 mg (USA recommendation) per day compared with 8.7 mg after menopause.

Haem iron vs non-haem iron

A plant-based diet has so many other health benefits that there is no reason to reach for a steak or liver to increase your iron levels. High intake of haem iron, found in meat, comes with undesirable effects on the human body, such as an increased risk of colorectal cancer. Plant foods have non-haem iron that may not get absorbed in as high amounts as the haem iron found in animal flesh and blood, but this is an advantage for us. Haem iron can cause inflammation and is linked to bowel, lung and pancreatic cancers and stroke.[12, 13]

Enjoy omega-3 fatty acids

Omega-3 and omega-6 fatty acids both play an important part in the menstrual cycle. Blood tests to check omega-3 fatty acid levels are not routinely recommended in the UK (see Chapter 33).

Eating soya can help regulate the menstrual cycle

The healthful plant-oestrogen content in soya works by displacing the excess unwanted oestrogens that come from our body fat or from hormones in meat and dairy and when eaten regularly, can help with weight loss.[14] Both these actions can have a beneficial effect on the menstrual cycle. We have dedicated Chapter 26 to soya myth-busting.

The role of ginger in heavy or painful periods

Oral ginger could be an effective treatment for menstrual pain, comparing favourably with a commonly used painkiller (mefenamic acid, an NSAID), based on the findings of a systematic review and meta-analysis in 2016 of a small number of studies.[15] Similar findings were observed in another trial in 2018.[16] A double-blinded randomised controlled trial using dried ginger significantly helped both with pain and heavy menstrual bleeding.[17] Taken regularly during a period, ginger seems to help by its action on prostaglandin synthesis and on inflammatory chemicals. It could, therefore, be a cheap and safer alternative with minimal side effects, especially if one wishes to avoid or cannot tolerate certain painkillers. However, these were all small studies and need to be replicated to be properly validated. In the meantime, it is certainly worth adding ginger for a few months in milder cases or alongside conventional medicines to see if it helps normalise flow. Ginger also helps with nausea, vomiting and diarrhoea that may be associated with periods. Spices are delicious and have so many antioxidant properties that it is always a good idea to add more of them to our diets.

I would suggest you start by enjoying ginger tea and adding fresh ginger when cooking regularly and then try ginger powder three times a day (one eighth to a third of a teaspoon) up to a maximum total of one teaspoon per day dissolved in water, as per the amounts used in the studies. This can be tried for about four consecutive days, commencing a day before the period starts, where possible, to see if it helps with the pain and the flow. Ginger capsules are more expensive while dried ginger powder or fresh ginger root will cost pennies.

Medical and surgical treatments for period problems in PCOS

Treatment for period problems in PCOS is highly effective with excellent outcomes, with a choice of oral medications, hormonal drugs, and surgical options after a fully informed discussion.

I must emphasise that diet should never be the only thing relied upon by those with heavy periods causing symptoms. If you have iron-deficiency anaemia on a simple blood test, you may need to take regular oral iron supplements, especially if pregnant or considering conceiving. I suggest a discussion with your healthcare professional first with regards to dosage and type of iron to take.

If there are no contraindications, medications to help with your bleeding and pain, such as anti-prostaglandins (ibuprofen) or antifibrinolytics (tranexamic acid) to reduce blood flow, may be prescribed to be used during your period.

Hormonal medications

If you are not trying actively for a pregnancy and there are no contraindications and you have been thoroughly advised, the Pill and other forms of hormonal contraception, including a progesterone-containing intrauterine coil (IUD), may be highly effective in managing your heavy or painful periods. The Pill or cyclical progesterone are also useful to manage missed or delayed periods and can be used to have a scheduled and more controlled monthly withdrawal bleed.

The Pill may be taken back-to-back, with a break every few months if desired, as there is no medical need to have a monthly withdrawal bleed and this is in fact preferred by many. However, if you notice spotting, finish the pack and have a bleed and start again. You will soon work out how many months you can go without spotting before you take a Pill break.

You must remember to take your Pill regularly, preferably around the same time each day to minimise spotting and for effective contraception. If you are concerned, or spotting persists, you should seek the advice of your doctor and also check you are up-to-date with your cervical screening if you have ever been sexually active.

Periods returning after the Pill

You do not need to have periods or withdrawal bleeds if you are on hormonal contraception. It may take a while for periods to come back for some people after stopping the Pill or hormone injections. This used to be known as 'post-pill amenorrhoea'. This is not a direct result of taking the Pill. Most women resume their periods within a few weeks, but this does depend on a number of factors, including what your previous cycles were normally like. If your periods were irregular prior to starting the Pill, they may go back to being irregular. Even if you had regular periods before you started the Pill, your periods may become irregular if you have gained or lost a significant amount of weight or had a stressful time coinciding with your Pill use. When you then come off the Pill, and note your periods are irregular, you may mistakenly think it is because you were on the Pill.

Seek help early

You may need to be referred by your family doctor to a hospital specialist for further tests and to discuss surgical treatment if there are other causes suspected for your heavy or painful periods.

Case study outcome: Keisha

My trained medical eye suspected Keisha was anaemic. In people with darker skin, it can be harder to assess anaemia, a state in which the level of haemoglobin in the blood is below the acceptable level. Doctors need to be more vigilant in people of colour, checking the palms, the eyelids, lips and inside the mouth for pallor rather than just checking for pale skin. Remember to mention specific symptoms such as tiredness, palpitations or feeling faint, and ask your doctor for a simple blood test to check for anaemia.

Keisha chose to go on cyclical hormone treatment (progesterone treatment) for a few months as well as iron supplements. She adopted a whole food plant-based diet over the course of three months with the help of a dietitian and was able to lose a significant amount of weight. Six months later, she had come off all medication and had taken up running as she felt full of energy. She was now having regular monthly cycles that were neither heavy nor painful. On a repeat blood test at six months and 12 months, she continued to maintain her iron levels on a healthy and varied plant-based diet.

The PCOS Myth Buster

Myth: A vegan or plant-based diet can stop your periods.
The facts: The long and short answer is that this is not true. Any diet that is restrictive in its food groups (fats, proteins, carbohydrates) can cause hormonal dysfunction through calorie restriction. Periods can stop due to eating disorders, low body fat stores, exercising too much, being under stress or eating a poor diet that is low in calories, whether it is vegan or not. We do not need animal products, ultra-processed foods, refined oils or fruit juices in our diets as these are not food groups. Eating a predominantly or exclusively whole food plant-based diet that is varied and has enough calories from all the major food groups supports regular menstruation.

PCOS POINTERS

- Infrequent ovulation in PCOS can cause delayed or missed periods.
- Heavy or prolonged periods can occur in PCOS.
- There may be causes other than PCOS if pain is a feature during your periods.
- Seek advice early if you are worried or if the problem persists longer than three months.
- Heavy periods are the commonest cause of iron-deficiency anaemia.
- Ginger can help reduce menstrual flow and period pain in some women.

Chapter 14

- Eat a varied, colourful plant-based diet with attention to iron-rich foods.
- You may benefit from iron supplements, with advice from your doctor.
- There are highly effective treatments available for heavy periods, so make an informed decision.

15

Getting pregnant
Fertility, preconception and pregnancy advice in PCOS

On receiving a diagnosis of PCOS, one of the fears you may have is that you can never get pregnant. Often, women tell me that is the only thing they remember, following their consultation with their doctor. This can contribute to a lot of anxiety but it is helpful to know there are a range of options out there for people with PCOS who are trying to conceive. While it is true that if you are living with PCOS it can be harder to get pregnant, I want to reassure you that most women with PCOS who wish to conceive do go on to have a baby. If you do have trouble getting pregnant, making positive changes to your lifestyle, and using fertility treatments as needed, can help you to significantly increase your chances of a successful pregnancy. This chapter doesn't make for easy reading but knowing the facts can help you make decisions early if having a biological child is something you would like.

Make lifestyle modifications as early as you possibly can, even years before you start to think of getting pregnant, as this can help not only with managing the other bothersome symptoms of PCOS but can also significantly reduce your risks of pregnancy complications, especially those associated with insulin resistance and body weight.

When it comes to planning for a baby, anxiety, depression and psychological symptoms of PCOS can impact your relationship, sexual intimacy and fertility treatment. Work on caring for your physical and mental health to the best of your ability. This should be with the help of the lifestyle changes we discuss throughout the book and by only ever seeking qualified medical advice rather than resorting to unproven and sometimes dangerous supplements and medications sold under the guise of 'natural' alternatives. Natural does not come in the form of a pill and natural does not always mean better.

Fertility and PCOS

Irregular cycles while trying to conceive

Irregular menstrual cycles such as missed or delayed periods suggest you are probably not ovulating regularly, making it harder but not impossible to fall pregnant. Fertility problems in PCOS usually arise from eggs not being released regularly from the ovaries (anovulation). PCOS is responsible for 80% of subfertility cases caused by anovulation.[2] Around 70-80% of those living with PCOS have difficulty in conceiving compared with 12.5% of those without the condition.[2, 3] However, do not assume you will definitely have problems falling pregnant and remember to use contraception when you do not wish to become pregnant.

There may be underlying thyroid problems in those with PCOS that can sometimes contribute to irregular menstrual cycles. The exact mechanism is not clear and long-term studies are needed to investigate this link further, especially to see if there is any effect on fertility. It is a good idea to have your thyroid checked if you have PCOS before you decide to try for a pregnancy.

Lifestyle changes can be more powerful than medications

Lifestyle modifications should always be recommended first to women with PCOS when compared with drugs such as metformin. This was the recommendation of a systematic review and meta-analysis published in 2020 that found the clinical outcomes, including improvements in frequency of menstrual periods and pregnancy outcomes, were not significantly different between lifestyle changes and metformin, an insulin-sensitising drug often used in PCOS, even though it is not officially approved.[6] Moreover, lifestyle modifications have been shown to have longer lasting benefits and only positive side effects. Metformin treatment has also not been shown to reduce pregnancy complications in PCOS.[7, 8, 9] Even if metformin is prescribed in certain specific situations, continue lifestyle modifications to get the maximum benefit.,

Advanced glycation end products (AGEs) and fertility

An accumulation of harmful inflammatory compounds called AGEs in the uterine tissue can have a negative impact on fertility in PCOS. Not only does it take longer to conceive but the uterus becomes inflamed, with inhibition of the implantation of a fertilised egg into the womb lining (see Chapter 12 for more on AGEs).

Fertility treatment if you have PCOS

If you have made all the possible changes to your lifestyle and haven't yet got pregnant, you may still need help with conceiving. You may require assisted conception and this is absolutely fine. It is important to make that decision early based on several factors. Women often blame themselves and feel they have failed, if they have not been able to conceive naturally. There should be no shame attached to asking for help.

The Pregnancy in Polycystic Ovary Syndrome (PPCOS) Study was a large prospective randomised controlled trial. It studied what clinical factors could predict a successful pregnancy outcome in women with PCOS. The study concluded that those with PCOS should be counselled early on in their fertility journey about their likelihood for live birth with simple first-line infertility therapy with the help of clinical parameters such as BMI (body mass index – see page 71), age, how long they had been trying to conceive and their excess hair growth score. Based on these scores, the study advised early referral for consideration of more advanced fertility techniques for those who were projected to have low likely pregnancy success rates.

I very briefly outline below some of the most common treatments, but every individual is different, with many factors affecting fertility and pregnancy outcomes.

Medical treatments

The first-line pharmacological treatments for inducing ovulation include oral medications like clomiphene citrate or letrozole treatment, with timed intercourse. There are several other effective medical treatments that are available to help you ovulate even when these first-line drugs have not been effective. These second-line treatments include hormones (for example, gonadotrophins) or keyhole ovarian surgery (laparoscopic ovarian drilling/diathermy). These techniques have good success, with live birth rates, but you should be fully informed and involved in all decision-making. Finally, there are assisted conception techniques that you might benefit from after discussion with a fertility specialist. The good news is that most women with PCOS will go on to have a baby although for some the journey may be long.

Alternative treatments

There is insufficient evidence to support the use of acupuncture to promote ovulation, pregnancy and live birth in PCOS according to the conclusion of a systematic review and meta-analysis of all published research. However, the review did find that acupuncture could promote the recovery of menstrual cycles and help down-regulate the levels of luteinising hormone (LH – see page 19) and testosterone in patients with PCOS. Acupuncture cannot be routinely recommended in the absence of robust trials.

Seeking help

Interestingly, studies have suggested there may be improved fertility with increasing age in PCOS. This is thought to be due to the reduction in the number of immature follicles that occurs naturally with age, making cycles more regular and ovulatory, increasing chances of spontaneous pregnancy. While this may be true, my advice is to seek medical help to discuss your options if you are not pregnant within six months of regular unprotected sex if you have PCOS and not wait for the 12 months that is advised to couples with no risk factors.

If you are above 35 years of age or have a pre-existing health condition such as endometriosis and/or fibroids, a history of infections such as chlamydia, chronic pelvic pain or you are struggling to get pregnant naturally, seek professional medical advice early. This is again so that you can have appropriate tests and treatment early or be referred for fertility treatment.

Egg freezing is an option for those with PCOS for the same reasons that apply to other women who wish to proactively increase their chance of pregnancy later in life. Similarly, egg donation comes with no increased risks of abnormal embryos if someone with PCOS wishes to donate eggs, although overall pregnancy rates are somewhat lower compared with those without PCOS (the 'control groups').

Preconception advice in PCOS

Make time for intimacy

Regular unprotected vaginal sex with a male partner offers the best chance for spontaneous conception. It can be more difficult to get pregnant if you are having delayed or missing periods as you might not be ovulating regularly. Having sex just around ovulation can be stressful and unpredictable, even with the help of expensive ovulation kits, which are also unreliable for those with PCOS. It is better to have unprotected sex every two or three days throughout your cycle, as it can be difficult to predict exactly when you ovulate in any given cycle.

Remember that even though the egg survives about 24 hours, sperm can remain active for two to three days and up to five days. You should track your menstrual cycles to know your pattern, with the help of a diary or an app on your smartphone. I still meet a lot of people who menstruate who do not know their period start dates; if this is the case for you this means when you do get pregnant, you might miss out on important tests in early pregnancy. If you are having pain during sex, do not ignore it, and seek help, as conditions like endometriosis can also cause fertility problems.

Preparing for a pregnancy

Leading a healthy lifestyle for both you and your partner and paying attention to all the six pillars of lifestyle can significantly improve your fertility chances. This is a good time to start optimising your diet and exercise so this healthier lifestyle becomes much easier when you are pregnant – if you think that is something you might want in the future (see Chapter 24).

It takes two

Subfertility is not always a woman's issue, with male factors accounting for a third of couples seeking help. Another third of couples trying for a pregnancy have both partners affected, so pre-conception advice should always apply to both. Some interventions can take months to achieve, such as folic acid supplementation, quitting smoking, avoidance of alcohol and certain medications, as well as optimising medical conditions and weight loss, so the earlier couples can get started to make positive changes, the better.

Supplements while trying to conceive

You should take a high-quality, medically-approved pregnancy supplement with all the recommended vitamins and minerals in the right dosage throughout pregnancy and during breastfeeding to ensure adequate intake of the important minerals and vitamins for a healthy pregnancy.

If you have a few months to prepare, start a prenatal supplement at least three to six months before, especially folic acid which greatly reduces a baby's risk of serious neural tube defects, such as spina bifida. Speak to your doctor as some situations call for higher than normal doses of folic acid, such as if you have type 2 diabetes, weigh more than a certain amount or have a family history of neural tube defects. If this is not possible, do start as soon as you find out you are pregnant, as the early weeks are critical for foetal development.

Smoking, caffeine and alcohol

Smoking and in fact, any substance use, has harmful effects on both the pregnancy and the foetus. There is also no safe level of alcohol consumption for a developing foetus so avoiding alcohol is the safest option in pregnancy and while trying to conceive. I suggest seeking help from your health professional if you think any of these apply to you.

New research suggests caffeine raises stillbirth risk in pregnancy, with a 27% increase in risk for each 100 mg consumed. This suggests that previously recommended safe limit guidelines of 200 mg (as little as two cups of instant coffee) may need to be reconsidered as per advice from the Royal College of Obstetricians and Gynaecologists (RCOG), UK. If you can significantly reduce and, if possible, completely cut out caffeine in the lead up to pregnancy, the cravings would have been dealt with by the time you are pregnant. Caffeine is not just present in coffee but also in tea, colas, dark chocolate and energy drinks, with the numbers easily adding up. There are excellent decaffeinated teas and coffees available that do not come with risks, although it's best to consume them outside of mealtimes as they can still affect iron absorption. With regard to herbal teas, not all are completely safe during pregnancy, especially if consumed in large quantities (see Chapter 27). Water remains the drink of choice.

Weight loss

Losing even 5-10% of your weight can help the return of regular ovulatory cycles, increasing the chances of falling pregnant.[1, 32, 34] If you have excess weight, it is better to lose what you can even before you consider ovulation induction therapy for better success. The approach to management of excess weight in those actively seeking pregnancy should always start with lifestyle changes (diet and exercise)[23] and, when necessary, weight loss surgery.[34] However, if you are 37 years or older, or because of your individual circumstances, ovulation induction fertility treatment may be offered either straightaway or after a short initial three-month attempt at weight loss with lifestyle. Lifestyle modifications should nevertheless continue side-by-side even when medical treatments are necessary (see Chapters 11 and 12). Sperm quality and erectile dysfunction also improve with weight loss in men.[24]

Check your environment

It is helpful to check your work and home environment, especially for identifying potential toxic exposures (including endocrine disruptors) such as lead, mercury, pesticides, household cleaning products, plastics used for storing food and water (avoid BPA-containing products), receipts, food labels, cosmetics, air pollution, infection risk and unsafe sources of water.

It is best to avoid many types of fish, including tuna and swordfish, and to limit fish such as salmon due to their potential mercury content.

There is no convincing evidence that exposure to common sources of electromagnetic field radiation, such as computer monitors, smartphones and microwave ovens, causes harm.

Stress and sleep

Having a regular sleep routine that prioritises restorative sleep of seven to nine hours every night, identifying your stress triggers and finding ways to manage your stress can help improve fertility and pregnancy outcomes. Ongoing stress and disturbed sleep are found to increase cortisol in the body, triggering insulin responses and insulin resistance if sustained (see Chapter 11).

Seeing a health professional before you are pregnant

Do remember to go prepared to your doctor with your medical history and questions to get the most out of your appointment (see Chapter 4). If you have a partner, involve them by taking them along or go with a trusted friend or family member who can be your second pair of ears. Your doctor should be able to advise you on further tests if needed, after a discussion and general examination, checking your weight, blood pressure and other risk factors. These often include swabs for infection (STI screening), HIV blood test, rubella immunity, full blood count to check for anaemia and thyroid and blood sugar tests. You may be referred for genetic testing and testing for blood disorders, tuberculosis and any other specialised tests that may be needed on an individualised basis. You should check you are up to date with necessary vaccinations before attempting pregnancy as well as your cervical smear.

If you identify as LGBTQIA+, you deserve a sensitive discussion without assumptions just as much as anyone else regarding pregnancy planning, contraception and prevention of infections. Seek out an empathetic healthcare professional as they are around. Sadly, in general, healthcare has not yet caught up to be equitable and this needs to change urgently, with education, training and policy changes.

Pregnancy and PCOS

Pregnancy risks

PCOS is a condition associated with low-grade, chronic inflammation, as demonstrated by higher levels of inflammatory markers such as C-reactive protein (CRP), which appears to worsen during pregnancy, possibly contributing to the excess risk of adverse pregnancy outcomes discussed next.

Miscarriage risk appears to be 20-40% higher than the baseline in the general obstetric population.[31] There are significantly increased risks of developing pregnancy-related diabetes (gestational diabetes), pregnancy-induced hypertension, pre-eclampsia, preterm birth and caesarean birth with PCOS when compared with the general obstetric population. In addition, babies appear to have a higher risk of admission to the neonatal intensive care unit.

Even in the absence of PCOS, excess weight is a risk factor for all these complications. Body weight seems to play a particularly important contributing role in many of the pregnancy risks seen in PCOS.[1, 34] A well-planned plant-based diet is an anti-inflammatory way of eating and is safe at all stages of pregnancy and during breastfeeding. It is endorsed by major dietetic organisations around the world.

Mental health concerns in pregnancy

There is little guidance available, either from national or international guidelines due to woefully inadequate research in this area, despite evidence to suggest that women with PCOS are at increased risk of developing perinatal mental health problems. In 2020, a large United States cohort study found women with PCOS at increased risk of both cardiovascular and psychiatric complications during the postpartum period. The researchers advised that PCOS should be recognised as an at-risk condition, recommending routine screening and early intervention to reduce complications.[38a] In another study from Australia, women reporting PCOS had higher prevalence of antenatal and postnatal depression and anxiety compared to women without PCOS.[38b] Prenatal psychological screening for women with PCOS should be implemented at a national level as a matter of urgency if we are to improve outcomes and reduce pregnancy and post-delivery complications. Healthcare professionals also need to improve at diagnosing PCOS, ideally even before pregnancy. A 2021 population-based cohort study of high-risk mothers in the USA found nearly 20% of women in this study sample who reported at least two of the PCOS symptoms had not received a clinical diagnosis for PCOS.[38c]

Gestational diabetes (GDM) is a warning for the future

The risks of GDM and type 2 diabetes appear to be increased in women with PCOS independent of body weight as indicated by body mass index (BMI).[41] Insulin resistance is present in around 65–80% of women with PCOS, independent of body weight, but is made worse if you do carry excess weight.[42] South Asian women are at particular risk of GDM, irrespective of BMI, as they often have an increased incidence of insulin resistance and at an earlier age (see Chapter 9).

Guidelines issued by the National Insitute for Health and Clinical Excellence (NICE) in the UK recommend that anyone with PCOS planning a pregnancy should be offered a 75 g oral glucose tolerance test (OGTT). If this is not performed preconception, it should be offered before 20 weeks' gestation. Furthermore, an OGTT should be offered to all PCOS patients at 24–28 weeks' gestation.

If you have PCOS, ask to be screened for gestational diabetes during pregnancy, as per your own national or local protocols, with referral to a specialist obstetric service if any abnormalities are detected.

GDM, once diagnosed in pregnancy, must be treated with medical nutritional therapy as advised by qualified dietitians and with self-monitoring of blood sugars. Moderate exercise should be actively encouraged unless you have received medical advice to avoid certain exercises. If lifestyle changes do not get blood sugar levels under control, insulin treatment is usually preferred over oral medications to improve pregnancy and neonatal outcomes in pregnancy.

Developing GDM in pregnancy is considered a marker or stress test as it puts you at a higher risk of developing GDM in the next pregnancy[32, 42] and is a predictor of developing future type 2 diabetes, type 1 diabetes, metabolic syndrome and cardiovascular disease. That is why it is advisable to be screened for type 2 diabetes 6-12 weeks after delivery and then to be rescreened every one to three years after.[43]

Future generations may also be at higher risk

Pregnancy appears to be a key window to optimise your cardio-vascular health and influence your child's lifelong cardiovascular health too. A multinational cohort study which included the UK, published in February 2021, showed children between the ages of 10 and 14 years whose mothers had poor heart health (BMI, blood pressure, glucose levels, cholesterol levels, smoking) at around 28 weeks of gestation also had worse cardiovascular health than controls. This is possibly due to epigenetic modifications inside the womb (see Chapter 2). All these risk factors are seen more often in mothers with PCOS so bringing in lifestyle changes as early and as much as you possibly can, even before you conceive, may help reduce risks to your unborn child (see Chapters 11 and 12).

Helping yourself

As the risks of pregnancy, delivery and neonatal complications are increased if you have PCOS, it is important to seek help from experienced health professionals as soon as you find out you are pregnant – preferably well before conception – so you can have the best possible pregnancy outcome. Hospitals should have established guidelines for when you are pregnant with PCOS, so problems can be addressed early and many of the associated complications prevented or managed appropriately.

Lifestyle changes have been shown to prevent or delay progression to type 2 diabetes and reduce cardiovascular risk for you[45, 46] and, possibly, for your child. Making changes in your diet and physical activity early can help reduce pregnancy complications.[32, 42]

Empowering yourself with information can help you to seek medical advice early and have better outcomes as many of these fertility and pregnancy-related issues have successful interventions and treatments available.

The PCOS Myth Buster

Myth: I can never have a baby because I have PCOS.
The facts: Even though PCOS is the commonest cause of subfertility, it is mostly due to anovulation which usually responds well to both lifestyle modifications and fertility treatment. Most women with PCOS do go on to have a baby but sometimes do need help with fertility treatment.

PCOS POINTERS

- Remember that most women with PCOS who wish to conceive do go on to have a baby.
- Irregular cycles are the main cause of subfertility in PCOS.
- Lifestyle changes can be powerful in improving both body composition and insulin resistance, helping with your fertility chances.
- Seek medical help if not pregnant within six months of regular unprotected sex if you have PCOS.Using fertility treatment if needed can help you to significantly increase your chances of a successful pregnancy.
- Try to plan your pregnancy, follow preconception advice, and take a medically-approved supplement including folic acid.
- The risk of pregnancy, delivery and neonatal complications can increase with PCOS, so it is important to seek help early in pregnancy.

Part Three

Managing PCOS (cont'd)

Section 3.2: Symptoms of androgen excess in PCOS

16

Spot the symptom
Acne

Like many skin conditions, acne can affect self-esteem and confidence, increasing feelings of social isolation. Many of my patients with PCOS tell me they feel very conscious of their skin a lot of the time, so much so that it affects their mood.

We usually associate spots and pimples with being a teenager. Acne affects 80-95% of adolescents in the west with most outgrowing their acne by their mid-twenties, responding well to general skincare advice and acne therapies. Women in general tend to suffer from acne more than men but are also more likely to seek help because of societal expectations.[1, 2, 3]

This is not the case for many people with PCOS-related acne that lasts well into adulthood, with many suffering extreme distress and anxiety when standard acne treatments fail to offer adequate relief. If you are spending more than an hour a day worrying about your skin, then I advise you to consider seeking medical help.

Adult acne

When acne persists beyond the age of 25 it is known as adult acne. If you are over the age of 25 or if you notice recurrent painful cystic acne that does not clear up quickly, you should ask your doctor to consider PCOS as a diagnosis even if you are under 25. This is even more important if you notice other signs of androgen excess, such as excessive facial or body hair growth, scalp hair loss or thinning and/or irregular periods, or also if standard treatment for your acne has not helped. Reactions to cosmetic products can cause adult acne and while there are many other causes, a thorough medical history by a qualified health professional can reveal an answer in most situations.

There are some serious causes of androgen-excess-related acne (see Chapter 6). If you notice a very rapid increase in severe acne, you must see your doctor urgently for tests and be considered for a referral to an endocrinologist.

PCOS-related acne

As hormone levels rise and fall at different stages of the menstrual cycle, most notice skin flare ups and oily skin in the run up to their period, but this can be much more pronounced if you have PCOS.

You may also notice most of your acne lesions tend to affect your chin, jawline, cheeks and upper neck, and over half of women with PCOS-related acne notice spots and lumps on the neck, chest and upper back.

Painful, inflamed cysts and hard nodules form beneath the skin which do not discharge and typically take a long time to resolve, often leaving behind scars and dark marks or patches (post-inflammatory hyperpigmentation). You may see excessive thick and dark hair growth in these same areas.

The cause of acne in PCOS

Acne is seen in at least a third of women with PCOS (20-40%), with the highest incidence of clinically significant acne in African

American, Hispanic and Indonesian women.[1, 4] Experts believe acne is related to several key factors, including excess sebum production by the sebaceous glands, blockage of follicles, excessive growth of the bacterium *Propionobacterium acnes* and inflammation.[5, 6] In PCOS, androgen excess and local androgen sensitivity are additional factors exacerbating all of the above to cause the symptoms of acne (see Chapter 6).

The increased levels of circulating or free testosterone in PCOS, and local skin glands being particularly sensitive to its effects (androgen sensitivity), are thought to increase the production of oily sebum by making the sebaceous skin glands bigger, which in turn interrupts the normal clearing of dead skin cells. Glands get blocked, skin bacteria flourish deep within the glands and this local inflammation makes hormonal acne in PCOS worse.

Androgen excess and local androgen sensitivity make acne worse in PCOS by:

- Excessive sebum production
- Blocking hair follicles
- Localised inflammation
- Overgrowth of bacteria.

Why a plant-based way of eating helps with acne

Until the early 20th century, diet was commonly used to treat acne but during the 1960s, the diet–acne connection fell out of favour. Over recent years, there is once again a growing body of evidence suggesting a relationship between diet and acne. Compared with other dietary factors, most research examines dietary glycaemic load (GL).[7] A low GL diet is typically low in saturated fat and high in whole grains, fruit and vegetables. In other words, a whole-food plant-predominant diet that is low in refined sugar and ultra-processed foods can help acne. A 12-week randomised control trial confirmed that a low GL diet made a significant difference in acne lesions as well as reducing insulin levels and body weight compared with those on a high GL diet.[8]

A relationship between chocolate consumption and incidence or severity of acne has not been proven[1, 9] and it is likely that the issue is with the sugar and dairy fat in the chocolate. Cacao is rich in magnesium so opting for a couple of dark chocolate squares with a high cocoa content of around 90% is the better option, or raw cacao nibs.

It is likely that the gut microbiome plays an important part in acne. Fermented foods rich in probiotics such as sauerkraut, miso and kimchi can help improve gut health by feeding our healthy gut bacteria. Probiotic foods have been found to reduce persistent pimples.[10, 11, 12, 13]

A review of all published research in 2020 suggested a whole food plant-based diet was beneficial for preventing skin ageing.[14] Soya also seems to be particularly good for the skin.[15]

Foods to avoid

Just as you want to choose whole plant foods regularly in your diet to reduce inflammation, you also want to reduce foods that promote inflammation. Ultra-processed foods such as cakes, crisps, biscuits, white bread, shop-bought desserts and fried foods are generally high in refined sugar, refined carbohydrates and unhealthy fats yet deficient in fibre. They also offer no health benefits. Instead, they actively contribute to worsening insulin resistance, weight gain and increased inflammation. Alcohol and caffeine can lead to

dehydration and skin flare ups. I suggest making water, unsweetened still or sparkling, your drink of choice.

There are some animal foods which contribute to oxidative
stress, increased AGE production and inflammation. Red and processed meats fall into this group and my advice to you is to steer
clear of these, whatever you may read on social media or in the
newspapers.

The role of dairy in acne

A review of 27 studies, published in the *Journal of the Academy of
Nutrition and Dietetics* in 2013, found fairly compelling evidence
linking dairy and acne.[7] The growth hormone and proteins (especially IGF-1) in milk are implicated in causing acne and acne flare
ups.

Studies were unable to determine the quantity of milk necessary to exacerbate acne. However, in a large study of over 47,000
women in the USA, those who drank two or more glasses of skim
milk a day were 44% more likely to have acne than those who did
not.[16] Researchers are not yet completely certain if the association
between dairy and acne is due to independent actions of the hormones in milk, the milk protein, the effect of milk on insulin and
IGF-1 concentrations or a combination of all these factors. We have
already discussed the known effect of insulin on the increase in
androgen levels.

It is certainly worth completely eliminating dairy for a period of
three to six months to see if your skin clears up. Just cutting out milk,
yoghurt and cheese is not always enough to see an improvement.
Dairy in its various forms is present in the most unlikely foods,
including strange ones like tinned tomato soup. It is also named
in several different ways so it is easy to be confused when reading
labels. Cow's milk along with milk from pregnant and lactating
goats, sheep, horses or camels are best left for their own offspring.

This is true for all milk and dairy products, including yoghurt, cheese, ice cream, ghee and all other products made with milk.

The role of lifestyle in acne

Some studies have found an association between stress and increased acne severity. Many aspects of modern life can have an impact on acne flare-ups by increasing inflammatory markers.[1, 17, 18] Prioritising sleep is also helpful, to reduce cortisol, often known as the stress hormone, raised levels of which can worsen stress and anxiety. Several studies have suggested a link between smoking and adult acne as well as an increase in non-inflammatory lesions.[19]

Supplements for acne

Essential oils and supplementation in the absence of deficiency have not been proven to help reduce acne breakouts.[20, 21] As available data are limited, spending money on expensive unproven supplements is a waste. I would suggest spending it on fresh and frozen produce, as you can get most vitamins, minerals and antioxidants. There are a few exceptions which we discuss in detail (see Chapter 27).

There are a few exceptions. I would recommend vitamin D supplementation throughout the year and getting your levels checked annually, if possible. An algae-derived omega-3 fatty acid supplement may also be considered on a plant-based diet as walnuts and flax seeds provide only some of the omega-3 requirements. Both these are important supplements in PCOS (see Chapter 27).

Managing acne with medications

The most common way acne is controlled is by lowering excess testosterone levels circulating in the body and skin with the help of the Pill, particularly one with a progesterone preparation that is better for the skin (with low androgenic potential). This may be combined with a low dose of a diuretic drug, such as spironolactone or another androgen blocker, to minimise the effects of testosterone, usually after a six-month trial of the combined oral contraceptive pill (COCP) if you are unhappy with the results. You may also be prescribed the androgen-blocking drug on its own, if you cannot take the Pill for any reason. None of these drugs can be prescribed if you are trying for a pregnancy. In individual cases, antibiotics or other medications, including topical and oral retinoids which are used to treat skin issues, may be prescribed by a qualified health professional.

It is so confusing with so many skincare products out there

It is really important to find a skincare regime that works for you. Some basic principles include gently cleansing your skin and removing makeup. It's advisable to avoid scrubbing the face with wash cloths or sponges which can spread infection. Instead, washing your face with lukewarm water twice a day and after removing makeup can be helpful. Over-washing can dehydrate the skin as can some skincare products. It is important to resist the temptation to touch your skin or squeeze or pick at your spots as this will increase local inflammation and spread infection.

Where possible, invest in cruelty-free oil-free or water-based makeup that is specifically labelled suitable for those with acne. Look for non-comedogenic skincare, which means products that do not contain ingredients that are likely to clog pores. For many, make up or skin camouflage (a specific skincare product) helps cover blemishes, discolouration and acne, which in turn can help in boosting confidence as many people with PCOS-related acne report feeling wary of social situations.[22] I do recommend you avoid make up if possible while at home to give your skin a break.

I suggest opting for a clean mineral sunscreen with a high SPF rather than a chemical sunscreen which can contain hormone disruptors such as oxybenzone, topping up regularly if out in the sun to prevent sunburn. A large wide-brim sun hat or scarf can also help protect your face, neck and scalp.

The PCOS Myth Buster

Myth: I thought dairy milk was good for our health?
The facts: There is no reason to include dairy in anyone's diet, including that of children, with cow's milk allergy being the most common serious food allergy in infants and young children and the most common single cause of fatal anaphylaxis.[23] Dairy consumption is significantly linked to some aggressive forms of prostate cancer and there is genuine concern that consuming dairy products may increase the risk of breast, ovarian and endometrial cancers. With regard to acne, it is certainly worth completely eliminating dairy for a period of three to six months to see if your skin clears up. It's a good idea to replace dairy with fortified plant milks and plant yoghurts.

PCOS POINTERS

- Consider PCOS if you suffer from:
  - Cystic acne that persists after the age of 25
  - Acne that does not respond to standard treatments or lifestyle modifications.
- Acne may be associated with excessive facial hair growth and often affects the jawline, back and chest.
- Dairy and dairy products are implicated as a causative factor in acne.
- A whole food plant-based diet can help acne symptoms.

17

Treating the root cause
Excessive facial and body hair growth

People with PCOS with androgen excess symptoms often admit to having a poor quality of life, with excessive facial and body hair growth often reported as the most distressing symptom.[1, 2] The costs of managing unwanted excessive face and body hair add an additional financial burden and stress for those with PCOS who are already dealing with the symptoms of androgen excess. This is perhaps why PCOS has been described as 'the thief of womanhood', with far-reaching consequences for everyone with the condition, whether or not they conform to 'feminine norms.'[3]

Hirsutism

The medical term for the excessive growth of darker, thicker and coarser hairs noticed by women on their face, neck, chest, tummy, lower back, buttocks or thighs is 'hirsutism.'[2] PCOS is the commonest condition associated with hormone-dependent excessive hair growth.

A family and genetic link to PCOS is known (see Chapter 2), which means there may be other family members with similar symptoms.

Hair growth on the face and back

Excessive hair growth is the most recognisable clinical sign in PCOS and suggests an increased production of androgens. About seven out of 10 women with excessive hair growth have elevated circulating free testosterone levels, even though in many, the total level of testosterone when measured in the blood is normal[4] (see Chapter 6). In those with normal testosterone levels on a blood test, the mechanism appears to be a heightened local sensitivity of the hair follicles (pilosebaceous unit) to increased amounts of androgens that are produced within the skin itself. This is known as androgen sensitivity.

You may notice thicker, darker hairs on your upper lip, chin, jawline and neck, in between your breasts, above and below your belly button, on your upper and/or lower back, buttocks and thighs. Not all these nine areas mentioned are affected in everyone.

Your doctor may check these nine areas for hair growth clinically and some may use scores for defining the severity of hair growth. There is a variation, with Han Chinese women with PCOS having the lowest rates of excessive hair growth compared to Hispanic, Black, Mediterranean or Middle Eastern women with PCOS, so scores may need to be adjusted accordingly.[5]

Specific type of hair growth

It is important to differentiate from other types of hair growth. An excess of soft, unpigmented androgen-independent hair, called 'vellus hair' or 'lanugo hair', may be seen in women with anorexia nervosa.

Excess hair distribution may be seen in some families and may differ depending on race. It is usually all over the body rather than in the specific pattern of hormone-dependent hair growth. This generalised excess growth of vellus hair is known as 'hypertrichosis'. Conditions such as malnutrition, an underactive thyroid and some oral medications, such as steroids, can cause a similar excess of hair growth. It is usually managed with regular hair removal methods.[4]

We live in a society where any amount of facial and body hair on women is considered unacceptable due to patriarchal beauty standards. If a woman finds these regular hairs bothersome, then this is referred to as unwanted hair and is not a sign of androgen excess. These regular hairs look and feel different to the PCOS hair growth pattern and respond very well to routine hair removal techniques.

Increasing age and menopause can also lead to increased facial and body hair because of changes in hormone levels.

If you have no other symptoms to suggest PCOS, then other causes should be explored. Sometimes, no cause can be found to explain increased hair growth. If you notice very rapid hair growth, you should seek urgent medical advice to rule out serious causes (see Chapter 6).

Solutions for excessive hair growth

As many of the symptoms of androgen excess in PCOS are visible to the outside world, it is not surprising that most women readily spend a fortune on treatments that often do not work as well as they do in those without the condition. Even so-called semi-permanent hair removal methods fall short of their promise when it comes to PCOS. Cosmetic therapies are often not reimbursed by health insurance or available on national health systems so, like many of my patients, you may run up large bills, without the positive outcome you hoped for.

It is important to find the hair removal technique that you can afford and one that suits you. It is helpful to remember no hair removal technique is perfect and you may need several top up treatments.

At the same time, addressing insulin resistance and losing weight, if you have excess weight, can help reduce androgen levels and excess hair growth. Be aware that medications used for reducing insulin resistance have limited benefit when it comes to reducing hair growth.

Spearmint tea is commonly used in Middle Eastern countries as a herbal remedy for women with excessive hair growth.[6] There is some evidence that it can help lower androgen levels. A randomised clinical trial of 42 women with PCOS and excessive hair growth found a reduction in free and total testosterone levels, and an increase in luteinising hormone (LH) and follicle stimulating hormone (FSH), when they consumed two cups of spearmint tea daily for a month.[7] While further studies are needed, it may be a good option for you. Spearmint tea is naturally caffeine-free, usually accessible and affordable, antioxidant-rich and has a pleasant, mild taste.

A combination of treatments

Excessive hair growth due to PCOS can be resistant to treatment so combined approaches work better. The best strategy involves removing existing hairs with cosmetic techniques and using lifestyle and medications to decrease androgen production to reduce the formation of new hair growth. Otherwise, you may find cosmetic treatments can fail.

It is recommended to wait at least six months before you consider changing treatments because of the length of the hair-growth cycle.[8] Treatment of hirsutism does respond very well to the Pill (COCP). The oestrogen in the Pill stimulates the liver to make a protein that binds testosterone (SHBG), thereby reducing the amount of testosterone that is exposed to the hair follicle. In some situations, adding an anti-androgen such as spironolactone alongside the Pill can help, especially when women are particularly bothered by their androgen excess symptoms. Otherwise, the Pill should be used as the first medication, with an anti-androgen added after six months if you are not happy with the initial cosmetic response.[9] These medications produce good results for many of my patients but cannot be offered to you if you are trying for a pregnancy or if you have any contraindications.

I encourage all my patients with PCOS to use lifestyle behaviour change, including exercise and diet, to help reduce androgen levels alongside conventional oral and/or topical androgen suppression medical treatments and cosmetic therapies, both short-term (shaving, waxing, threading, bleaching, chemical depilation and plucking) and longer-term (electrolysis, laser and intense pulse light therapy) for the best results.[10]

The PCOS Myth Buster

Myth: I have heard I have to let the hair grow out for the doctor to make an assessment.
The facts: No, you do not need to do this at all. Self-treatment sometimes can limit clinical assessment but should not affect treatment. Your description of your hair distribution and type of hair should be enough for your doctor to make a diagnosis, even if you have already removed the hair.

PCOS POINTERS

- The medical term for excessive facial and body hair growth is 'hirsutism'.
- Excessive facial and/or body hair growth is the most recognisable sign in PCOS.
- Androgen excess or local androgen sensitivity can cause hairs to be thicker and darker.
- Addressing weight and insulin resistance through lifestyle can help slow hair growth.
- Cosmetic hair removal can be expensive and may not deliver the results expected.
- Find an affordable technique that suits you when considering short-term and longer-term treatments.
- Androgen suppression with the Pill and/or androgen blockers can be helpful but persist for six months to see the effects.

18

It's not all down the drain
Female-pattern hair loss

Hair loss is distressing for most people at any age. This can be particularly hard for women with PCOS as they tend to be younger than average when first noticing hair loss and thinning. They may also be struggling with unwanted weight gain as well as trying to manage excessive body and facial hair growth and acne, the other symptoms of androgen excess in PCOS. This can result in severe psychological distress that often gets overlooked by health professionals, who sometimes just focus on treating physical symptoms.

Female-pattern hair loss (FPHL)

Hair loss from the scalp has been referred to as alopecia or androgenetic alopecia. While these terms may have been acceptable previously in medical discussions, there is already enough stigma attached to women's health, and especially to the symptoms of androgen excess (see Chapter 6). We should all be making a conscious effort to avoid terms such as alopecia and replace it with FPHL or 'female-pattern hair loss'.[1]

Typically, the hair loss in most FPHL spreads out from the middle of the scalp, starting at the top of the head. In most people with

PCOS, the frontal hairline tends to remain intact despite general hair thinning and hair loss.[2, 3] The scalp remains normal but the hairs gradually become smaller, shorter and lighter until eventually the follicles may shrink completely and stop producing hair.[4]

FPHL is usually seen with increasing age as women approach menopause and is often hereditary.[5] In more recent times, hair thinning and hair loss are becoming a common complaint at a younger age, perhaps due to a combination of lifestyle factors, such as stress, diet and alcohol, with the increasing prevalence of PCOS also a contributing factor.

In women with PCOS, FPHL is seen at an earlier age and is hormone (androgen) dependent, although other underlying factors, such as stress, can make it worse.

Hair loss due to PCOS

It is thought 20-30% of women with PCOS have evidence of FPHL, with the vast majority also showing signs of excess facial and body hair growth and/or acne.[6, 7]

If you experience only isolated hair loss, other causes should be explored with your doctor as it is unlikely to be PCOS. Hair loss in teenagers with PCOS is unusual so again your doctor should consider other causes, rather than immediately labelling it as PCOS.

Hair loss is often multifactorial, meaning caused by several things. Detailed medical history and examination by your doctor are therefore important to make sure the right diagnosis is reached, as it is only then that the right treatment can be offered. If you notice extreme hair loss without an obvious explanation, check in with your doctor urgently so the more uncommon but serious causes of FPHL can be ruled out as discussed previously (see Chapter 6).

The assessment of FPHL is essentially by observation by your health professional. Hair loss on the scalp is usually assessed visually. The 'pull test' as the name implies is not helpful.[8]

Supplements and hair loss

It's helpful to check levels of vitamin D (see Chapter 27) and supplement adequately. Blood tests to measure levels of ferritin (stored iron) are helpful as these deficiencies can contribute to increased scalp hair loss, with or without PCOS.[1] In general, however, there is no evidence for supplementing with unproven supplements, in the absence of deficiency.[9] For many women, healthy iron and ferritin levels can be achieved with a well-planned plant-based way of eating, including foods such as beans, soya, lentils, chickpeas, kale, broccoli, quinoa, cashew nuts, chia and flax seeds, and dried apricots. Some of you may need iron supplements, especially if you are iron deficient either because of heavy periods or a poor diet, both of which need to be addressed for a better quality of life.

Some people with PCOS may benefit from a trial of zinc supplements, especially if their regular diet is lacking in zinc-rich foods, such as oats, legumes, nuts and seeds.

As with all supplements, over-supplementing with over-the-counter medications should be avoided as some supplements carry the risk of worsening hair loss or even of toxicity[10] (see Chapter 27).

Helping yourself

Addressing all aspects of PCOS offers the best hope of success as hair loss can be difficult to treat as an isolated symptom. There is no cure for FPHL, so all efforts must be made to manage symptoms early and try and slow down hair loss. I suggest addressing all aspects of lifestyle, especially stress and sleep. Make a concerted effort to eat a diverse range of whole plant foods, including foods rich in key micronutrients, such as iron and zinc, supplementing if needed with professional help, especially with vitamin D.

It is normal to lose up to 150 hairs in a day and as hair loss is usually gradual, a significant amount of hair thinning may have occurred before you first notice it. Having a good hair-care regime, such as using a conditioner and a wide-toothed comb to prevent unnecessary hair loss, is useful. You should keep an eye on the amount of hair you lose when you brush or wash it. It is also helpful to avoid touching and pulling on your scalp hair.

If possible, protect your scalp from sunburn by applying sunscreen or a head cover (scarf, hat or a wig).

Early intervention by your doctor to find other underlying causes of FPHL or contributing factors in PCOS can help reassure you that all is being done. A referral to a trusted and qualified hair loss specialist (trichologist) to manage hair loss will help avoid unnecessary and unproven treatments.

The PCOS Myth Buster

Myth: Tying back my hair has no effect on hair loss.
The facts: Traction alopecia is a form of hair loss at the front hairline, usually as a result of chronic tension on the hair. While you may be able to reverse this initially, hair loss can become permanent so it is a good idea to avoid tight braiding or ponytails.[11] Try swapping hair ties for scrunchies.

PCOS POINTERS

- FPHL (female-pattern hair loss) is the preferred term rather than alopecia.
- FPHL can be difficult to treat.
- Protect your scalp from sunburn.
- Supplements such as vitamin D, iron and zinc may help alongside a well balanced plant-based diet.
- Reduce insulin resistance and androgen levels through lifestyle.
- Stress management and adequate good quality sleep are important.
- Consulting a qualified hair loss specialist can help avoid unproven treatments.

Part Three

Managing PCOS (cont'd)

Section 3.3: Addressing lesser known symptoms of PCOS

19

Making your peace with PCOS
Anxiety, depression, sexual problems and mood disorders

PCOS and mental health

Many of my patients are surprised to hear that their anxiety and other mood symptoms may be linked to their PCOS. Please do not feel resigned about such symptoms, as there is a great deal that can be done to help with mental health issues in PCOS. The vast majority of anxiety and depressive disorders associated with this condition are mild (50%) to moderate in nature and are treatable.[1] There is little doubt that much more research and funding are needed into mental health to help clarify some of the increased risks noted in people living with PCOS. The important thing is for you and your health professional to recognise there is an issue, so you can understand more about your situation and be supported to access help early if you need it from those qualified to do so.

Anxiety, depression, disordered eating, daily fatigue and reduced sexual and relationship satisfaction are all symptoms seen more frequently in those living with PCOS, with one study suggesting depression was four times higher than in those without PCOS.[2, 3] At least one in three people with PCOS experience symptoms of anxiety and one in four suffer from depression, with a higher risk of suicide.[1] The psychological impact of PCOS remains poorly recognised by the medical community and public awareness also needs to be raised urgently at the same time. Those with PCOS are at an increased risk of psychological and behavioural disorders, including bipolar disorder and obsessive-compulsive disorder (OCD),[4] while experiencing a poorer quality of life.[5, 6] Adolescents with PCOS also have higher rates of moderate to severe anxiety and depressive symptoms compared with their peers.[7] In a study involving nearly 17,000 women with PCOS, an increased risk of ADHD and autistic spectrum disorder in their children was noted compared with controls.[8]

Sexual function in PCOS

While studies on sexual functioning (for example, orgasm completion, pain, sexual desire) in PCOS show mixed results, ranging from no significant reduction to moderate impairment, there is good evidence that feelings of inadequacy in social and sexual situations are frequent and considerably correlated with the degree of excess hair growth.[9] Women with excess hair can feel inhibited, ashamed of their body hair and less 'feminine', which compromises their sexual confidence. Focusing only on sexual dysfunction means that this aspect of the quality of sexual life goes unaddressed. It may be difficult to openly discuss sexuality with your healthcare professional but asking for a referral to a psychologist or psychosexual counsellor can help improve your situation.[10]

The cause of mental health issues in PCOS

We don't know the exact cause of anxiety and depressive symptoms in those with PCOS. They can appear independent of body weight, subfertility or androgen excess symptoms.[11, 3] However, it is likely that the combination of the chronic, complex and frustrating nature of PCOS and living with acne, excessive hair growth, subfertility, menstrual irregularities and/or excess weight contributes to mood disorders.[7] Additionally, changes in self-image from PCOS-related symptoms may negatively influence sexuality.[12, 13]

Screening for mental health is urgent in PCOS

More than 95% of those living with PCOS are dissatisfied with the emotional support and counselling they receive.[14] This needs to change.

It is important to raise awareness among both the public and all health professionals about these lesser known PCOS symptoms. It would be very helpful if a system were in place to routinely screen for anxiety and depression as well as for eating disorders, sleep issues and sexual dysfunction in everyone with a diagnosis of PCOS, including teenagers and young people. This screening, according to the Androgen Excess and PCOS Society, should take place at the time of diagnosis of PCOS.[7, 15] In my experience of talking to patients, this screening rarely happens. However, screening alone does not improve outcome and your doctor should have a system in place for appropriate referral and treatment by those who are qualified to do so.[3, 14]

If your health professional's assessment points to the physical symptoms of PCOS as the main reasons for your anxiety and depression, more than one treatment option may be offered at the same time. An example would be the Pill and anti-androgen treatment prescribed at the same time for particularly bothersome acne or hair growth. It is important to be aware that the Pill may be associated with mood changes in some, especially teenagers, so an open conversation and careful observation (keep a diary) are advised in these situations when prescribing the Pill, if this is considered the most suitable option for you. Lifestyle modifications and dietary changes should be discussed in a compassionate manner with you, so you feel motivated to make changes rather than judged, as this can be counterproductive. If you find your healthcare professional is not helpful or overly judgemental with regard to lifestyle modifications and dietary changes, then it is important to seek a second opinion.

If initial treatment of both physical or mental symptoms does not make a significant difference, it is really important that your doctor considers referring you to the appropriate specialist for further assessment and treatment. A scientific review of relevant medical studies showed a lack of benefit when it came to the use of antidepressants as a first line of treatment for depression and other mental health symptoms in those with PCOS,[2] so a full, informed discussion must take place with you before you are prescribed these medications. Therapy for psychosexual issues or cognitive behaviour therapy (CBT) can be helpful for many as the first or only option. These therapies provide space for confidential discussions which address negative thinking patterns and equip you with coping strategies.

Improving emotional well-being

Tell your doctor if you are suffering from low mood or any of the symptoms discussed here, even they do not ask you, as you may benefit from a referral to a therapist. NHS waiting times can be long and may not be easily accessible, so talk to your GP or specialist to see if they can expedite referral or refer you privately to a trusted therapist, if this is something you can afford. Some providers offer a sliding scale depending on your income. CBT is the most popular option. Find a therapist who suits your needs best so you can gain the most from your sessions. By seeking help for your PCOS symptoms early, appropriate medical treatment can be started sooner rather than later. Managing symptoms of weight gain, acne and increased hair growth can help improve how you feel about yourself. If you are worried about fertility, remember most women with PCOS do go on to conceive.

You may wish to join support groups so you can talk to people going through similar issues. Eating ultra-processed foods that promote inflammation can also negatively impact your mood, so consider replacing these foods with more colourful fruit and vegetables, rich in micronutrients and antioxidants, that can help reduce inflammation. Regular exercise, especially outdoors and in natural light, can help release endorphins and lift mood. Restorative sleep, managing stress through mindfulness and other techniques and avoiding alcohol and caffeine can all make a significant difference to how you feel. Aim to address all six pillars of lifestyle as best as you can by all the ways we have suggested previously (see Chapters 11 and 12).

The PCOS Myth Buster

Myth: I have heard that medications are the best way to manage my anxiety.
The facts: Cognitive behavioural therapy (CBT) is more effective than medications for most people, although some will benefit from medication too. Lifestyle changes can also be helpful, especially exercise, diet, sleep and addressing stress triggers, avoiding alcohol, caffeine and smoking. Please see our list of resources (page 381) for organisations providing information and support around mental health.

PCOS POINTERS

- Anxiety, depression and sexual dissatisfaction are seen commonly with PCOS.
- Feelings of inadequacy in sexual and social situations in PCOS appear to correlate with the degree of excess hair growth.
- All health professionals should be made aware of these symptoms of PCOS.
- Treatment of physical symptoms of PCOS can help improve mental health.
- Tell your doctor if you are struggling with your mental health even if you are not asked specifically.
- Ask for a referral to a specialist so you can receive the correct treatment for your symptom(s).
- Cognitive behaviour therapy (CBT) is usually more effective than medications for most people.
- Addressing all six lifestyle pillars can help improve mood.

20

Healing the war with your body
Disordered eating in PCOS

People often do not link their binge-eating to their missing periods or to their PCOS, as most health professionals and the public remain unaware of the link between disordered eating and PCOS. There is currently little public education about this important issue.

Eating disorders (EDs) come with a very real emotional and physical cost to the person as well as to their family and wider society, significantly impacting quality of life. It is therefore crucial we care as a community about eating disorders in people with PCOS, raising awareness so help may be accessed early as these are treatable conditions. More research and funding in this area are urgently needed.

Yo-yo dieting

Body image is defined as the way a person may feel, think about and view their body, including their appearance, and is influenced by many factors. Lower self-esteem from physical symptoms of PCOS and psychosexual problems can lead to negative body image and feeling unattractive with a loss of feminine identity. While most women in the general population are unhappy with their body, this feeling is heightened in those living with PCOS. Feeling judged because of body weight or body size dissatisfaction can trigger a lifelong cycle of 'yo-yo dieting', with cycles of starvation and binge eating, in those with PCOS. Therefore, it is important to identify and address these emotional issues early.

Eating disorders in PCOS

A systematic review and meta-analysis, published in 2020, of 36 studies involving nearly 350,000 women, reported that women with PCOS, when compared with those without PCOS, were more likely to display a higher prevalence of EDs, such as binge eating disorder (BED), which is binge eating without purging, and bulimia nervosa (recurrent episodes of binges with compensatory behaviours such as self-induced vomiting or over exercising) rather than anorexia nervosa.[2] These eating disorders often go unrecognised and as this aspect is usually not considered by the doctor, you may never get asked about it. The focus is usually just on body weight and weight loss as most individuals with BED are in the excess weight range (as are many with PCOS) and on physical symptoms, meaning mental health often gets overlooked. Moreover, many people with PCOS and EDs are unaware of the cause for their distress, not realising that their eating and weight-related thoughts and behaviours may be unusual.

The link between PCOS and binge eating is poorly understood but androgen excess, insulin resistance, mood symptoms and body image issues are all likely to play a part.

EDs characterised by bingeing symptoms, particularly BED, have an increased risk of medical complications also associated with excess weight, such as type 2 diabetes, cardiovascular disorders and fertility issues.

The link between androgen excess and eating disorders in PCOS

Anxiety, depression and mood symptoms (see Chapter 19) are all increased in the presence of disordered eating in PCOS and may result in disrupted relationships, isolation and family stress.[4] A study found increased androgen sensitivity in PCOS might promote bulimic behaviour since androgens have appetite-stimulating effects and can impair impulse control.[5] The combined prevalence of EDs was as high as 36% in those with excessive hair growth symptoms in PCOS.

An anti-diet approach

As there is an increased risk of disordered eating in people with PCOS, restrictive or fad diets such as low-carb or low-fat diets can be potentially triggering for some, even if they achieve their weight loss goal. Even a plant-based approach may hinder your management, if underlying mental health issues and eating disorders are not explored or addressed. Proper medical nutrition planning by qualified dietitians and nutritionists with a special interest in PCOS can help you achieve sustainable weight loss without resorting to extreme measures or restrictive dieting. It is better to focus on having an overall healthy dietary pattern while addressing mental health issues with the other lifestyle pillars (see Chapter 11). Accomplishing a 'healthy' weight should not be at the cost of psychological well-being.

Periods and disordered eating

If you remember (see Chapter 1), hormones released from our brain control our periods. When calorie intake drops below a critical level, the signals from the brain often stop the production of the hormones in our ovaries, as they are not considered essential for survival. A pregnancy is not in our interest in a famine or an eating disorder, so periods often stop or become infrequent.

You deserve to be treated non-judgementally and with empathy

You can achieve long-term success with managing all aspects of your condition with the support of healthcare professionals who understand the various mental health and physical barriers in PCOS. They should take the time to listen with empathy and no judgement while asking questions to help recognise and address the obstacles faced. This can be extremely rewarding for both you and your doctor when you see the results.

Some initial questions by your doctor to check for body image concerns alongside a thorough interview about your medical symptoms can be invaluable, allowing for an urgent referral to an age-appropriate eating disorder service with your consent.

You may feel there is stigma in seeing a therapist. There should be no stigma attached to receiving the right care and no one should be made to feel this way, especially as early referral to a qualified therapist or psychologist in appropriate situations is invaluable in helping you address body image issues.

The PCOS Myth Buster

Myth: Eating disorders are not seen in Black or minority communities.

The facts: This is not true as all populations are at risk of eating disorders. However, disordered eating and eating disorders may not be picked up as often in people of different ethnic and racial groups, those at higher body weights, or LGBTQIA+ individuals and this is also true for those living with PCOS. The reasons are complex but include lack of inclusive care, pervasive stereotypes about eating disorders as well as stigma attached to these conditions, making it harder for people to seek help.

PCOS POINTERS

- There is a higher prevalence of disordered eating and eating disorders (EDs) in people with PCOS (binge-eating and bulimia).
- Many people with PCOS are unaware of their EDs.
- Excess hair growth is associated with higher risk of EDs as androgen sensitivity increases appetite and results in poorer impulse control.
- Mood symptoms, including anxiety, are more commonly associated with EDs in PCOS.
- Periods may stop or become irregular with EDs.
- Negative body image is common in those living with PCOS.
- An anti-diet approach is helpful for successful management of PCOS.
- People with EDs deserve to be treated with empathy and non-judgement; they are not their illness.

21

From counting sheep to a good night's sleep
Disturbed sleep

Sleep is critical for our hormonal health and disturbed sleep can be related to PCOS. A lack of deep restful sleep can result in androgen excess, fluctuations in both blood sugar and cortisol levels and worsening of insulin resistance in those with PCOS. If you have been diagnosed as being in the excess weight range or are insulin resistant, this carries the highest risk of sleep disorders, although you can be in the normal BMI range and still suffer from sleep apnoea.

In people with PCOS, glucose tolerance appears to be related to severity of sleep-disordered breathing. Disturbed sleep alters hormones that regulate appetite, such as ghrelin and leptin. This can lead to one choosing more calorie-dense nutrient-poor foods, such as sugary refined foods, fat-laden pizzas and burgers, which further worsen blood sugars and sleep patterns.

Sleep disorders in PCOS

Sleep disturbances in PCOS are unfortunately under-recognised and under-reported. Insomnia and obstructive sleep apnoea (when breathing stops and starts during sleep) are in fact common in PCOS.[6] Snoring, excessive daytime sleepiness and morning headaches are all indicators of sleep apnoea for which you need to be referred urgently by your health professional to a sleep medicine clinic for further tests and treatment.[7] This is because there is a link between obstructive sleep apnoea and long-term health problems, including cardiac issues.[6]

Helping yourself

The first step is to recognise that you have trouble with sleep and bring it to the attention of your doctor. You must seek urgent help if you think you have sleep apnoea.

You may wish to try and incorporate all or as many of the steps for sleep hygiene into your life as possible (see the sleep section in Chapter 11). Lifestyle changes and cognitive behaviour therapy for insomnia (CBT-I) should be tried before sedatives.

We tend to underestimate the power of sleep, especially in modern life, often because of a fear of missing out. If you already suffer from disturbed sleep, I urge you to pay particular attention to this pillar now, as the repercussions of poor sleep are long lasting, increasing your risks of type 2 diabetes, heart disease, cancer and dementia.

You may also notice disturbed sleep from worrying about acne, excessive hair growth, fertility or body image issues or the stress of the long-term implications of PCOS, so addressing these may help with better sleep.

Prioritise your sleep, ensuring you get seven to nine hours of restorative sleep by avoiding stimulants as well as bright lights a few hours before bedtime. Going to bed at the same time every day and sleeping in a darkened cool room, perhaps with an eye mask, can make a difference to the quality of your sleep. You will find regular exercise, exposure to morning daylight, eating your evening meal at least a couple of hours before bedtime and choosing foods that cause less disruption to your blood sugars, can all help. I also suggest finding ways that help you to unwind, perhaps with a warm bath, caffeine-free herbal tea, reading a book or meditating.

The PCOS Myth Buster

Myth: Sleeping five to six hours is normal.
The facts: Getting restful sleep for seven to nine hours each night is essential for health, with teenagers needing eight up to 10 hours every night. Sleep is an essential lifestyle pillar and lack of it can cause severe hormonal disruption.

PCOS POINTERS

- Restorative sleep of seven to nine hours every night is critical for our hormonal health.
- Sleep disturbances, including insomnia, in PCOS are under-recognised.
- Obstructive sleep apnoea, including snoring and excessive daytime sleepiness, is common in PCOS.
- Lifestyle changes and cognitive behaviour therapy for insomnia (CBT-I) should be tried before sedatives.
- Seek help early.

22

It's getting hot in here
PCOS and menopause

Despite half the population facing this natural life stage and with PCOS affecting at least one in 10 women, there has been little research into how PCOS affects the menopause or the lead up to the menopause. All over the world, menopause occurs around the age of 51 years. It is defined as the end of menstrual cycles and is diagnosed after 12 months without a period. Menopause may not always bring an end to all your PCOS issues.

The three criteria that are normally used to diagnose PCOS (Rotterdam Criteria – see page 40) all change with the onset of menopause.[1] In menopause, the ovaries shrink in size naturally, ovarian egg follicle numbers decrease and periods stop. Even without PCOS, many postmenopausal women notice thicker facial and body hair growth and scalp hair loss and thinning. Acne is reported by 15% of women over the age of 50, making it harder to work out exactly how PCOS affects the menopause.[2]

Interestingly, in those with PCOS, periods may become more regular after the age of 40[3, 4] and PCOS appears to delay menopause by two years on average for reasons that are unclear.[1, 5, 6, 7, 8] Women with PCOS have fewer hot flushes and night sweats compared with controls. The premenopausal difference in the waist to hip ratios also disappears as postmenopausal women without PCOS also tend to gain weight around the middle.[5, 9]

In a 30-year longitudinal cohort study published in 2021, those with PCOS continued to have higher androgen levels, declining into the normal range by the age of 81 years, and although levels were lower than previously, symptoms such as increased facial and body hair growth did not decrease.[5, 6, 10]

Postmenopausal women with PCOS have higher blood sugars, blood pressure (hypertension) and lipid levels (triglycerides) than 'controls' (those without PCOS), as well as raised levels of an inflammatory marker called high sensitivity C-reactive protein (CRP). Despite this, there is no obvious increase in cardiovascular events, and mortality appears no different compared with women without PCOS.[11, 5] There seems to be a lower incidence of underactive thyroid issues in those with PCOS in the menopause for reasons that are unclear.[5, 9] I discuss the longer-term risks of PCOS in Chapter 23.

How to help yourself

If you are menopausal and have never been diagnosed with PCOS, a long history of irregular cycles or anovulatory subfertility may help give your doctor a clue. You may continue to experience signs of androgen excess (excessive facial or body hair, acne or female-pattern scalp hair loss) so do make it a point to highlight your previous medical history and current symptoms so your doctor can offer you options.

Unless you notice rapid onset of symptoms which require urgent medical attention, routine testing for androgens or other hormone levels in postmenopausal women is unhelpful and unreliable.

Paying careful attention to all six lifestyle factors can help you eliminate or improve many of the symptoms associated with menopause and PCOS. By adopting a whole food plant-predominant diet, you will be able to address the insulin resistance, high tri-glyceride levels, raised blood pressure and excess weight gain seen in menopause (see Chapters 11 and 12). Avoiding alcohol, ensuring restful sleep, incorporating strength training at least twice a week along with stress management, will together enable you to enjoy this stage in your life. Menopause is a wonderful time to take a fresh look at your life and prioritise your own needs.

The PCOS Myth Buster

Myth: PCOS symptoms will disappear with the onset of menopause.
The facts: There is not a lot of research available on what happens during and after menopause with PCOS. Hot flushes do seem to be fewer compared with women without PCOS ('controls'). It does, however, appear that symptoms of androgen excess may persist. In particular, increased hair growth and risks of hypertension, abnormal blood sugar and lipids are higher than in those without PCOS.

PCOS POINTERS

- More research is needed into menopausal symptoms in PCOS.
- Periods often become more regular after the age of 40.
- Menopause appears to be delayed by two years.
- Hot flushes appear to be fewer than in controls.
- Androgen excess symptoms may persist into menopause.
- It is important to be mindful of the long-term risks of PCOS and bring in lifestyle changes as early as possible.

23

Living longer, living better
Long-term consequences of PCOS

Women all over the world are living longer. The life expectancy of women in 2020 in the UK was 83.3 years, 84.7 in Canada, 81.7 in the USA and 88 in both Japan and Hong Kong. In India, women now live for 71.8 years and in all these countries, men tend to live a few years less. Within each country, there are significant differences based on socioeconomic and ethnic groups. I tell my patients with PCOS that by bringing in lifestyle changes as early as they can, future problems may be averted.

Health span, not lifespan

Is it enough if we just live longer, or do we want these extra years also to be free of chronic diseases and illness, such as type 2 diabetes, heart disease, cancer and dementia? Rather than focusing only on life expectancy and the years we are alive (our lifespan), perhaps we should perhaps use the term 'health span'. Chronic lifestyle diseases result in deaths which could have been prevented, lifelong disability, compromised quality of life and astronomical, unsustainable healthcare costs. PCOS is a complex chronic condition.

The aim should be to improve quality of life and prevent serious complications such as type 2 diabetes or cancer.

The long-term risks associated with PCOS

All the risks described below are either preventable or can be managed successfully to maintain your quality of life. The key is to make positive lifestyle changes as early as possible alongside western medical therapies when indicated.

Most of the risks described with PCOS seem to be related to increased body weight, which affects many living with PCOS. The risks for those with healthy body weight and PCOS remain undetermined. Overall, mortality rates in all those living with PCOS is not increased compared with the general population,[1] but it must be remembered that the general population in most countries is not metabolically healthy either.

The main underlying abnormality that leads to long-term problems appears to be insulin resistance with raised insulin levels.

Metabolic syndrome

Characterised by increased blood pressure, high blood sugar, excess body fat around the waist and abnormal cholesterol or triglyceride levels, metabolic syndrome affects a third of those living with PCOS. It is associated with increased risks of cardiovascular disease, type 2 diabetes, cancer, sleep apnoea and psychological problems.

Type 2 diabetes

More than half of all women with PCOS develop type 2 diabetes by the age of 40.[2] There also appears to be a more rapid progression from impaired glucose tolerance to type 2 diabetes in PCOS, and at an earlier age compared with the general population.[3, 4]

There is a 10-20% increased risk of impaired glucose tolerance (which means blood sugars are above normal levels, but not high enough to warrant a diagnosis of type 2 diabetes) and type 2 diabetes in PCOS. This risk is even higher if you carry your weight around your middle, have a history of gestational (pregnancy-related) diabetes, a family history of diabetes or are from certain ethnic backgrounds, such as South Asian (five-fold increase in Asia).[2, 5]

Cardiovascular disease

An excess risk of heart disease in women with PCOS is not well established. Cardiovascular risk markers such as abnormal lipid profiles, type 2 diabetes, insulin resistance, high blood pressure, central obesity and pro inflammatory markers like CRP are higher in those with PCOS compared with controls, but it is not clear if this risk translates into clinical heart disease as one gets older.[3] High androgen levels and low sex hormone binding globulin (SHBG) levels have also been linked to increased cardiovascular risk in both premenopausal and postmenopausal women with PCOS.[3, 5] Much more research is needed in this area of cardiovascular health in PCOS. Until then, as heart disease remains one of the top killers in all countries, it is sensible to make your risk as low as possible, irrespective of your family history, for better health outcomes. Remember, genes are not our destiny (see Chapters 2 and 10).

Endometrial cancer

A longstanding history of infrequent periods (at intervals of more than three months) or absent menstrual periods can increase the risk of the lining of the womb overgrowing (endometrial hyperplasia) or even of womb (endometrial) cancer, especially if you have excess weight.[1, 3, 4] We know that those with PCOS are approximately two to six times more likely to develop womb cancer than those without the condition.[5] However, the overall risk of womb cancer remains relatively low.[1, 4] There does not appear to be an association between PCOS and breast or ovarian cancer and no additional surveillance is currently suggested.[5, 6] We know that regular consumption of soya can reduce the risk of endometrial cancer.[7, 8]

Non-alcoholic fatty liver disease (NAFLD)

NAFLD is a condition where increased levels of fat within the liver can impair its proper functioning. Although women with PCOS appear to be at increased risk for NAFLD, there are no clear guidelines on which screening tests to use and what medical therapies work best. It is currently recommended to use lifestyle modifications as the main approach for managing this condition, often associated with increased body fat or type 2 diabetes.[5]

Osteoarthritis

There is also evidence showing that women with PCOS have both a higher prevalence and a higher risk of developing osteoarthritis, the most common form of arthritis. In a large prospective study in Denmark, women with a PCOS diagnosis had both a higher prevalence and accelerated onset of osteoarthritis in both weight- and non-weight-bearing joints, when compared with age-matched controls. While multiple risk factors for osteoarthritis include female sex and obesity, the study results indicated that body weight alone is unlikely to explain the accelerated development of osteoarthritis in women with PCOS.[9]

COVID-19 risk

Women with PCOS are considered typically to belong to an age and sex group which should be at lower risk (relatively young and female) for severe COVID-19.[10] There now appears to be an increased risk of catching COVID-19 infection with PCOS. A large population-based retrospective cohort study carried out during the pandemic found 51% of those with PCOS had an increased risk of COVID-19 infection compared with controls.[11] The study looked at more than 21,000 women with PCOS in a primary care setting and compared them with more than 78,000 controls. Even after known risk factors such as insulin resistance, weight and androgen excess had been adjusted for, there appeared to be inherent PCOS-specific factors putting someone with PCOS at 26% higher risk. PCOS is associated with impaired glucose regulation, excess weight and androgen excess, most of which overlap with COVID-19 comorbidities. Some of the possible associations in PCOS, such as low vitamin D levels, gut bacteria imbalance (dysbiosis) and increased chronic inflammation, are also possible reasons for increased susceptibility.

Reducing the risk of catching Covid-19

If you are living with PCOS, do call the attention of your doctor to your increased risk, get vaccinated if eligible and specifically adhere to infection control measures during the COVID-19 pandemic. This is also an opportunity to address your PCOS by managing insulin resistance, excess weight and androgen excess through a plant-predominant anti-inflammatory diet and healthy lifestyle (see Chapters 11 and 12).

Helping yourself

Prevention is the best cure. There is a lot of truth in this old saying. Start by making small changes so that over time, a healthy way of living becomes a way of life.

Lifestyle changes, especially diet and exercise, can make a significant difference to improving insulin resistance and androgen levels and normalising blood sugar levels, blood pressure and body fat composition. All these are the major risk factors for developing problems both in the short and longer term when you are living with PCOS. A lifelong commitment can prevent many of these conditions completely or at least make them much more manageable. See Chapters 11 and 12 and Part 4 of this book to find out how you can make positive changes to your lifestyle.

Early detection and treatment of impaired glucose tolerance with lifestyle changes, and medications when needed, are crucial to prevent further health complications. You should speak to your doctor and ask to be screened for type 2 diabetes regularly (every one to three years), especially if you have any additional risk factors.

Aside from lifestyle modifications, to reduce your risk of womb cancer you should consider having a withdrawal bleed at least every three to four months, usually with progestogens if you have very infrequent periods. If you have prolonged bleeding or if you are not having periods at all, you should see your doctor urgently for a pelvic ultrasound scan as a thickened womb lining may suggest an abnormality that will need to be assessed with a biopsy and other tests to rule out hyperplasia or cancer.

The PCOS Myth Buster

Myth: I am destined to develop diabetes due to my PCOS and my family history.
The facts: As we have said many times before in this book, genes are not our destiny. We may be more or less predisposed to develop certain conditions, but these are broadly defined probabilities rather than a certainty. There is plenty of scientific evidence that making changes to your diet and other aspects of your lifestyle can help prevent chronic conditions like type 2 diabetes, or halt them in their tracks. It is never too late to take positive steps to improve your health.

PCOS POINTERS

Long-term risks of PCOS include:
- Metabolic syndrome
- Type 2 diabetes
- Increased risk for cardiovascular disease
- Non-alcoholic fatty liver disease (NAFLD)
- Womb (endometrial) cancer
- Increased risk of COVID-19.

Remember:
- Health span is more important than lifespan
- Addressing lifestyle factors early can help prevent and manage the longer term risks of PCOS.

Part Four

The 21-day PCOS programme

with Rohini Bajekal, Nutritionist

Part preface – Rohini's story: From self-loathing to self-acceptance
Introduction: How to live PCOS free – PCOS FREE: An eight-step plan to transform your life

Rohini's story
From self-loathing to self-acceptance

It took many years before I confronted the possibility that I could have PCOS. It's testament to the complex nature of this condition that for a long time I had no idea what was wrong with me. At school, I had suffered with premenstrual syndrome (PMS) and painful periods. As a result, I started taking the contraceptive pill. It made a huge difference to my quality of life in the last few years of school.

Anxiety and over-thinking

While growing up, I ate mostly home-cooked food with lots of beans, dal, vegetables, fruit and nuts. I had been an ethical vegan since I was a teenager, but once I started university at Oxford in 2007, I struggled to find vegan options. I drank sugary soya caramel lattes daily. Bourbon biscuits and chips with lashings of ketchup were my go-to foods when hungover. As the only woman and person of colour studying my subject at my college, I sometimes felt like the odd one out. On nights out, I would drink to excess, which was normalised at university. This gave me a short-lived confidence boost, which never lasted long. I often felt low for days after and my anxiety would worsen. Come the next week, the same cycle would continue again. I would pick myself up by drinking coffee or eating sugary sweets to concentrate in lectures. When experiencing bouts of anxiety, I wouldn't leave my bedroom unless I had a class. This cycle of baseline anxiety and short-lived substance-fuelled confidence seemed inescapable. However, over time, and with the support of friends and a course of cognitive behavioural therapy, I began to break the cycle of over-thinking.

Losing my locks

My first major flare-up came during final exams, a particularly stressful time at university. My hair began falling out and I developed moderate cystic acne, a type of inflammatory acne that causes painful breakouts deep in your skin. My mother, Dr Nitu Bajekal, mentioned it could be PCOS but I wasn't ready to confront this possibility. I also mistakenly thought PCOS only affected people with excess weight. I continued to take the Pill and a few months after I left university and moved to London to work in public relations, the hair loss stopped. I put it down to the stress and exhaustion of Finals and put it out of my mind.

Seeking answers

Over the next few years, a recurring pattern emerged. My symptoms would flare up whenever my stressful lifestyle and work caught up with me. I often sacrificed my sleep due to constant fear of missing out on social life and I don't remember ever feeling truly energised. I tried coming off the Pill a few times but could not deal with the accompanying return of acne and excess hair growth. By the time I experienced another severe acne outbreak in late 2013, I had become so self-conscious about my skin that I would routinely cancel social engagements. I saw a naturopath as well as a dermatologist and tried everything from antibiotics to prescription skin creams and laser therapy, but nothing seemed to make much of a difference. At the time, I had started exercising with some regularity and noticed that alcohol and sugary processed foods exacerbated my skin issues. However, I had little understanding of nutrition at the time and couldn't establish a deeper link.

Letting go of my inner critic

A turning point in my PCOS journey came when I had the opportunity to move to Mumbai, India, in 2014, to join a healthy juice start-up as Brand Manager. Navigating the move to another country by myself inspired a new sense of self-confidence. I swapped shop-bought sandwiches for home-cooked food. I also found that alcohol and caffeine did not feature as much in my social life in Mumbai, with boozy nights out and hangover brunches relegated to my London past. Cutting down my intake of both made such a difference that I slept nine hours a night. My anxiety seemed to have settled entirely and I felt free of my inner critic for the first time in years.

Healthy mind and body

By the time I met my now-husband at a party celebrating Holi, the festival of colours, I was feeling far more confident. While dating, we often went to the gym together and I began lifting weights for the first time in my life. I slept well, looked after myself and started eating lots of fresh local fruit. A side effect of this was that I lost weight while eating an abundance of home-cooked plant-based Indian food such as dal, brown rice and vegetable dishes. I went to the bathroom daily after having experienced constipation throughout my life. Most importantly, I felt energetic and happy.

Surprising blood sugar levels

After having noticed first-hand the impact of lifestyle on my personal wellbeing, I started reading about nutrition to find answers. I came back to the UK to study a Master's in Nutrition and Food Sciences in 2016. I had started including some eggs and fish in my diet after returning to the UK. During this time, I had my HbA1c measured (a marker used to measure long-term blood glucose levels) as part of an assignment. It showed that I was pre-diabetic. Needless to say, this was a real shock. I hadn't considered the possibility that I could be close to chronic illness. I worked out regularly and felt great but my blood tests simply did not match up.

A few months later, my father successfully put his type 2 diabetes in remission with a healthy plant-based diet. I felt inspired by him and did the same to tackle my underlying insulin resistance. It helped that I was able to reconnect with veganism as an active ethical stance, which gave me a deeper sense of purpose and inner peace.

Getting a diagnosis

The pre-diabetic results were a wake-up call. After finally acknowledging that I might have PCOS, I saw an endocrinologist in 2018 who confirmed the diagnosis. With my mother's support, I spent the next year acquainting myself with the complexity of the condition and the importance of addressing all aspects of my lifestyle. I have since committed to managing my PCOS by focusing on all six pillars of health. We will discuss these in the chapters to come.

Living PCOS free

As PCOS is a chronic lifelong condition, understanding my body and individual triggers has been key for me. Avoiding alcohol and caffeine has really helped me along with enjoying a healthy plant-based diet pattern. Sleeping well and managing stress have a huge role along with being kinder to myself. I include movement in my day and go for long walks, practise yoga or go to a fitness class with a friend. Learning to set healthy boundaries has also helped my relationships to flourish.

I have regular menstrual cycles with normal markers on blood tests and am now off the Pill. I still experience flare ups of symptoms such as acne whenever I neglect self-care, particularly during stressful life events. It has been humbling to balance the realisation that while I am managing my symptoms, it is still a journey and I must be gentle with myself as I undertake it.

I truly feel that without PCOS, I might not have been motivated to sustain a lifestyle that has transformed my mental and physical health. As a nutritionist and lifestyle medicine professional, I now feel incredibly privileged to be able to help others achieve a greater sense of wellbeing in their lives.

Rohini Bajekal
Nutritionist and Board-Certified Lifestyle Professional

Introduction

How to live PCOS free
PCOS FREE: An eight-step plan to transform your life

So far, this book has focused on educating you about the building blocks of your reproductive and endocrine health, learning what drives PCOS as well as how it manifests in different people. Let us now shift our attention to our real focus: managing this condition in our daily lives.

PCOS FREE is an eight-step plan to help you take control of your PCOS and achieve a greater sense of wellbeing in your everyday life. The advice given throughout this book is encapsulated in this acronym and can be adapted to your individual lifestyle.

By following the eight steps in PCOS FREE, you can find your way back to being your happy and vibrant self. The eight steps are:

Plant predominant

Community

Optimism

Self-care

Fun

Rest

Exercise

Empower

P is for PLANT PREDOMINANT

Eating more plants is the foundation of PCOS FREE. Basing your meals around whole grains, beans, fruit, vegetables, nuts and seeds offers mental and physical benefits in both the short term and the longer term. When you focus on what you're bringing in rather than what you're removing, this becomes a joyful process. Think abundance rather than deprivation. Focus on adding more colour to your plate and try to eat mindfully without guilt or shame.

Tips:

- Snack on fruit with some nuts or simply add an extra serving of greens to your meals such as a handful of kale in a curry.
- Get more in touch with the food you eat by growing your own herbs on your windowsill.

C is for COMMUNITY

Connecting with others is a fundamental part of emotional and physical wellbeing.[1] Living with PCOS can be an isolating experience, especially when you are dealing with anxiety that can make social encounters stressful. Focus on the quality of your relationships rather than the quantity and those who accept you for who you are. It can be easy to cancel social engagements when you are struggling with PCOS symptoms but spending time with others makes us healthier and happier.

Tips

- If you are more outgoing, cultivate new ways to meet people, such as joining a local sports team, volunteering for a cause you believe in or learning a new language.
- You may prefer to engage in quieter activities such as walking with a friend, taking part in a book club or joining a PCOS support group online.

O is for OPTIMISM

Optimism reflects the belief that the outcomes of events or experiences will generally be positive. It is associated with engaging in healthy behaviours, such as prioritising sleep, and may even help you live longer. It's even associated with a reduced risk of certain conditions, such as anxiety and cardiovascular disease.[2] By reading this book, you have opened yourself up to learning and to new possibilities. Reframe PCOS to see it as an opportunity or challenge rather than as a life sentence.

It's important to emphasise that optimism is not toxic positivity, the belief that no matter how painful or difficult a situation is, you should maintain a positive mindset, which leaves you feeling invalidated and guilty. It is not possible for everything to be great all the time, so allow yourself to process emotions rather than suppressing them, and develop healthy coping strategies.[3] On a day-to-day basis, try to adopt an outlook that gives you hope for the future.

Tips

- The words you tell yourself on a daily basis are as important as the food you eat. Practising positive affirmations on a daily basis allows you to move away from negative or self-critical thoughts.

- Keeping a gratitude diary helps you to notice the things that go right in your everyday life, whether big or small, and to challenge pessimism.

S is for SELF-CARE

Taking care of your own needs is an essential part of *Living PCOS Free*. Self-care may include deep breathing, running in nature or having a long bath. It may involve setting healthy boundaries with others or simply saying 'no'. A self-care practice can help you better manage PCOS symptoms, such as anxiety or sleeping issues, allowing you to be more in tune with your mind and body. However, self-care should always come from a place of love rather than punishment. This is why our 21-Day PCOS Programme is centred around self-care and nurturing yourself. Self-care can be about small habits that you do to feed yourself emotionally, spiritually and physically. Whether it's a daily activity or a monthly practice, these regular practices in your 'self-care toolbox' can help you feel better.

Tips

- If you're not sure where to start, try developing the habit of taking a break from screens for a weekend or adopting a morning yoga or stretch routine which can be relaxing.
- Create a calming atmosphere at home before engaging in a self-care activity, such as turning down the lighting, grabbing your favourite blanket and putting on some music.

F is for FUN

Having fun is an essential part of being human and it may look different for everyone. PCOS symptoms can make it difficult for you to live in the present moment and even rob you of joy at times, but finding a way to enjoy the little things can make life better. Children and companion animals can bring out the fun, imaginative side of us that we often forget as we get older. Playful activities release endorphins, stimulate the brain and help us be creative. Growing up does not mean that you have to be serious all the time.

Tips

- Find moments to have fun, in whatever way that means to you. Whether it's an adventure in nature, watching comedy or playing boardgames with friends, cultivate a sense of curiosity, fun and light-heartedness in your life.

- If you find that your life feels overly scheduled, try revisiting an activity you loved as a child, such as painting by numbers or colouring in, doing a puzzle or flying a kite.

R is for REST

Making time for mental down-time is as important as physical rest and relaxation. You may automatically think of rest as sleep and, while quality, restful sleep is essential for good health, rest can take a variety of forms. Whether you're walking outside, meditating or simply having a day in your pyjamas to 'do nothing', it all helps. Rest can also lower levels of cortisol, the stress hormone, which studies show are higher in those living with PCOS. Looking at everything through a lens of productivity and output can take its toll on our mind and body and is contrary to the evidence that shows that rest is a basic human need – one that improves health, immunity and satisfaction.

Tips

- Carve out time in your schedule to prioritise rest and relaxation. Take regular breaks from screens and social media to reconnect with yourself, nature and loved ones.

- Find what works for you and listen to cues from your body to prevent feelings of overwhelm and burnout. Make sure you challenge any feelings of guilt that come up while resting or the notion that you could be doing something else. Allow yourself to truly 'switch off'.

E is for EXERCISE

Moving your body regularly and on a daily basis is a core part of *Living PCOS Free*. Exercise can be an excellent outlet for stress relief and enjoyable once you find an activity and rhythm that work for you. Embrace moving your body to feel energised and strong and improve your mood. Regular movement can help increase your body's sensitivity to insulin[4] as well as improving many other health markers and reducing anxiety and depression.

Tips

- Mix it up with both strength training and cardio sessions and ensure you don't overtrain by making time for rest.

- Try to walk as much as possible, and ideally outdoors in nature, to reap even greater mental health benefits. If you spend most of your working day sitting down, make movement a part of your routine in other ways - walking while taking a phone call or climbing stairs count too.

E is for EMPOWER

Empower yourself by taking control of your own life and your health as it's never too early or too late. Remember that no one knows your body better than you. You are enough, just as you are, so trust yourself and remain open-minded. Anything is possible.

Tips

- Empowering yourself is a lifelong process.
- Trust your instincts but reach out when you need to and seek medical advice.

24

Mind the gap
How to transition to a plant-based way of eating

Bring in whole plant foods

A dietary pattern centred around whole plant foods, rich in fruit, vegetables, whole grains, legumes, nuts and seeds, is one of the healthiest choices you can make.[1] So far, we have discussed the many benefits of a plant-based diet for managing PCOS and how it can meet nutritional requirements at all stages of life, from birth to old age. However, when it comes to making the switch, it is helpful to learn practical ways to introduce more plant-based foods into your diet. Understanding the nutrition basics and common challenges makes this way of eating enjoyable and sustainable in the long term.

There is no one right way to make the transition to a plant-based diet. Some people feel ready to make the shift overnight whereas others prefer gradually to include more plant-based foods in their diet over time. The latter may allow the gut microbiome to adapt to the increase in fibre and lessen side effects such as bloating. Making gradual, consistent changes will also help you build confidence in your plant-based cooking.

All healthy dietary patterns require consideration, so do not let the idea that you need to 'plan' a healthy plant-based diet put you off. As many of us did not grow up eating a lot of plant-based foods, it takes time to reimagine your plate without basing meals around animal products. Learn from the many cuisines that have been prioritising plants for thousands of years, such as African, Indian, Chinese and Mexican. Swap or 'crowd out' animal foods and ultra-processed foods for plant-based ingredients which are nutrient-dense and tasty. This means swapping meat, dairy, fish and eggs for protein-, iron- and zinc-rich plant foods such as beans, lentils, tofu and tempeh. Soya is versatile and has many health benefits (see Chapter 26).

Don't be too restrictive

Experiment with new recipes to expand your plant-based meal repertoire and try stews, curries and colourful stir-fries. You will discover the incredible diversity that exists within plant-based eating.

It is also a good idea to avoid being too restrictive to ensure this way of eating is sustainable for you. For example, plant-based meat alternatives may be especially helpful for some people as they can provide familiarity in terms of texture and flavour, are convenient to prepare and are often fortified with key nutrients such as B12. Where possible, aim to base most of your meals around whole plant foods which tend to be more beneficial for health, the environment and your wallet. A 'food first' approach is recommended rather than lots of unnecessary and expensive supplements, but it's especially important to ensure a reliable source of vitamin B12 on a plant-based diet (see Chapter 27).

Gluten-free diets

Gluten is a protein naturally found in many grains, such as wheat, rye and barley. It is in common foods such as cereals, bread, pasta, table sauces and even beer. Studies on whole grains show that they reduce the risk of a number of chronic diseases, including type 2 diabetes,[2] suggesting that those consuming gluten-free diets are at a possible disadvantage and may risk nutrient deficiencies.[3]

Coeliac disease is an autoimmune condition that affects around 1% of the population. There is no cure but gluten must be eliminated from the diet to avoid a variety of serious health problems.[4] To date, there's no substantial evidence to suggest that PCOS is associated with coeliac disease.[5] Despite the buzz on social media and current wellness trends, there's no reason to remove gluten-containing foods from your diet unless you have coeliac disease or non-coeliac gluten sensitivity (NCGS).[6]

NCGS refers to a reaction to gluten leading to wide-ranging symptoms that are not caused by an allergic or immunologic response. The symptoms of intolerance vary and may include bloating, joint pain, depression and diarrhoea.[7,8] Although NCGS appears to be more common than coeliac disease, its true prevalence is unknown. I would advise you to keep a note of your symptoms and work with a qualified health professional if you are planning to follow a gluten-free diet. Many gluten-free products have poor nutritional value,[9] but it is possible to thrive if you include naturally gluten-free whole grains such as quinoa, red rice, amaranth, buckwheat, millet and, if tolerable, oats.

Remember your 'Why?'

As you bring in changes, remind yourself that it's okay to slip up – all-or-nothing thinking doesn't help. Whether you have gone plant-based for health, the environment or animal welfare, it's important to remember your 'Why' to stay on track. Some people benefit from watching documentaries about the environment, meeting people who share their values or writing down daily health goals to strengthen resolve. If you would like to adopt a plant-based lifestyle but need individual support, reach out to a qualified nutritionist or dietitian who understands plant-based nutrition and can guide you. Everyone can benefit from nutrition advice, but it can be especially helpful in PCOS or if you have a medical condition such as coeliac disease or a history of disordered eating, or are planning a vegan pregnancy.

What to eat

Figure 6: *Whole plant foods*

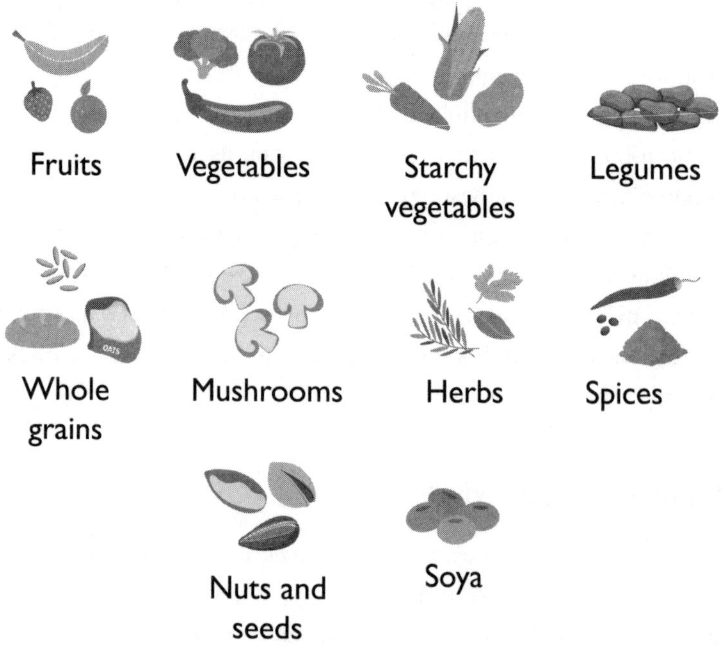

Fruits

Vegetables

Starchy vegetables

Legumes

Whole grains

Mushrooms

Herbs

Spices

Nuts and seeds

Soya

Whole grains

In general, all whole grains are nutritious. However, the more heavily processed the grain, the lower the nutritional value, and the higher the glycaemic index (GI). Swap out refined grains for mostly intact whole grains, such as brown rice, millet, buckwheat, amaranth or quinoa, as they are higher in fibre, protein and micronutrients than refined versions. For example, if you usually have puffed wheat or quick cook oats for breakfast, try oat groats (intact whole grains) or steel-cut oats (cut whole grains). Wholewheat pasta, legume pasta (such as edamame or chickpea pasta) and wholemeal bread are all good additions too but are made from ground grains and are more quickly absorbed into the bloodstream than their whole counterparts. Colourful whole grains, such as red quinoa and red rice, typically contain more beneficial phytochemicals and antioxidants than their beige counterparts.[10]

Legumes

'Legume' is a general term used to describe the seeds of plants from the legume family, which includes beans, peas, lentils and peanuts. These are some of the most healthful and sustainable protein sources on the planet. All varieties, including green peas, chickpeas, black beans, soya beans, lentils, tofu and tempeh, are rich in protein, fibre, vitamins and minerals. Tinned or canned goods are fine for convenience but try and opt for BPA-free canned or jarred versions.

Beans and lentils contain a good mixture of fibre and complex carbohydrates, providing a slow release of energy, stabilising blood sugar levels and keeping you full for longer.

Fruit and vegetables

A diet rich in fruit and vegetables can lower the risk of the most common chronic diseases. Fruit and vegetables are bursting with thousands of plant compounds known as phytochemicals and should ideally be included in every meal. Keep a diverse mix of both fresh and frozen produce to hand for tasty, colourful meals. The darker the colour, the greater the concentration of phytochemicals so opt for dark kale rather than iceberg lettuce. Berries, citrus and dark leafy greens are especially nutritious.

Nuts and seeds

Enjoy a variety of nuts and seeds as they are a powerhouse of nutrition and are even associated with a lower risk of developing cardiovascular disease.[11] Walnuts, chia, hemp and flax seeds are all rich in alpha-linoleic acid (ALA), an essential omega-3 fatty acid, while cashews and sunflower seeds are a great source of zinc. Store these in the fridge or freezer to extend shelf life and prevent rancidity.

Herbs and spices

Whether dried or fresh, herbs and spices are packed with antioxidants with anti-inflammatory properties. They make it easy to create flavourful plant-based meals while decreasing the need for added salt, oil and sugar.

Other useful staples

Other staples in your diet may include calcium-fortified plant milks and yoghurts (such as soya milk), vinegars and other fermented foods, high quality oils such as extra virgin olive oil and condiments such as nutritional yeast, tamari, tahini, mustard and miso.

Our five top tips for transitioning to a plant-based diet

1. **Focus on protein-rich foods.** Getting enough protein is not an issue if you are eating a variety of plant-based foods and getting enough calories. However, if you are excluding beans, lentils and soya from your diet or you are undereating, you are more likely to struggle. Add tofu or tempeh into stir-fries, base meals around lentils and beans and replace dairy with fortified soya milk.
2. **Enjoy omega-3 rich foods daily.** Choose 1-2 tablespoons of ground flaxseeds or chia seeds, 30 grams of walnuts or 3 tablespoons of hemp seeds every day. These foods are also high in fibre.
3. **Focus on complex carbohydrates.** Don't be scared of 'carbs' and enjoy mostly intact whole grains such as quinoa and red rice, as well as starchy vegetables cooked with the skin on, such as potatoes and sweet potatoes.
4. **Look at the big picture.** No single food has the ability to make or break your health. Enjoy a variety of plant-based foods and develop and nurture a positive mindset and approach to eating.
5. **Take it at your own pace.** You know your body best. Learn the nutrition basics, supplement appropriately and enjoy the journey. Be patient and you will reap the benefits.

Figure 7: *The* Living PCOS Free *Plant-Based Plate*

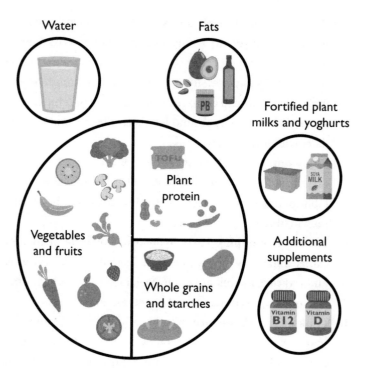

The PCOS Myth Buster

Myth: I will be constantly bloated on a plant-based diet.
The facts: Irritable bowel syndrome (IBS) symptoms such
as bloating are commonly experienced by those living
with PCOS.[12] Avoiding foods that are high in fibre is not
a good solution in the long term as this means removing
health-promoting foods from your diet which may compromise the health of your gut microbiome. Our recipes in
Living PCOS Free are rich in fibre and contain a variety of
legumes, all excellent for gut health. Bloating and digestive

issues can be a particular issue for those transitioning from a standard western diet to a whole food plant-based diet, rich in fibre. Over time, most people find that they are less or not at all bloated on a plant-based way of eating. If your symptoms do not improve, it's important to consult your doctor so that you can rule out conditions such as inflammatory bowel disease and coeliac disease.

Our 10 top tips to avoid bloating on a plant-based diet

1. **Introduce beans and lentils gradually. Start with smaller lentils first.** When introducing fibre-rich food, it's best to take it slowly so your gut bacteria, which play an important part in digesting your food, can adjust to the increase in dietary fibre. Start with a tablespoon of lentils at a time and build up the amount over the course of a few weeks or months.

2. **Rinse canned beans and lentils thoroughly.** Ensure you thoroughly drain and rinse canned pulses to remove the aquafaba, the liquid containing indigestible carbohydrates. This can lead to gas-induced discomfort.

3. **Soak beans and lentils overnight and sprout before cooking them.** Soak beans and lentils for six to 10 hours to reduce their cooking time, drain the soaking water and rinse and ensure you cook them thoroughly. Sprouting legumes (and whole grains) before cooking them is an excellent way to increase their nutrient value, including protein digestibility.[13] If you undercook beans and lentils, the lectins present will not break down and this can lead to gastric distress in some cases, with nausea, vomiting and diarrhoea. Cook them until they're so soft you could easily mash them.

Canned and jarred pulses are pre-cooked so there is no need to cook them again.

4. **Avoid ultra-processed foods, excess caffeine and alcohol.** Ultra-processed foods, alcohol and caffeine can all trigger digestive symptoms. Try to limit their consumption, keeping a food diary to note how you feel when you consume them.

5. **Eat mindfully and chew each mouthful thoroughly**. Digestion starts in the mouth so keep your phone away and enjoy your food without the distraction of a screen. Sit at the table and chew your food well. In general, it takes around 20 minutes to feel full once we start to eat.

6. **Enjoy herbs and spices.** Herbs and spices such as turmeric, mint, fennel and cumin may help with digestion and taste delicious in a soup, curry or dal. Peppermint is another great digestive aid as is kombu, a Japanese seaweed.

7. **Try asafoetida.** This spice, often known as *hing* in India, helps minimise bloating and gas. Add a small pinch to dal or curries.

8. **Grate ginger into meals or sip on ginger tea.** Ginger relaxes the muscles of the digestive tract and has anti-inflammatory properties, helping with period pain, nausea and cramps. Grate one or two tablespoons into your bean and lentil dishes or enjoy it as a tea. You can use either fresh grated ginger or the powdered form.

9. **Drink plenty of water as you increase the fibre in your diet.** Drinking plenty of water helps fibre do its job and crowds out sugar-sweetened beverages. Aim for eight glasses a day, although the amount you need depends on a number of factors including your activity levels, size, age and the climate.

10. **Remember that farting is a normal bodily function.** We really need to normalise regularly passing gas, which is a

sign that your digestive track is working as it should. Some bloating, especially in the lead up to your period, is nothing to worry about but do seek medical advice for persistent issues that affect your quality of life.

The PCOS Myth Buster

Myth: Seed cycling will balance my hormones.
The facts: Seed cycling is an alternative medicine practice which claims to regulate reproductive hormones throughout the menstrual cycle. It involves eating four different seeds (pumpkin, flax, sesame and sunflower) at different times of your cycle. There are, in fact, no scientific studies on seed cycling, or any evidence to support the belief that cycling these seeds actually regulates hormones or menstrual cycles. The kernel of truth is that these seeds are highly nutritious, a great source of vitamins, minerals and polyunsaturated fatty acids. An overall healthy plant-predominant diet can help support hormone function and a variety of seeds may be enjoyed as part of this, providing there are no allergies. While seed cycling is perhaps less overtly damaging than other wellness myths, it can be time-consuming and expensive, overcomplicating a healthy diet. It may also provide false hope for people trying to manage hormonal conditions.

PCOS POINTERS

Six top tips for transitioning to a plant-based diet:
- Focus on the big picture and aim to base most meals around whole plant foods.
- Focus on protein-rich plant foods, especially beans.
- Enjoy daily omega-3-rich foods such as ground flax seeds.
- Ensure a reliable source of vitamin B12.
- Focus on complex carbohydrates such as sweet potatoes.
- Make consistent changes and take it at your own pace.

25

Skip the SOS for PCOS
Salt, oil and sugar

Skipping the SOS means minimising added salt, oil and sugar in your diet. Salt, oil and sugar are often viewed as essential for delicious food but the recipes in *Living PCOS Free* are packed with flavour with minimal use of oil. The flavour comes from the use of herbs, spices, aromatics such as garlic and ginger, and other plant foods which have nutritional benefits. The aim is not to demonise salt, oil or sugar, which are generally fine in small amounts, but rather to provide suggestions for prioritising nutrient-dense foods, which it is especially important for people with PCOS to do.

For people with a history of disordered eating, it might not be appropriate to focus on reducing or eliminating added sugar or oil. It is more important to prioritise your wellbeing over restriction. You can adapt our recipes to suit your preferences too.

Don't be so salty

Salt has an essential role in the body, including in transporting water and in transmitting messages between our brain and the rest of our body. However, those of us eating a regular western diet are getting far too much of it, with the average person in the UK consuming

8 grams (g) of salt every day.[1] The World Health Organization (WHO) recommends that adults consume no more than 5 g on a daily basis. Diets high in salt can cause raised blood pressure, thereby increasing the risk of heart disease and stroke.

In the UK, around 75% of the salt we eat is added during food manufacturing,[1] so simply eating more whole plant foods is a great way to reduce salt intake. Skipping high sodium foods such as crisps, stock cubes, cheese and processed meat, and limiting plant-based foods that are high in sodium such as olives and pickles, can help further reduce salt in the diet. It's a good idea to read the label as foods that are marketed as healthy, such as certain pasta sauces and breakfast cereals, are often high in salt.

In most of the recipes in *Living PCOS Free*, we use fresh and dried herbs, spices, citrus, vinegars, pepper and mustard as the main seasonings, so you need to add less salt. If desired, we recommend adding salt at the table using a salt mill to get the flavour.

Why cooking with less oil is a good idea

Over 70% of the world's population is now living with excess weight. Oils are a dense source of calories with one tablespoon of oil containing around 120 calories. In general, choosing whole food sources of fats which come with fibre, unlike their oils, is preferable, especially if you are planning to lose weight in a healthful way.

Chemically speaking, free oils are chains of carbon found in a purified state. The extraction process removes most of the other ingredients of the whole food. As a result, oils do not have the abundance of phytonutrients, vitamins and minerals that occur naturally in whole plant foods such as nuts and seeds.

Olive oil

A clear exception is authentic cold-pressed extra-virgin olive oil (EVOO), but it tends to be expensive and harder to find. EVOO and canola oil contain monounsaturated fats (MUFAs) and poly-unsaturated fats (PUFAs), with studies showing health-promoting benefits for the brain and the heart. These oils are always preferable to eating butter, ghee and coconut oil which are high in saturated fat, or trans fats found in ultra-processed foods, all of which may slow blood flow for hours after a fatty meal. Animal-derived fats and tropical oils such as coconut oil raise LDL cholesterol consistently, as well as the risk of cardiovascular disease. Studies consistently show that swapping saturated fat in the diet with the monounsaturated fat from EVOO lowers cholesterol levels, thereby improving heart health.

Cooking with oils heated to high temperatures can release advanced glycation end products (AGEs). We know that AGEs can adversely affect the ovaries, creating hormonal disruption, especially in those with PCOS (see Chapter 12). While olive oil is suitable for sautéing, rapeseed or avocado oil are better options for cooking at higher temperatures due to their higher smoking points, but they should still be kept to a minimum.

Modest amounts of oil can be added if you wish, especially if this improves your enjoyment of food and cooking. However, for most people there is no evidence to suggest that oils have to be an essential part of their diets. High quality cold-pressed extra-virgin olive oil (EVOO), used raw or in low-temperature cooking, may be useful. It can be an especially helpful addition to the diet for those who find it hard to maintain weight or for those who would like to gain weight, as well as for children. Hemp seed oil, flaxseed oil or walnut oil are some other omega-3-rich options.

Healthy whole fats

There is a distinction between oil and healthy fats, the latter of which are essential for everyone. Fat can help with the absorption of certain nutrients, such as fat-soluble vitamins A, D, E and K. Nuts, seeds and avocados provide healthy unsaturated fats, without one needing to reach for the oil. There is greater fat absorption from nut butters, such as almond butter, than from the whole nut. Eating whole plants is therefore generally preferable because of the fibre content, which traps all of nature's healthful antioxidants. Adding or removing oil should never be a source of anxiety or stress as it can lead to a restricted dietary pattern and distract from the overall importance of eating a healthy, plant-predominant diet.

How to get started with oil-free cooking

We encourage people to learn by starting to gradually reduce the oil they use to cook with by half every week until they are using little or none. Alongside this, we advise learning to cook, sauté and roast with hot water, apple purée, vinegar, stock or wine, all of which can be great substitutes depending on the meal.

If you want the flavour of oil in certain dishes, we suggest adding a few drops of cold-pressed oil to a dish after it has been cooked or prepared. For example, add EVOO to a salad, a few drops of mustard oil to Bengali dishes or sesame oil to Chinese dishes. You will be surprised how good your dishes can taste with little or no oil. Our flavoursome and hearty recipes will get you started on your journey.

You don't need sugar to be sweet

In recent years, almost every ill has been blamed on sugar, accompanied by a great deal of fearmongering in the media. However, it is true that added sugars are simply not necessary in a healthy dietary pattern and the amount we are currently eating as a population is excessive. Free sugars (which means sugars added to food or drinks, and sugars found naturally in foods such as brown sugar, honey, maple syrup, agave and unsweetened fruit and vegetable juices) should not make up more than 5% of the calories you get from food and drink each day. An exception to this is whole fruits and vegetables. The idea that fruit has too much sugar is misleading as whole fruits come packaged with fibre, vitamins, minerals and water unlike their juiced counterparts. We explore this in more detail in Chapter 12.

Diets high in added sugar are especially harmful to people with PCOS, as they are linked to type 2 diabetes, high triglycerides, heart disease and weight gain. As insulin resistance is often a hallmark of PCOS, eating fewer simple sugars and refined carbohydrates can help you achieve better blood glucose control, reducing your risk of type 2 diabetes and helping you to manage your weight.

Women with PCOS are also at greater risk of periodontal disease, also known as gum disease.[2] The science is clear that a high intake of free sugars is associated with periodontal disease, independent of traditional risk factors.[3] It is therefore important to crowd out foods which often contain a high amount of sugar, oil and salt, such as biscuits, cakes, ice cream and chocolate bars, as well as sugary foods, including sugar-sweetened beverages and sweets. Sugar is also found in surprisingly high quantities in certain savoury foods, such as pizza, table sauces, low-fat yoghurts, ready meals and many breakfast cereals. Do brush your teeth twice a day with a fluoride toothpaste, floss regularly and attend dental hygiene appointments, especially during pregnancy.

In the recipes in *Living PCOS Free*, we try to sweeten dishes using fruit by adding applesauce, mashed banana or perhaps a small amount of dried fruit, all of which include some fibre and other nutrients. Where we do use small amounts of maple syrup, which has a lower glycaemic index (GI) than table sugar, we keep this to a minimum.

Beverages to reduce sugar cravings

A liquorice, fennel or spearmint tea may also curb sugar cravings. While small amounts of liquorice are safe to eat, you should avoid large amounts as liquorice can raise blood pressure. Avoid liquorice root in pregnancy as it may be linked to child development issues.[4] Another tip is to try a cup of hot lemon and ginger tea or cinnamon tea and add a tablespoon of apple cider vinegar. Start with a teaspoon if you don't like the taste of vinegar.

If you usually drink fizzy drinks with your meals, try a sparkling water, slice of lemon and flavoured infused vinegar, such as raspberry vinegar. Due to their acetic acid content, vinegars can be helpful in reducing glucose and insulin levels after a meal, suggesting they may positively impact glycaemic control.[5]

An overall healthy dietary pattern

Remember, what we do consistently is what contributes far more to our overall health and wellbeing than what we consume at the occasional meal or special occasion. Each meal, especially those shared with others, is an opportunity for connection, joy, pleasure and nourishment. Most importantly, the food you eat should not be a constant source of stress or anxiety.

The PCOS Myth Buster

Myth: You should limit the amount of fruit you eat if you have PCOS.

The facts: Fruit is one of the healthiest foods that people with PCOS can eat and this common misconception shows the danger of reducing foods to their individual nutrients rather than looking at the whole package. Fruit comes packaged with beneficial phytonutrients, fibre and water and has consistently been shown to reduce the risk of type 2 diabetes, even with high fruit intakes.[4] The fibre present helps slow the absorption of fruit sugar (fructose) in the bloodstream, which is why juices which contain minimal fibre should be limited. Even fruits such as bananas and mangos are considered low GI and are in the medium glycaemic load (GL) range. Pairing them with some soya yoghurt or a few nuts will further reduce the glycaemic response. The main reason we don't recommend eating only fruit-based diets, such as fruitarian-style diets, for PCOS, is that you would miss out on all the other nutritious plant-based foods, such as beans, and it would be much harder to achieve certain nutrient intakes, such as protein. Although it's a great source of fibre, dried fruit should generally be limited to a serving a day as it's a concentrated source of energy in a small package. However, all whole fresh or frozen fruit is health-promoting and, of all fruits, berries pack the greatest antioxidant punch.

PCOS POINTERS

- Use salt, oil and sugar (SOS) as flavourings rather than main features of any dish.
- Experiment with herbs, spices, flavoured vinegars, and lemon juice as alternatives.
- If you choose an oil, choose cold-pressed extra virgin olive oil over most other oils.
- Eat a variety of whole fruits as they are full of fibre and micronutrients. Try to replace sugar and sweeteners with whole fruit, mashed banana, applesauce, dates or fresh or dried fruit when you can in cooking and baking.
- Adopt a diet rich in whole plant foods with minimal added salt, oil or sugar.
- Eating whole plant foods with healthy unsaturated fats promotes good health, especially when replacing saturated (mostly animal-derived) fats and trans fats.

26

Soya: Healthy or not?
The role of soya in PCOS

Soya (or soy as it is known in North America) is not only safe but has a positive role in managing your PCOS. We want to reassure you, with the help of the scientific evidence, both of the safety and the many health benefits of soya. Having read this chapter, we hope you will feel confident about adding unprocessed or minimally processed soya products to your diet regularly, whether you have PCOS or not.

A magic bean

Soya deserves a special mention, even though it is technically classified as a legume. Think of it as a magic bean, not unlike Jack and the Beanstalk's magic beans.

All plants contain all nine essential amino acids – building blocks that our body cannot make and which must come from external sources.[1] What makes soya remarkable is that it contains all nine in a similar proportion to animal protein, making it a high-quality protein source but without any of the undesirable effects of animal foods.[2] Soya is low in the undesirable saturated fats found in high amounts in animal products. It is a rich source of fibre, healthy PUFAs (polyunsaturated fats) and resistant starch and a good source of vitamins and minerals such as calcium, iron, potassium, folate and magnesium.

Soya and hormones

With hundreds of scientific studies resulting from over 30 years of rigorous research on soya, and more than 2000 soya-related peer-reviewed articles published every year, the message is clear: soya is a healthy addition to any dietary pattern. Unless one is allergic, eating soya is healthful for every age and for all genders.[3] Soya plays an especially beneficial role in reproductive health, including PCOS.

A great many of the misconceptions about soya stem from the fact that it contains phytoestrogens (plant oestrogens) which resemble the oestrogen hormone found in our body but with much weaker oestrogen activity. These plant compounds occur naturally in other plant foods but are found in higher quantities in soya.

The phytoestrogens that are best known are *isoflavones* found in soya beans, chickpeas, beans, fruit and pistachio nuts, and *lignans* found in flaxseeds, sesame seeds and whole grain cereals.[4]

Soya isoflavones mimic oestrogen in some tissues of the body, while in others they have an anti-oestrogen effect. This dual action, known as a 'selective estrogen [oestrogen] receptor modulator' (SERM) effect is responsible for many of the positive health benefits of soya that are separate from its other properties of being rich in fibre and protein.[5]

Soya does not affect fertility

Despite the misconceptions, reproductive health is not adversely affected by soya in men or women and it may actually help improve fertility levels. Asian countries have historically consumed soya as part of healthful dietary patterns for thousands of years, without an adverse impact on male or female fertility. Consuming soya or soya-based formulas from infancy also has been shown to have no negative effects on general or reproductive health.[6] There is some evidence from studies of women going through fertility treatment that isoflavones aid fertility and improve birth rates.[7]

All clinical studies have shown that isoflavones have no negative effect on sperm concentration or quality. Studies in humans consistently show that eating soya foods does not raise oestrogen levels, disrupt hormonal balance or reduce testosterone concentrations in men.[3, 8]

A slimmer waist in those with PCOS

When consumed regularly, soya has been consistently shown to help with the symptoms of PCOS and improve many of the metabolic markers seen in the condition.[9, 10] A randomised controlled trial, published in 2018, looked at the effect of dietary soya intake on weight loss, glycaemic (blood sugar) control, lipid profiles, biomarkers of inflammation and oxidative stress, and triglycerides. It showed that consuming soya helped counteract hormone disruption and resulted in weight loss among patients with PCOS.[9]

Soya helps build bone and reduces cancer risk

There are many other health benefits of including soya bean products in your diet if you have PCOS. Soya, when consumed regularly, is known to promote bone health and reduce the risk of osteoporosis.[11, 12]

When started early in childhood or young adult life, consuming as little as one portion of soya daily may reduce breast cancer risk.[13, 14, 15] In women, soya foods appear to increase the length of the menstrual cycle by one day, although ovulation is not prevented. This minor effect on menstrual cycle length could help to decrease breast cancer risk, although more research is needed to confirm this.[16]

The risk of other cancers such as colorectal, liver and ovarian cancers, is also lower in those who consume soya regularly, as is the risk of prostate cancer in men.[13, 6]

Soya is good for the bowel including in those with inflammatory bowel conditions such as ulcerative colitis.[17] There are heart benefits too, with fermented versions of soya such as tempeh being particularly cardio-protective.[18, 3] As gut health is often compromised in PCOS, and heart disease and certain cancer risks may be increased in those with PCOS in later life, it makes sense to add soya regularly to your daily diet.

Recommended servings of soya

Whatever your diet, you should aim to consume two portions of whole or minimally processed soya foods daily. One portion is a 250-ml cup of soya milk or soya yoghurt, or 80 g, which is roughly a handful, of tofu, tempeh, edamame beans, natto or mature soya beans. We suggest rotating the types of soya bean products, so you get to eat a variety throughout the week along with other colourful plant foods. Some people with higher calorie needs, such as athletes, can benefit from eating up to four portions of soya a day.

Two servings of these traditional soya foods per day provide around 15–20 g protein and approximately 20–50 mg isoflavones, with the protein in the soya representing around 20–25% of your total dietary protein intake.[19, 3, 20]

Processed forms of soya

We are often asked about the type of soya one should consume. It is preferable to include whole or minimally processed soya products daily rather than highly processed alternatives. It is fine to enjoy the occasional soya sausage or soya-based plant-based meat alternative, especially for children and older adults, as they are a good protein source. They can add fun and familiarity to a plant-based diet at parties and picnics. It is also a useful addition for those transitioning to a plant-based way of eating. However, they can contain higher levels of salt, sugar and saturated fat, although far less than a traditional pork sausage. In general, however, if you have PCOS, we encourage you to enjoy less processed soya most of the time.

We also do not have enough information yet to recommend what are known as 'soya protein isolates', such as protein powders, as a rule for the average person or in PCOS. They may mimic animal whey protein with its effect on insulin-like growth factor (IGF1), which promotes the growth and development of bone and tissue but in excess may worsen diabetes and promote the growth of certain cancers.[20]

Fortified vs organic soya products

In the UK, we would recommend choosing fortified soya products such as calcium-set tofu and calcium-fortified soya milk, as these are good sources of an important nutrient. Calcium from soya is just as well absorbed as from dairy products, with soya milk having the added advantage of being vitamin-D enriched, which is not the case for cow's milk in the UK. Calcium-set tofu contains approximately 400 mg of calcium per 100 g. It also contains magnesium, another useful nutrient for healthy bones. Increasing the intake of dietary fibre and magnesium has been shown to help in reducing insulin resistance and high androgen levels in women with PCOS[15]

At present, organic soya milk is not usually fortified in the UK, so we recommend choosing fortified products over organic, as the benefits are greater in this situation and the products are more affordable too. Edamame beans come in pods like peas, so choosing organic is not really needed. In the UK, almost all soya for human consumption comes from Asia and is not genetically modified.

Soya allergy

Compared with allergy to milk, eggs, peanuts and fish, soya allergy is less common in the UK. Only a tiny proportion of adults are allergic to soya – that is, no more than 0.5% of the population. Compared with 20-30 in 1000 children with dairy allergies, only 3-4 in 1000 children are allergic to soya.[21] Some reports suggest that children with soya allergy have a good chance of outgrowing it but how often this occurs is not clear. If allergies are suspected; it is important to see your doctor as some food allergies can be serious.

Soya and thyroid issues

Coexistent thyroid dysfunction is not a contraindication for consuming soya in the amounts we have recommended above.[22] However, you do need to check with your doctor if you are in any doubt.

The general recommendation is to consume your thyroid medication (usually levothyroxine) 30–60 minutes before breakfast or four hours after the last meal.[23] You should also ensure adequate iodine intake through a supplement if needed (150 mcg) as most standard western diets are deficient in iodine.

Plant-based diets without soya

You can still thrive with PCOS on a plant-based diet, rich in other beans and lentils, even if you cannot have soya. However, do not deny yourself the benefits of this wonderful bean, unless you are allergic to it. If you have gut health issues or an intolerance or sensitivity to beans rather than a true allergy, consider reintroducing it slowly over time, ideally with the help of a nutrition professional.

Soya and the environment

The demand for soya is not being driven by those eating plant-based diets. Over 70% of soya grown in the Amazon is used to feed farmed animals whereas only around 7% is used for human consumption in foods such as tofu and tempeh. This non-genetically modified soya is still produced mostly in Asia as well as in the USA and Europe. The answer is not to stop eating soya but to significantly reduce our consumption of animal products.

The Worldwide Fund for Nature (WWF) estimates we each consume on average, 61 kg of soya per year, which is more than 1 kg a week. Most of this soya is being consumed indirectly by us as it is fed to animals. The production of one litre of cow's milk requires more than 22 times more water and 12 times more land than one litre of soya milk, while generating three times more greenhouse gas emissions.

Originally from southeast Asia, the soya plant is a nitrogen-fixing legume first discovered for human use around 5000 years ago. Soya is now primarily used for animal feed and some biofuels. Its cultivation is a major driver of deforestation in the Amazon basin, with animal agriculture, including animal feed, responsible for 80-85% of soya production. Chicken and eggs have the heaviest soya footprint, followed by pork and farmed salmon. Much of the controversy arises as a result of genetically modified (GM) soya monocrops grown primarily in the United States, Brazil and Argentina. The United Nations estimates a need for new land by 2028, almost twice the size of Switzerland, in order to grow soya for animal feed.

The PCOS Myth Buster

Myth: Soya will mess with my hormones
The facts: This is one of the most common myths around. Long-term observation studies have confirmed no negative effect on reproductive health in either men or women. Sperm counts, hormone levels and fertility rates are not affected negatively by soya.[3, 24] The most detailed review of research published to date, looking at 417 reports including clinical studies, systematic reviews and meta-analyses, concluded that soya or isoflavones could not be labelled as endocrine disruptors, with likely protective effects on both the breast and the uterus.[23] The saturated fat and oestrogen hormones found in animal products are more likely to cause hormone disturbances. When soya replaces dairy and red or processed meat, it is likely to provide even more health benefits for the prevention of chronic diseases and certain cancers.

PCOS POINTERS

- Soya reduces insulin levels, can help with weight loss and improves many of the symptoms and metabolic markers of PCOS.
- Soya has a beneficial role in reproductive health and does not affect the fertility of any gender.
- When consumed regularly, soya can reduce the risk of several cancers.
- There is no need to avoid soya if on thyroid medications.
- Soya is safe for all ages as part of a varied diet unless one is allergic to it.
- Soya is a good source of healthy plant oestrogens, fibre, protein, fats and other nutrients.
- Soya is best eaten in a minimally processed form, such as edamame beans, tofu, tempeh and soya milk.
  Two 80-g portions of soya are recommended daily for an adult.

27

Food first approach
The role of supplements in PCOS

Supplements are big business. In the UK alone, the nutritional supplement market is projected to reach over £10.5 billion ($15 billion) by 2023, with continued growth expected. There are thousands of supplements on the market specifically targeted at women with PCOS, often supported with little evidence and surrounded by marketing hype. This is especially true when it comes to PCOS and fertility, with unsubstantiated claims around supplements, such as the ability for them to 'cure PCOS'. While there are some supplements that may be helpful for women with PCOS, we recommend adopting a 'food first' approach, with adequate supplementation as required.

The medicine is in the food

There is nothing radical or new about a food first approach, which looks at optimising health through daily nutritious food. The food and drink we consume daily affect our health now as well as in the longer-term. By meeting our nutrient needs through a variety of whole plant foods, we can obtain major macronutrients as well as essential vitamins, minerals, fibre and water. These foods also contain thousands of beneficial micronutrients, such as carotenoids, flavonoids and polyphenols.

A helping hand

There are a few situations where we may not be able to obtain all our nutrients from food, and different variables may be at play. These include certain medical conditions, certain medications, limited access to healthy foods, allergies and intolerances, soil quality and even how much sunlight we get. Supplements do have a role to play here and, in some cases, may have life-changing benefits. For example, taking a folic acid supplement before conception reduces the risk of spina bifida and other neural tube defects in infants. It's therefore important not to conflate what is 'natural' with what is optimal for health. We will explore some of the helpful supplements for PCOS in this chapter.

Seek individualised advice

It is best to consult with your healthcare professional regarding the best supplements for you, especially if you are taking prescription medication, considering conceiving, are pregnant or breastfeeding, or if you're seeking advice for your child.

The role of supplements in PCOS

There is some evidence for certain vitamin or mineral supplements having some benefit in symptom relief, including insulin resistance and androgen excess, for those with PCOS. Published studies are of variable quality, and robust enough evidence to recommend routine use is lacking for most supplements. An individualised approach is advised if supplements are to be added, as we have said, but our recommendation is to address most deficiencies first through a varied plant-based diet.

Vitamin D

Vitamin D is a fat-soluble vitamin and, as its synthesis occurs in our skin on exposure to sunlight, it is technically a hormone. Sunlight is very variable depending on where you live and cannot be relied on for vitamin D synthesis completely. Vitamin D deficiency is common in women with PCOS. There is some evidence that vitamin D supplementation may improve reproductive function and insulin sensitivity.[1, 2] After an initial blood test to measure levels, the advisable dosage of vitamin D3 can vary between 400 and 2000 IU per day (that is, 10-50 micrograms (mcg)), taken with the largest meal of the day, especially in the winter months. If higher doses are needed, they should be used only under medical supervision to avoid vitamin D toxicity.

In addition to supplementing, enjoy direct sunshine between the hours of 11:00 am and 3:00 pm on your arms, legs or back for 15-45 minutes, depending on the colour of your skin; 30-45 minutes are needed for darker skin. Apply sunscreen after the recommended timing for sun exposure, taking care to avoid sunburn. Choose a mineral sunscreen over standard sunscreens as there appears to be better protection from ultraviolet radiation, checking it is approved as UVA (EU standard). Aim to strike a balance between protecting yourself from the sun and getting enough vitamin D from sunlight.

Most foods are poor sources of vitamin D, including eggs and mushrooms, and so should not be relied on as your only source. In a vegan diet, the main sources of vitamin D are fortified dairy-free milks and yoghurts, providing an average of 1.1 mcg per 100 ml/g, and fortified breakfast cereals.

B vitamins in PCOS

Folic acid or 'folate' (the natural form of vitamin B9), vitamin B6 and vitamin B12 have significant roles in the regulation of homocysteine. Elevated levels of homocysteine appear to have a role in worsening of insulin resistance and in an increased risk of cardiovascular and reproductive symptoms in PCOS. Broccoli, green leafy vegetables, green peas, soya, chickpeas, kidney beans and other legumes are good sources of folic acid and B6, so include them in your diet regularly.

Vitamin B12

Vitamin B12 (cobalamin) is a water-soluble vitamin and essential nutrient which helps keep the body's nerve and blood cells healthy and plays a part in forming DNA, the genetic material in all cells. Vitamin B12 deficiency may take several years to manifest as the body has stores which last a while, and symptoms can range from fatigue to permanent neurological damage. Vitamin B12 deficiency can also cause a type of anaemia known as megaloblastic anaemia. Independent of the anaemia, B12 deficiency can damage the nervous system, which is serious. Although B12 is found in meat, dairy and eggs, it is actually made by bacteria in soil and water. This supplement is essential if you are on a plant-based diet at any age given the lack of plant sources of B12.

The recommended daily intake (RDI) of vitamin B12 is 1.5 mcg for both men and women, though pregnant and breastfeeding women have higher needs. It is advised to take a vitamin B12 supplement in a dosage of 25-100 mcg daily or 2000 mcg /week of cyanocobalmin (more shelf-stable and cheaper than methylcobalmin) if you are under 65 years old. Even in omnivores, supplementation is worth considering in people above the age of 50 as ageing is an important risk factor for B12 deficiency.

If taken less frequently than daily, higher doses are required. Only 10 mcg of a 500 mcg B12 supplement is absorbed in people without a deficiency, hence the need for higher supplement doses than the body's daily needs of the vitamin.

Vitamin B12 is better absorbed in smaller, frequent doses. This is because B12 binds to a substance called intrinsic factor released in the stomach. This process is easily overwhelmed if there is one big dose, rather than being divided over two separate meals. Only enough intrinsic factor is excreted per meal to absorb 2-4 mcg of B12. If you choose to obtain B12 from enriched foods, like yeast extract, fortified meat alternatives or nutritional yeast, then servings should ideally be eaten three times a day.

Vitamin B12 injections raise levels more quickly and may be needed if a deficiency is diagnosed. Some people cannot absorb vitamin B12 due to certain digestive conditions and therefore need injections under the guidance of a health professional.

Vitamin B12 supplements are generally safe but too high a dose may cause side effects, such as dizziness, headaches, nausea and vomiting. Vitamin B12 supplements can also interact with other drugs, such as metformin for diabetes and vitamin C among others, so it's wise to check with your doctor if in any doubt.

Iodine

A trace element, iodine, is an essential component of our thyroid hormones. PCOS is associated with increased prevalence of thyroid issues, including autoimmune conditions, so having your iodine levels and your thyroid function checked and taking medications and/or a supplement may be helpful if advised by your doctor.[3]

Salt in the UK is not iodised, and neither are the fancy rock salts often used nowadays. Seaweed and sea vegetables, such as nori and dulse, are good iodine sources, but they contain varying amounts and can be unreliable. Iodised salt is also a good source, but we have already discussed how one should try and minimise salt in general.

The daily requirement for iodine is about 150 mcg per day; if you are concerned you are not getting the required amount in your diet, you may wish to take a supplement. However, too much iodine can be a problem just as too little can. In some people with inadequate iodine intake, overconsumption of raw cruciferous (cabbage-family) vegetables may block the thyroid gland's ability to absorb iodine.

Omega-3 fatty acids

Omega-3 fats are a type of polyunsaturated fat. They are essential fats, which means our body cannot make them on its own and we need them to survive as they are involved throughout the body at a cellular level and are important for brain health.

We get the omega-3 fatty acids we need from the foods we eat. The form of omega-3 typically found in plants is called alpha-linolenic acid (ALA) and is needed to make two other omega-3 fats. These two long-chain fatty acids that have the most direct health benefits are eicosapentaenoic acid (EPA) and docosahexaenoic acid (DHA). They are found in algae and plankton which are eaten by fish which is why fish are a rich source of EPA and DHA.[4]

As some people don't convert ALA from food substances very efficiently, it may be worth considering an algae-derived omega-3 supplement (EPA plus DHA) of 250-1000 milligrams (mg) daily. In addition, consider including 1-2 tablespoons of ground flaxseed powder daily and/or of chia seeds (soaked) daily and/or six walnut halves daily and/or ¼ cup hemp seeds, all of which are good sources of ALA.

Based on current evidence, omega-3 fatty acids may be recommended for the treatment of PCOS in those with insulin resistance as well as high LDL cholesterol and triglycerides.[5] Omega-3 fatty acids and 400 IU of vitamin E co-supplementation for 12 weeks in PCOS women in a randomised controlled trial significantly improved markers of insulin resistance and levels of total and free testosterone.[6] Long-term benefits beyond six months of treatment remain unknown.

Chromium

Supplementation with chromium has also been shown to significantly improve the chances of ovulation and reduce androgen excess and menstrual dysfunction in PCOS.[7, 8] It can also improve glucose control if abnormal but does not help in those with normal glucose tolerance.[9]

A dietary supplement with the minimum recommended intake of the trace mineral chromium (RDA 25 mcg/day) may be helpful under guidance. We do not yet know the effects of taking high doses of chromium.

Zinc

Supplementation may have some potential for improving abnormal lipid levels and insulin resistance in PCOS, as seen in some studies.[8] Plant-based sources of zinc include beans, chickpeas, lentils, tofu, walnuts, cashew nuts, ground flaxseed, chia seeds, hemp seeds, pumpkin seeds and quinoa.

Inositol

One of the key ingredients in a diet that emphasises whole grain intake, legumes and nuts in place of refined carbohydrates is inositol hexaphosphate. Myo-inositol is a naturally occurring sugar in fruit, beans, grains and nuts that can improve insulin resistance. Inositol (myo-inositol and di-chiro inositol) is a nutritional supplement.

A meta-analysis of 10 randomised controlled trials revealed that myo-inositol alone, or combined with DCI (D-chiro-inositol), improved the metabolic profile of women with PCOS, also increasing SHBG when supplementation lasted for at least 24 weeks.[10] In other clinical trials, inositol has been shown to improve insulin action, decrease androgen levels and improve ovulatory function in both lean and obese women with PCOS.

The benefits of metformin in PCOS appear at least partly to be due to increasing inositol availability.[11] Myoinositol with folic acid taken for three to six months has shown some promising results in helping women ovulate and is thought to work by reducing testosterone/insulin levels, although it cannot yet be routinely recommended.

In a systematic review published in 2018, inositol appeared to regulate menstrual cycles, improve ovulation and induce metabolic changes in PCOS, but evidence was lacking for pregnancy, miscarriage or live birth.[12]. Inositol supplementation during pregnancy, often combined with folic acid, has been studied as both potential prevention and treatment for gestational diabetes mellitus. While there are some data to suggest a reduction of gestational diabetes risk in PCOS, inositol in any form should still be considered experimental until more evidence becomes available. However, as it appears to have few side effects and is widely available at low to moderate cost, a discussion with your healthcare team on an individual basis is recommended.[13]

Melatonin

Melatonin is best known as a sleep aid, and it is both a hormone and an antioxidant. Secreted by the pineal gland, it regulates circadian rhythms, reproduction and the sleep cycle. Women with PCOS have been found to have low levels of melatonin. There is some evidence that supplementation may improve egg quality and maturation of the immature eggs and reduce oxidative stress and inflammation. Taking inositol along with melatonin may improve fertility even more than taking melatonin alone. More studies on melatonin are needed and it is not currently recommended in pregnancy. You can support production of melatonin through a healthy lifestyle, but if you choose to supplement, it is best to consult a healthcare professional.

Supplementation while on the Pill

Based on a detailed review of the effects of oral contraceptives on nutrient status, we recommend taking a multivitamin supplement containing B complex vitamins, folic acid, vitamins B12, C and E and minerals including zinc, magnesium and selenium.[13a]

A word about over-supplementation

A multivitamin cannot in any way be a substitute for a well-balanced plant-predominant dietary pattern. Some supplements, such as of vitamin A, can also have adverse health effects, acting very differently when they are isolated in supplement form, compared to when they are consumed as part of a whole food. A few herbal supplements have been studied and may help in improving menstrual dysfunction and insulin sensitivity associated with PCOS, but research evidence is not strong enough to recommend these routinely.[14]

Preconception and pregnancy supplementation

You should take a medically approved pregnancy supplement with all the recommended vitamins and minerals in the right dosage throughout pregnancy, after delivery and during breastfeeding to ensure you have adequate levels of all the important minerals and vitamins. For example, ensure you are taking 400 mcg folic acid and at least 25 mcg vitamin D (1000 IU) daily.

If you have a few months to prepare, start a prenatal supplement at least three to six months before conception. Otherwise, start as soon as you find out you are pregnant as the early weeks are critical for foetal development.

Folic acid and folate

Make sure you take 400 mcg of folic acid every day, rather than any other form often marketed as more natural, as folic acid is the only one proven to reduce neural tube defects in the foetus. Try to consume plenty of green leafy vegetables, beans, broccoli, avocados and peas, which are good dietary sources of folate. You will need to take a higher dose of 5 mg of folic acid in certain situations – for example, if you have a family history of spina bifida spinal defects, have a BMI over 30, are on certain medications, or have coeliac disease or type 2 diabetes.[15]

Iodine

Seaweed as a source of iodine is unpredictable in pregnancy and some varieties, such as hijiki, contain too much iodine which can be toxic. It is best avoided unless you are used to consuming it and know what you are doing.

As many prenatal supplements contain little to no iodine (essential for brain, nervous system and thyroid development in the foetus), it is important to supplement with 200 mcg of potassium iodide daily rather than relying on food sources.

Omega-3 fatty acids

A scientific review of relevant medical studies in 2018 looking at 70 randomised controlled trials in middle- and high-income countries, found increasing omega-3 long chain polyunsaturated fatty acids intake during pregnancy, either through supplements or in foods, may reduce the incidence of premature birth and low birthweight. Women who take these supplements during pregnancy were also more likely to have longer pregnancies.[5] Another earlier systematic review concluded that there was no conclusive evidence to either support or refute omega-3 long-chain polyunsaturated fatty acid supplementation in pregnancy as a way of improving cognitive or visual development in offspring.[16]

Until more conclusive evidence is available and as there are currently no UK recommendations for omega-3 supplements in pregnancy, if you do not eat fish for any reason (eat a completely whole food plant-based diet because you are vegan, for cultural reasons or you don't like the taste), it is prudent to take 500-1000 mg of algae-derived omega-3 supplements. Ideally, you should start these three to six months before conception and continue throughout pregnancy and breastfeeding, whilst reducing your intake of omega-6 fatty acids that are typically much higher in a standard western diet that includes ultra-processed foods. ALA is found mainly in flax seeds, walnuts, chia seeds, edamame, oatmeal and green leafy vegetables, for example, and although it should not be relied on completely in pregnancy, these foods should be included regularly as part of a healthy diet.

Over-supplementation in pregnancy

You should also avoid megavitamins, non-essential dietary supplements and herbal preparations given that the risk to the foetus from these substances is not fully known. For example, doses of vitamin A of more than 5000 IU can cause birth defects. You should avoid eating liver for the same reason,[15, 17] although plant-based food sources of beta-carotene, converted to vitamin A in the body, do not carry risks.

Food first

There is a great deal of confusion around supplements, but this is definitely an area which is not one-size-fits-all. The supplement industry is also largely unregulated so there can be a great variation between brands, with quality issues, including fillers. Exercise caution if something seems too good to be true, as there is truly no substitute for a healthy diet. Certain supplements can however be beneficial, especially when added to a overall healthy diet pattern.

The PCOS Myth Buster

Myth: A plant-based diet is dangerous because it lacks vitamin B12.
The facts: This is not true. You do need to supplement with vitamin B12 if you are on an exclusively plant-based diet, but provided you do so, it is one of the healthiest choices you can make. Vitamin B12 is made by bacteria in the soil and we need supplements as humans cannot make vitamin B12 themselves. Food sources of vitamin B12 are generally unreliable apart from certain fortified foods. Vitamin B12 is often added to animal feed as most animals are now reared in factory farm settings. Ensuring a good source of vitamin B12 is non-negotiable on a plant-based diet and supplements are relatively cheap and easily available.

PCOS POINTERS

- Adopt a 'food first' approach.
- There is no substitute for a healthy plant-predominant diet.
- Supplement under medical guidance.
- Vitamin B12 supplementation is essential if you are on a plant-based diet.
- Vitamin D, iodine and algae-derived omega-3s should be considered.
- Inositol, chromium and zinc may be helpful for PCOS in some cases.
- There are specific supplements, including folic acid, that are important in pregnancy.

PCOS POINTERS IN PREGNANCY

- Choose a medically approved prenatal and pregnancy supplement with folic acid, starting three to six months before trying to conceive if possible.
- Only choose medically approved folic acid pregnancy supplements over other folate supplements.
- Supplementation with iodine, vitamin D and omega-3 helpful after discussion with your health professional.

28

Daily affirmations for PCOS

Affirmations are powerful and positive simple statements that can help us challenge negative thought patterns. Affirmations can decrease stress, increase well-being, and make us more open to behaviour change.[1] Women with PCOS are more likely to experience self-esteem issues, including problems with body image[2] (see Chapter 20). Positive affirmations can help strengthen self-worth over time, often by giving individuals a broader view of the self and focusing on core values such as kindness and compassion. Research also shows that positive affirmations can activate the reward system in the brain, which can have an impact on the way we experience both emotional and physical pain.[1]

Developing an affirmation practice

There is no right or wrong way to begin an affirmation practice. Starting slowly and building up to a consistent daily practice is a good strategy. Try not to skip days if possible.

- Say aloud an affirmation when you wake up to set a positive intention for the day, or when you get into bed at night.
- Repeat each affirmation out loud around five to 10 times. Focus on the words as they leave your mouth and believe them to be true.

It may take time to notice a shift in your mindset or behaviours so be patient with yourself. Try to think of affirmations as a step towards change, rather than the change itself. For example, 'I deserve to nourish my body' might guide you to a daily habit of eating fresh fruit and vegetables. While you are responsible for making the change yourself, the affirmation might provide a starting point.

Feeling authentic

If you feel a bit awkward at first, consider writing down your affirmation several times in your journal or diary. I have provided a mix of affirmations below, and in our 21-Day Programme (page 315), for inspiration, but affirmations tend to provide the most benefit when they are specific to you. If an affirmation feels inauthentic or focuses on a statement you don't believe to be true, it may have little benefit. An affirmation should speak directly to you and be relevant. For example, if you are going through fertility issues, an affirmation such as 'I feel supported and loved through my fertility journey' may be especially helpful. You can create your own affirmations that are meaningful to you, addressing particular concerns or worries you may have.

Thirty daily positive affirmations for PCOS

1. My mind and body are strong and resilient.
2. I listen to my body and take things at my own pace.
3. I trust my body and that it knows what it's doing.
4. With every no, I'm creating space for yes.
5. My self-care is important and worth making time for.
6. I give myself permission to rest.
7. I deserve to nourish my body.
8. I move my body to look after myself.
9. I love moving my body in ways that I enjoy.

Chapter 28

10. I am powerful and can do anything I put my mind to.
11. I am as kind and loving to myself as I am to others.
12. I release negative thoughts from my mind and attract the good.
13. I am strong. I am worthy. I am enough.
14. I am listening to my inner voice.
15. I am worthy of love and acceptance.
16. I am thankful for the positive things in my life.
17. I release all of my worries.
18. I treat my body with respect and compassion.
19. I am stronger today than I was yesterday.
20. I am healing every day.
21. I know that I am not my PCOS; it does not define me.
22. I am patient and kind to myself every day.
23. I am at home in my body.
24. I let go of all fear and replace this with love.
25. I speak to myself as I would to a close friend.
26. I can challenge my negative thoughts with positive ones.
27. I trust myself. I trust my body.
28. I am beautiful on the inside and it shines through on the outside.
29. My life is what I make of it. I have all the power.
30. I am more in tune with my body than I have ever been before.

29

Self-care activities

Self-care is all the steps you take to take care of yourself so you can stay physically, mentally and emotionally well. This is highly individual and only you can decide what kind of self-care is best for you. The beneficial effects of self-care include improved well-being and lower morbidity (levels of illness), mortality and healthcare costs.[1] However, we must emphasise that self-care is not the solution for serious medical conditions such as depression and it is important to seek medical advice in these situations.

Health literacy as self-care

The International Self-Care Foundation includes health literacy as a pillar of self-care. This means that any step you take towards better understanding health information that helps you make appropriate decisions about your own health and well-being counts as self-care too.[2]

Self-care challenges

The performance of self-care behaviours can be influenced both positively and negatively by the attitudes of others. Research also shows that people face various challenges that interfere with their ability to adopt these self-care behaviours, including chronic disease and disability.[3] While the term 'self-care' suggests it is about the individual taking actions, we also need families and the wider community, especially healthcare professionals, to truly prioritise it as a vital element of health.

Self-care looks different for everyone

It's a good idea to have a wide variety of self-care activities to draw on when you need to. Self-care can look different for every person and differ from one day to the next. For example, you might feel like an active form of self-care, such as hiking, one day but, on another day, a relaxing form of self-care, such as meditating, might be best for you. I have suggested some self-care activities below but you may have a completely different idea of what self-care looks like for you. Don't compare yourself to others as what is relaxing for one person might be highly stressful for another and vice versa. We are constantly evolving so it's a good idea to try something new if your current self-care practices are no longer serving you.

Thirty self-care activities for PCOS

1. Meditating
2. Deep breathing
3. Forest bathing (shinrin-yoku)
4. Mindfulness
5. Yoga
6. Moving your body in nature
7. Gardening
8. Daydreaming
9. Listening to music
10. Guided imagery
11. Having a long bath

Chapter 29

12. Self-massage with lotion or oil
13. Putting on a face mask
14. Cooking one of your favourite meals
15. Cuddling with a companion animal or a loved one
16. Switching off from digital devices
17. Praying
18. Making a cup of tea
19. Baking
20. Knitting
21. Sketching, painting or colouring in
22. Having an orgasm
23. Singing
24. Playing a musical instrument
25. Writing in a gratitude journal
26. Reading for leisure
27. Listening to a podcast
28. Playing boardgames
29. Watching a familiar show or movie
30. Therapy.

30

Forms of movement

Physical activity has become the most documented and acknowledged health advice in relation to both staying healthy and regaining health physically and mentally. Moving your body regularly is a key pillar in managing the symptoms of PCOS (see Chapter 11), for the maintenance of health and for reducing the risk of long-term issues associated with the condition.

Joy as a driving force

The term 'exercise' doesn't necessarily conjure up feelings of joy as it is often associated with diet culture, fitness trackers and calorie counting rather than an activity that encourages a positive experience. Joy and passion are the strongest driving forces of physical activity, with studies highlighting the importance of supporting people to find a kind of physical activity that they like.[1] In other words, the best form of movement is the one that you will do consistently and enjoy. Below are some examples of forms of movement that might be enjoyable to you and make you feel good.

Thirty forms of movement for PCOS

1. Walking
2. Hiking

3. Jogging
4. Running
5. Cycling
6. Strength training with weights or bodyweight exercises
7. Pole dancing
8. Playing football
9. Tennis
10. Badminton
11. Swimming
12. Salsa dancing
13. Boxing
14. High intensity interval training (HIIT)
15. Trampolining
16. Climbing
17. Skipping
18. Hula hooping
19. Inline skating
20. Netball or basketball
21. Surfing
22. Rowing
23. Trampolining
24. Pilates
25. Yoga
26. Martial arts
27. Sexual activity
28. Solo dance party in your bedroom
29. Cleaning your living space
30. Gardening.

31

The plant-based PCOS pantry

The list below is a shopping list to help you get started with a plant-based lifestyle. You certainly don't need to buy every item on the list but once you have a few staples in your pantry, you'll be able to create healthy, quick and tasty plant-based meals. This list is also not exhaustive as there are thousands of foods around the world that can be enjoyed as part of culturally diverse plant-based diets.

Non-starchy vegetables

Beetroot

Bell pepper

Bok choy

Broccoli

Cabbage

Carrot

Cauliflower

Celery

Chilli

Courgette

Cucumber

Fennel

Garlic

Ginger

Kale

Lemon

Lettuce

Microgreens

Mushrooms

Onion

Peppers

Radish

Rainbow chard

Rocket

Spinach

Swiss chard

Tomato

Watercress

Starchy vegetables

Butternut squash
Peas
Potatoes

Sweet potato
Yam

Fruit

Apples
Apricots
Bananas
Blackberries
Blueberries
Cherries
Jackfruit

Mangoes
Oranges
Peaches
Plantain
Plums
Raspberries
Strawberries

Dried fruit

Apricots
Figs
Mulberries

Goji berries
Dates
Raisins

Frozen foods

Frozen fruit (berries, pineapple etc)
Frozen vegetables (peas, spinach, kale, sweetcorn etc)

Plant-based protein sources

Beans (cannellini, chickpea, kidney, edamame etc)
Chia seeds (milled to ensure you absorb omega-3 fats)
Edamame beans
Flaxseeds, milled
Hemp seeds
Hummus (homemade ideally)

Lentils (beluga, puy, red lentils, yellow lentils etc)
Meat alternatives (occasional)
Nuts (Brazil nuts, walnuts, cashews, almonds, pine nuts etc)
Quinoa
Seeds (pumpkin, sesame, sunflower, poppy)
Tempeh
Tofu

Fermented foods

Kimchi
Miso
Sauerkraut

Dairy alternatives

Choose ones which are fortified and free from added sugar.
Plant-based milk alternatives (soya, oat, cashew, hemp etc)
Plant-based alternatives to yoghurt (soya, almond, oat etc)

Whole grains

Amaranth
Bread (whole wheat, whole grain sourdough)
Buckwheat
Bulgur
Farro/wheatberries
Freekeh
Kamut
Millet
Noodles (buckwheat, brown rice, sweet potato)
Oats (groats, steel-cut, rolled)
Pasta (wholewheat, brown rice pasta, lentil pasta, edamame bean)
Pot barley
Popcorn
Rice (red rice, black rice, brown rice, wild rice)
Rye berries
Sorghum
Spelt
Teff

Condiments

Maple syrup

Mustard

Nori flakes

Nutritional yeast (fortified)

Oils (extra virgin olive oil,
    flax oil, walnut oil)

Soya sauce

Tamari

Vegetable stock (low-sodium)

Herbs and spices

Asafoetida

Basil

Bay leaves

Black pepper

Cacao powder

Cayenne powder

Chilli powder

Cinnamon (choose
    organic Ceylon)

Cloves

Coriander powder

Cumin powder

Curry powder

Dill

Fenugreek powder

Garlic powder

Onion powder

Oregano

Paprika, smoked

Paprika, sweet

Star Anise

Turmeric

Vanilla powder

Fresh herbs

Basil

Chives

Coriander

Dill

Mint

Parsley

Rosemary

Sage

Thyme

Wheatgrass

32

The 21-day programme for living PCOS free

When making lifestyle changes, it can be difficult to know where to start. Our 21-day programme for living PCOS free is a quick and easy guide if you aren't sure how to start incorporating the principles discussed throughout this book. I often say to my clients that you won't know how good it feels until you see it for yourself. Over the course of three weeks, you will try our delicious and nourishing plant-based recipes (pages 325-372), prioritise self-care, move your body and practise daily affirmations. In the first week, the time commitment is shorter; this then increases over the following two weeks to allocate more time for each activity until they form a natural part of your routine.

Please note that this plan is not a substitute for individual medical and nutrition advice and guidance. Do consult your health professional if you have any concerns.

When it comes to making our recipes, the vast majority of ingredients can be found at UK supermarkets. Depending on where you live, there are several online converters for recipe units and cooking ingredients.

Our recipes have been created over the years in our family kitchen and generally do not need precise measurements. Many of the recipies can be modified to suit your dietary preferences or to substitute ingredients that are available to you. There may be some trial and error initially but cooking by instinct can be hugely enjoyable. Don't forget to tag us @drnitubajekal and @rohinibajekal on social media and to use the hashtag #LivingPCOSFree as we would love to see your creations.

Listen to your body

It is impossible to create a plan that is tailored for everyone so listen to your body and adapt the plan to suit your lifestyle and starting point. For example, if you are very active, you may require larger portions or extra snacks with your meals. We also recommend enjoying additional portions of fruit and vegetables, such as a hearty green salad prior to the main meals. You do not, of course, need to follow the plan exactly as it is laid out. Perhaps try including one of our plant-based recipes every day or whatever you feel is manageable for you. Batch-cooking the recipes is a great option, so you enjoy leftovers the next day or freeze the soups, dals and stews for later. When eating plans become complicated, they become harder to stick to. If you already exercise, build on what works for you and what you enjoy. Most importantly, try and dedicate this time to focusing on the areas that you feel need most attention in your life.

Eat in line with your circadian rhythms

Our hormones love routine. Try to have set meal times daily, with a hearty breakfast soon after waking, a good-sized lunch and a smaller dinner. If you feel you need a snack, try to choose fresh fruit with nuts or one of the snack options in the list of recipes. Research shows that eating larger breakfasts and lunches is more beneficial for those with insulin resistance than a greater number of meals and snacks spread throughout the day.[1] In other words, breakfast like a king, lunch like a prince and dine like a pauper. This helps nurture your circadian rhythms and regulate your internal body clock. Aim to have your last meal by 7:00 pm in the evening, if possible, to allow for a gentle overnight fast. This is not a form of caloric restriction but rather a pattern in which you adjust your meal timings to support your body's natural rhythms, thereby improving metabolism and digestion.

The 21-day meal and lifestyle plan for living PCOS free

Week One

Day	Affirmation	Movement	Self-care
Monday	'My mind and body are strong and resilient'	Jog/run (15 minutes)	Meditation (15 minutes)
Tuesday	'I listen to my body and take things at my own pace'	HIIT (15 minutes)	Self-massage with favourite lotion (15 minutes)
Wednesday	'I am beautiful on the inside and it shines through on the outside'	Strength training (15 minutes)	Deep breathing exercises (15 minutes)
Thursday	'I move my body to look after myself'	Yoga (15 minutes)	Meditation (15 minutes)
Friday	With every no, I'm creating space for yes	HIIT (15 minutes)	Deep breathing exercises (15 minutes)
Saturday	'My self-care is important and worth making time for'	Strength training (15 minutes)	Writing in a gratitude journal (15 minutes)
Sunday	'I am as kind and loving to myself as I am to others'	Cycling on an indoor bike or outdoors (15 minutes)	Meditation (15 minutes)

Week One

Breakfast	Lunch	Dinner	Drink
Overnight oats with stewed mixed berries	Miso noodle vegetable soup	Greek bean stew	Spearmint tea
Steel-cut oats with sliced banana	DIY bowl with homemade tahini dressing	Green pea min-estrone soup	Sunshine turmeric shot
Applesauce granola	Baked sweet potato, guaca-mole and black bean salad	Baked tofu, broccoli and red pepper stir-fry	Spearmint tea
Turmeric tofu scramble	DIY bowl with homemade tahini dressing	Butternut squash soup with baked tofu croutons	Ginger turmeric tea
Spiced cinnamon and apple porridge	Almond butter noodles with tofu and vegetables	Eat out or order in with friends	Spearmint Tea
Turmeric tofu scramble	Tangy tomato sweet potato chickpea curry	Macaroni and cheese with steamed greens	Sunshine turmeric shot
Baked banana and berry porridge	Tomato onion dal with brown rice with cucumber mint raita	Pinto bean chilli with red rice quinoa	Green smoothie

Week Two

Day	Affirmation	Movement	Self-care
Monday	'I am powerful and can do anything I put my mind to'	Jog/run (20 minutes)	Meditation (20 minutes)
Tuesday	'I feed my body nourishing food'	HIIT (20 minutes)	Putting on a face mask (20 minutes)
Wednesday	'I can challenge my negative thoughts with positive ones.	Strength training (20 minutes)	Deep breathing exercises (20 minutes)
Thursday	'I know that I am not my PCOS; it does not define me'	Yoga (20 minutes)	Meditation (20 minutes)
Friday	'I love moving my body in ways that I enjoy'	HIIT (20 minutes)	Deep breathing exercises (20 minutes)
Saturday	'I am at home in my body'	Strength training (20 minutes)	Writing in a gratitude journal (20 minutes)
Sunday	'I am strong. I am worthy. I am enough'	Cycling on an indoor bike or outdoors (20 minutes)	Meditation (20 minutes)

Week Two

Breakfast	Lunch	Dinner	Drink
Overnight oats with stewed mixed berries	Miso noodle vegetable soup	Indian red lentil dal and rice with beetroot rocket salad	Spearmint tea
Steel cut oats with sliced banana	DIY bowl with home-made tahini dressing	Green pea min-estrone soup	Sunshine turmeric shot
Applesauce granola	Greek bean stew	Baked tofu, broccoli and red pepper stir-fry	Spearmint tea
Turmeric tofu scramble	DIY bowl with home-made tahini dressing	Tomato onion dal with beet-root rocket salad	Ginger tur-meric tea
Spiced cinna-mon and apple porridge	Baked sweet potato, gua-camole and black bean salad	Eat out or order in with friends	Spearmint tea
Turmeric tofu scramble	Pinto bean chilli with red rice quinoa	Macaroni and cheese with steamed greens	Sunshine turmeric shot
Chickpea-flour pancakes with coriander	Red lentil ragù with wholewheat spaghetti	Green pea min-estrone soup	Green smoothie

Week Three

Day	Affirmation	Movement	Self-care
Monday	'I treat my body with respect and compassion'	Jog/run (30 minutes)	Meditation (30 minutes)
Tuesday	'I am thankful for the positive things in my life'	HIIT (30 minutes)	Having a relaxing bath (30 minutes)
Wednesday	'I trust myself. I trust my body'	Strength training (30 minutes)	Writing in a gratitude journal (30 minutes)
Thursday	'My life is what I make of it. I have all the power'	Yoga (30 minutes)	Meditation (30 minutes)
Friday	'I release all of my worries'	HIIT (30 minutes)	Deep breathing exercises (30 minutes)
Saturday	'I am stronger today than I was yesterday'	Strength training (30 minutes)	Doing a jigsaw puzzle (30 minutes)
Sunday	'I am at home in my body'	Cycling on an indoor bike or outdoors (30 minutes)	Meditation (30 minutes)

Week Three

Breakfast	Lunch	Dinner	Drink
Overnight oats with stewed mixed berries	Miso noodle vegetable soup	Greek bean stew	Spearmint tea
Steel-cut oats with sliced banana	DIY bowl with homemade tahini dressing	Green pea minestrone soup	Sunshine turmeric shot
Applesauce granola	Tangy tomato sweet potato chickpea curry	Baked tofu, broccoli and red pepper stir-fry	Spearmint tea
Turmeric tofu scramble	DIY bowl with homemade tahini dressing	Butternut squash soup with baked tofu croutons	Ginger turmeric tea
Spiced cinnamon and apple porridge	Baked sweet potato, guacamole and black bean salad	Eat out or order in with friends	Spearmint tea
Turmeric tofu scramble	Indian red lentil dal and rice with balsamic-drenched soya aubergine	Pinto bean chilli with quinoa and red rice	Sunshine turmeric shot
Baked banana and berry porridge	Red lentil ragù with wholewheat spaghetti	Edamame and lentil khichadi	Green smoothie

After the 21-day programme

By this point, hopefully you will be feeling great inside and out and finding it easier to make lifestyle changes a part of your everyday life. Introduce these habits into your life and you'll build on the foundations to manage your PCOS now and in the future, to live as long and healthily as possible.

33

Recipes for living PCOS free

Breakfast

Applesauce granola
Overnight oats with stewed mixed berries
Baked banana and berry porridge
Chickpea-flour pancakes with coriander
Spiced cinnamon and apple porridge
Steel-cut oats with sliced banana
Turmeric tofu scramble

Main courses

Macaroni and cheese with steamed greens
Tomato onion dal with brown rice
Butternut squash soup with baked tofu croutons
DIY bowl with homemade tahini dressing
Miso noodle vegetable soup
Greek bean stew
Edamame and lentil khichadi
Indian red lentil dal and rice
Green pea minestrone soup
Red lentil ragù with wholewheat spaghetti

Pinto bean chilli with red rice quinoa

Baked sweet potato, guacamole and black bean salad

Tangy tomato sweet potato chickpea curry

Almond butter noodles with tofu and vegetables

Baked tofu, broccoli and red pepper stir-fry

Side dishes

Balsamic-drenched soy aubergine

Cucumber or sweetcorn mint raita

Beetroot rocket salad

Paprika hummus

Snacks, drinks and desserts

Green smoothie

Sunshine turmeric shot

Ginger turmeric tea

Cacao, date and almond balls

Apricot, tahini and coconut balls

Banana, oat and walnut cookies

Breakfast

Applesauce granola

Serves 10

4 cups rolled oats
1 cup mixed raw nuts (almonds or hazelnuts work well)
½ cup mixed raw seeds (sunflower seeds, pumpkin seeds etc)
1 tsp ground cinnamon (or spices of choice)
1/3 tsp salt
1 tsp vanilla extract
3 tbsp maple syrup (or sweetener of choice – this is optional
    and you can use more apple purée instead)
1 cup unsweetened smooth apple purée
½ cup dried cranberries (or other dried fruit of choice)
Optional: Add chia seeds, hemp seeds, dried blueberries or
    more unsweetened dried fruit after the granola is out of the
    oven.
To serve: soya or other plant-based yoghurt and extra fresh
    fruit.

1. Preheat a fan oven to 160ºC and line a baking tray with parch-
    ment paper or use a silicone baking mat.
2. In a large mixing bowl, combine the oats, nuts and seeds.
3. Add the ground cinnamon or any other spices, such as ginger
    or nutmeg, the salt, vanilla extract, maple syrup and apple
    purée.
4. Stir the mixture thoroughly so it is evenly coated.
5. Spread the mixture evenly on the lined baking tray or silicone
    mat and put it in the oven.
6. Bake for around 30-40 minutes, checking on it halfway and
    tossing well. It should be golden brown but not burnt.

7. Remove from the oven when it is fully dry and has formed chunks. Add chia or hemp seeds if desired. Store in an airtight container for up to five days.
8. Serve with soya yoghurt or soya milk (or plant-based yoghurt or milk of choice).

Top tip: Aim to include a handful of nuts and seeds daily as they are a great source of healthy unsaturated fats.

Overnight oats with stewed mixed berries

Serves 2

1 cup rolled oats (often called 'jumbo' or 'old-fashioned' oats)
1½ cups fortified soya milk
1 tsp ground cinnamon
½ tsp vanilla extract
1 cup frozen mixed berries
1 tbsp maple syrup (optional)
To serve: ground flax seeds; 2 tbsp walnuts, broken into pieces

1. Mix the oats, soya milk, cinnamon and vanilla extract in a bowl. The oats absorb some of the plant milk overnight so don't worry if it looks too wet.
2. Store covered in the fridge for at least four hours or preferably overnight. It can stay in the fridge for a couple of days if you prefer to make a bigger batch.
3. In a pan, heat the frozen mixed berries with a couple of table-spoons of water and the optional maple syrup or sweetener of choice.

4. Serve the stewed berries on top of the overnight oats and add extra ground flax seeds and/or walnuts for an omega-3 boost.

Top tip: Oats are an excellent source of dietary fibre including beta-glucans and resistant starch, with overnight oats having higher amounts of the latter. Resistant starch helps to improve digestion, increasing feelings of satiety and fullness and even lowering blood sugar after meals.[1]

Baked banana and berry porridge

Serves 4-6

½ tsp oil for greasing the pan (or line with parchment paper for oil-free)
2 tbsp ground flaxseed + 6 tbsp warm water
2 cups whole rolled oats
1 cup walnuts, chopped roughly
½ cup almonds, chopped roughly
1 tsp baking powder
1 tsp ground cinnamon
½ tsp salt
1 cup fortified soya milk (or plant milk of choice)
6 tbsp apple purée
1 tsp vanilla extract
Sweetener such as date syrup (optional)
1-2 bananas, chopped
1½ cups fresh/frozen mixed berries
To serve: soya or other plant-based yoghurt and extra fresh fruit

1. Preheat a fan oven to 170ºC and lightly grease a 20x20-cm (8×8-inch) baking tray (or line with parchment paper)

2. Mix the ground flaxseeds and warm water in a bowl and leave to stand until they form a gel-like consistency.

3. Keeping around half a cup of the nuts aside for later, in a large bowl, mix the oats, remaining nuts, baking powder, cinnamon and salt.

4. To the bowl with the flaxseed mixture, add the soya milk, apple purée and vanilla extract. Add in the extra sweetener if you require for taste. Whisk thoroughly.

5. Pour the contents of the bowl with the wet ingredients into the dry ingredients and stir to combine. Add in half of the mixed berries. Mix to combine.

6. Add slices of banana to the bottom of the baking tray. Pour the mixture into the baking tray and decorate with extra slices of banana, berries and the half cup of nuts you kept aside.

7. Bake for 40-50 minutes until the top is crispy but not overly brown and the middle nice and thick.

8. Cool for 15 minutes before serving with a dollop of fortified soya (or other plant-based) yoghurt and extra fresh fruit.

Top tip: All berries are high in antioxidants and micronutrients. Frozen work just as well as fresh and may even be more nutritious as the berries are packed at their prime.

Chickpea flour pancakes with coriander

Makes 6 pancakes

1 cup room temperature water (plus more water if needed)
1 cup chickpea flour (can also use gram flour - adjust water as
    you might need less)
¼ tsp turmeric
¼ tsp cumin seeds
½ tsp salt
1 medium red onion, finely chopped
1-2 green chillies, finely diced (optional)
1 medium-sized tomato, finely chopped
1 big handful coriander leaves and stalks, finely chopped
Olive oil (optional)
To serve: Hot sauce or homemade chutney (optional)

1. Mix the chickpea flour with 1 cup of water in a bowl, pref-
    erably using a whisk to ensure there are no lumps. As it will
    be quite thick, add water until you get a smooth, pourable
    consistency that is not too liquid.
2. Add the turmeric, cumin seeds, salt, onion, chillies, tomato
    and chopped coriander. Also add around 1 tsp olive oil if you
    don't have a good non-stick plan. Let the batter rest for a few
    minutes.
3. Oil the pan if needed but keep it to a minimum; this is not a
    necessary step if you have a good non-stick pan.
4. Using a ladle, pour enough batter to make a pancake. Spread
    it around so it is not too thick or it won't cook.
5. Once the edges of the pancake look cooked after a few min-
    utes, flip it over just as you would a regular pancake. Cook for
    another few minutes until ready.

6.   Use up all the batter to make six pancakes. Serve with home-made coriander and mint chutney, hot sauce or even soya yoghurt.

Top tip: Chickpeas are versatile and can be used in sweet and savoury dishes. Hummus, chickpea flour and aquafaba can be used in a variety of dishes. Chickpeas can be sprouted before they are cooked too and added to salads, increasing the nutritional content. They are a great source of soluble fibre and phytoestrogens as well as folate and other B vitamins, iron and phosphorus.

Spiced cinnamon and apple porridge

Serves 1

1 cup (85 g) rolled oats (or 3/4 cup cooked steel-cut oats)
250-300 ml fortified soya milk (or plant milk of choice)
1 tsp ground cinnamon
½ red apple, grated or diced finely into matchstick pieces
2 tbsp flaxseed powder
Optional: 1 chopped date, chopped walnuts and/or drizzle of almond butter

1.   Pour the oats, plant milk, cinnamon and apple into a pan and simmer until the mixture thickens, usually after around 5-10 minutes.
2.   Serve with flaxseed powder.
3.   Add a chopped date, drizzle of almond butter or some walnut halves for crunch.

Top tip: Cinnamon can help with lowering blood sugar and insulin levels.

Steel-cut oats with sliced banana

Serves 2

1 cup steel-cut oats (sometimes called 'pinhead oats'), soaked
   overnight and rinsed
2-3 cups water
1 cup fortified soya milk (or other plant milk of choice)
1 tsp ground cinnamon
4 tbsp flaxseed powder
To serve: 1 large banana, sliced

Optional preparation: For a shorter cooking time and to improve the nutritional value of the porridge, soak the steel-cut oats overnight. If you skip this step don't worry as the oats will take around 15 minutes longer to cook and you will just need more water.

1. Bring two cups of water and the oats to a boil in a saucepan. Once boiling, reduce to a gentle simmer so that the water doesn't spill over the sides of the pan; there should just be a bubble or two ever few seconds.
2. Simmer for around 20 minutes, checking every so often to add more hot water if needed. Stir once in a while scraping the bottom to ensure that the oats are not getting stuck.
3. Cook until the oats are very creamy; the longer you cook them, the creamier and easier to digest they will be.

4.   Add in one cup of soya milk (or plant milk of choice) a minute before you take the porridge off the heat, along with the cinnamon.

5.   Turn off the heat and allow to cool for a few minutes

6.   Serve, adding 2 tbsp ground flax seeds per person, the slices of banana, and a drizzle of nut butter if you like. If you like a sweeter porridge, mash in an overripe banana while it cooks rather than at the end.

7.   You can batch cook this porridge without the milk and store it in an airtight container in the fridge to enjoy for up to three days. Add extra plant milk when you reheat a portion.

Top tip: Flaxseeds are a rich source of lignans (plant oestrogens) and help to reduce breast cancer risk as well as providing healthy omega-3 fats.[2]

Turmeric tofu scramble

Serves 4

1 tsp dried basil
1 tsp cumin seeds or cumin powder
1 tsp turmeric powder
1 pinch pepper powder
1 large, finely chopped onion
1-2 finely chopped green chillies
2 chopped medium-sized tomatoes
1 cup frozen green peas
1 cup fresh spinach/kale or 1 small cube frozen spinach
1 400-g block tofu
1-2 tbsp soya sauce

1 pinch kala namak (black salt) for eggy sulphurous taste (optional)

1 tbsp tomato paste or ketchup or sriracha (optional)

To serve: Fresh basil or coriander leaves for garnish

1. In a hot pan, dry-roast the basil, turmeric and cumin until you can smell the spices but avoid burning them.
2. Add the onion and chillies and sauté until they are pink and translucent.
3. Add 1-2 tbsp hot water instead of oil to cook the onion if needed.
4. Add the tomatoes and sauté for 3-4 minutes.
5. Add the frozen peas and frozen spinach, cover and cook for 4-5 minutes on medium heat.
6. Add the block of tofu (crumble it with your hands in a separate dish or grate it) and mix thoroughly.
7. Cover and cook for 2-3 minutes.
8. Add the soy sauce and black salt and cook for another couple of minutes, mixing thoroughly.
9. Add the fresh spinach if using and the ketchup/sriracha tomato paste and mix.
10. To serve, garnish with herbs. This recipe can be enjoyed on its own or as a side dish or in a wholemeal wrap.

Top tip: Tofu is a minimally processed product made from soya beans and is a complete protein with good amounts of all nine essential amino acids.

Main courses

Macaroni and cheese with steamed greens

Serves 6

Steamed greens
2 bags greens, such as spring greens, kale, savoy cabbage or a
  mixture
2-3 tbsp water
½ lemon, juiced

1. Rinse and drain the greens and remove any tough bits such as
    thick stalks.
2. Slice the greens into thin ribbons and sauté with a 2-3 tbsp
    water.
3. When the greens are soft, add the lemon juice to taste, or
    a splash of apple cider vinegar if you don't have any fresh
    lemon.

Macaroni and cheese
600 g (roughly) wholewheat macaroni (or gluten free)
1 yellow onion, finely diced
3 cloves garlic, crushed and finely diced
1 tsp extra virgin olive oil (optional)
1 cup cashews, soaked for at least two hours and drained
2 cups potatoes, peeled and roughly chopped
1 cup carrots, peeled and roughly chopped
3 tbsp lemon juice
1½ cups unsweetened fortified soya milk (or other)
1 tsp Dijon mustard
8 tbsp nutritional yeast
1 tsp mixed Italian herbs

½ tsp garlic powder

½ tsp smoked paprika

½ tsp ground black pepper

1 tsp salt

1-2 tbsp extra virgin olive oil (optional)

Optional toppings:

2-3 pickled jalapeños (or to preference), diced

Handful fresh basil leaves

½ cup panko breadcrumbs (or gluten free)

¼ tsp salt

1 tbsp extra virgin olive oil (EVOO)

1. Preheat a fan oven to 180ºC.
2. Boil the potatoes and carrots for about 10 minutes or until tender. Drain and set aside.
3. Add the onion, garlic and 1 tsp olive oil to a large baking dish and put in the oven for 10 minutes.
3. Cook the macaroni according to instructions until just al dente. Drain and set aside.
4. In a large blender, add the cashews, potatoes, carrots, lemon juice, soya milk, mustard, nutritional yeast, herbs, spices and extra virgin olive oil. Blitz then taste and adjust the seasoning.
5. Add the cooked pasta to the baking dish (with the garlic-onion mixture) and toss so the onion and garlic are well distributed.
6. Pour the 'cheese' sauce on the pasta. It should be thoroughly coated. (Store any leftover sauce in the fridge for a couple of days.)
7. If wanted, add the jalapeños and basil leaves on top of the cheesy pasta mix.
8. In a separate bowl, mix the breadcrumbs with olive oil and salt and distribute evenly on top of the pasta.
9. Bake in the oven until the top is golden brown for 20 minutes.

10. Serve with the steamed greens.

Top tip: Butternut squash is packed with beta-carotene, a nutrient that the body converts to vitamin A and which helps to maintain healthy eyes.

Tomato onion dal with brown rice

Serves 4-6

Brown rice
2 cups brown rice
4 cups water

1. Thoroughly rinse the brown rice in a sieve.
2. Add to the stove, bring to the boil and then lower to simmer.
3. Cook for around 20 minutes with the lid on, on a low heat, checking occasionally.
4. Eat immediately or cool and then refrigerate (eat within a couple of days).

Tomato onion dal
2 cups dried mung lentils, rinsed and drained (also called 'split yellow peas' or 'petite yellow peas')
2 green chillies, slit
1 onion, chopped finely
3 fresh tomatoes, diced
4 cm (1½ inches) fresh ginger, diced finely
3 garlic cloves, grated or crushed or chopped finely
1 tsp turmeric
1 pinch black pepper

1 pinch asafoetida (*hing*) (optional)

2 tsp black mustard seeds

2-3 curry leaves (fresh or dried – available from Indian stores and some supermarkets)

2 big handfuls spinach leaves, chopped (use frozen if needed)

Bunch coriander, chopped including stems

1 lemon, juiced

1. Heat a deep pan and dry-roast the mustard seeds, turmeric, black pepper and hing, taking special care not to burn these spices.
2. Add the curry leaves, garlic, ginger and chilies with a splash of hot water. Sauté and add the onions. Sauté for a couple of minutes on a medium heat, adding additional splashes of hot water to deglaze the pan if needed – don't add too much.
3. Add the tomatoes, stir and cover and cook for 5 minutes.
4. Add the rinsed and drained mung lentils after the tomatoes have cooked, along with 6 cups water. Simmer for 30 minutes and check on it periodically to see if more water is needed. The lentils should be soft – as an example, they should be easy to mash when done.
5. Turn the heat off and add in the spinach and most of the coriander, including coriander stems (full of flavour). They'll wilt in the residual heat. (Reserve some of the coriander for garnish.)
6. Allow to cool slightly and serve with the fresh lemon juice (or add the juice to the pan once cooled to retain the vitamin C, which is destroyed by heat).
7. Serve with the brown rice or quinoa or enjoy on its own as a soup. Garnish with fresh coriander.

Top tip: Avoid burning spices as blackened foods and deep-frying increase toxic products called AGEs (advanced glycation end products). These cause damage to blood vessels and hasten aging of the ovaries, especially in PCOS where the ovaries seem to be particularly sensitive. Animal products, especially barbecued meat, have the highest level of AGEs. Cooked chicken has more AGEs than fried potatoes. Steaming and boiling create the least AGEs in food.

Butternut squash soup with baked tofu croutons

Serves 4

1 red onion
1 tsp cumin seeds
½ tsp turmeric
2 bay leaves
4 garlic cloves, crushed and or diced
1 red chilli, finely diced (optional)
10 mm fresh ginger, diced finely
1 medium-sized butternut squash, 3 cups cubed
2 large carrots, diced
1 cup split red lentils, rinsed
6 cups vegetable stock (either shop bought or homemade)
½ tsp dried basil
½ tsp smoked paprika
1 pinch black pepper
1 tsp salt (optional)
1 block of tofu (roughly 250 g) (smoked tofu tastes really good), blotted dry and diced into cubes

1. Preheat a fan oven to 180°C.
2. In one teaspoon of olive oil (or water if oil-free), sauté the red onion, cumin seeds, turmeric and bay leaves, for a couple of minutes being careful not to let it burn.
3. Add the garlic and chilli and sauté for another few mins, adding a splash of water to prevent it sticking.
4. Add the ginger, butternut squash and carrots and coat well with the spices.
5. Add the lentils, vegetable stock, basil, paprika, black pepper and salt to the pan and bring to the boil.
6. Cover and simmer on a low heat for 30 minutes until the butternut squash and lentils are soft.
7. Meanwhile, after blotting the tofu dry, chop it up into small cubes and pop in the preheated oven for 10-15 minutes to firm up.
8. Once the soup has cooled for a bit, blend using an immersion blender or add to a strong blender. I do it in a couple of batches. Add a splash of water if you prefer it less thick.
9. Serve hot with the baked tofu 'croutons'.

Top tip: Aim to eat 80 g (a small handful) of tofu a few times a week as one of your two portions of soya per day. Tofu is an excellent source of protein, calcium, iron and a number of other micronutrients. It's low in saturated fat and free of cholesterol, while being rich in healthy fats, both monounsaturated and polyunsaturated.

DIY bowl

Serves 1

1 cup fresh leafy greens such as spinach leaves or kale plus a generous sprinkling of fresh herbs (basil/parsley/dill/coriander)

1 cup other vegetables such as, stir-fried mixed vegetables

½ cup legumes such as marinated chickpeas, baked tofu, black beans or sprouted lentils

½ cup whole grains or potatoes such as brown rice, baked sweet potato wedges, quinoa

3 tbsp healthy plant-based fats such as avocado slices, raw nuts and seeds or creamy nut or seed-based dressing

Optional:

1 tbsp fermented foods such as kimchi or sauerkraut

1 handful sprouts such as broccoli or alfalfa

1. Assemble your bowl keeping a theme in mind – for example, an Asian-inspired bowl could have baked tofu, stir-fried green vegetables, brown rice, kale, satay-based sauce and kimchi.

2. Store components separately in the fridge to enjoy at another time, including the homemade tahini dressing (below).

Top tip: Fermented foods such as sauerkraut and kimchi are rich in probiotics – beneficial microorganisms that help grow the healthy bacteria in your gut and reduce inflammation. This may help with digestion and better nutrient absorption.

Homemade tahini dressing

Serves 2

½ cup light sesame tahini
2 cloves garlic, minced
1 tsp garlic powder
4 tbsp apple cider vinegar
1 medium-sized lemon, juiced
1 tsp sriracha (optional if you like heat)
Water, as needed for desired consistency
1 handful fresh parsley leaves, chopped finely
Salt and fresh black pepper to taste

1. Whisk the tahini, fresh garlic, garlic powder, apple cider vinegar and lemon together or use a blender. Add the sriracha.
2. Add water to thin to achieve the consistency you like.
3. Add the parsley leaves and serve on salad.

Top tip: Tahini is a sesame seed paste that is a good source of calcium as well as being packed with healthy fats. Apple cider vinegar, along with other vinegars, can be effective in reducing glucose and insulin levels after a meal, suggesting they may help glycaemic control. [1]

Miso noodle vegetable soup

Serves: 2 (or 4 small portions)

1 large red onion, diced
4 cloves garlic, crushed and diced

1 hot red chilli (optional)

1 tbsp grated ginger

2 cups chestnut mushrooms, sliced (or mixed mushrooms if you prefer)

1 red bell pepper, diced

1 400-g block pre-cooked tofu, marinated and diced into cubes (or marinate and bake at home)

3-4 cups low-sodium vegetable stock

1 tbsp dark brown miso paste

1 tbsp rice vinegar

3 pak choi, trimmed and chopped

1 tbsp sesame seeds

1 tbsp dulse or nori flakes

200 g soba (buckwheat) noodles

1. Sauté the onion in a little hot water (or oil if you prefer) for a couple of minutes, then add the garlic and chilli. Add a splash of hot water to deglaze the pan if necessary.

2. Add the mushrooms and sauté until they turn slightly brown, then add the pre-cooked marinated tofu, red pepper and ginger.

3. Mix the miso paste thoroughly with ¼ cup hot water until dissolved. Pour it into the pan. Stir for a minute.

4. Add the vegetable stock, rice vinegar and simmer for a few minutes.

5. Add the pak choi.

6. In the meantime, boil water in a separate pan and, once boiling, add the buckwheat noodles. Simmer for 5 minutes, then remove from the heat and immediately rinse with cold water so they don't stick together.

7. Add the noodles to the miso soup and stir for a minute. Then turn off the heat.

8. To serve, sprinkle the sesame seeds and dulse flakes on top.

Top tip: Minimally processed or whole soya is a great addition to our diet and is suitable for all ages. Relatively unprocessed soya products are better, such as edamame beans, mature soya beans, tofu, tempeh, soya curls, miso and natto with soya sausages and soya meats best reserved for treats.

Greek bean stew

Serves 4

1 tsp extra virgin olive oil, or 1 tbsp vegetable stock if oil-free
1 medium onion
2 cloves garlic, crushed or and diced
1 red chilli, diced finely
2 carrots, diced
1 400 g can chopped tomatoes in tomato juice
1 tbsp concentrated tomato paste (or ketchup)
1 red bell pepper, diced
1 stick celery, diced
1 veggie stock cube
1 bay leaf
½ tsp ground cinnamon
1 tsp dried basil
½ tsp pepper
1 tsp salt (optional)
1 400 g can cannellini beans or a similar white bean
1 bunch spinach leaves, chopped
To serve: 1 cup quinoa, cooked in 2 cups water

1. Finely dice all the vegetables into small cubes.
2. Sauté the onion, garlic and chilli for 2-3 minutes until softened in 1 tbsp olive oil (or vegetable stock).
3. Add the carrots.
4. Add the chopped tomatoes, tomato paste and stock cube together with the bay leaf, cinnamon, basil, pepper and salt, as desired.
5. Add the red bell pepper, celery and a splash of water if the mixture is too thick.
6. Simmer for around 10 minutes until the vegetables are al dente.
7. Add the cannellini beans and simmer for 5 minutes, adding some water if needed.
8. Turn off the heat and add in a bunch of chopped spinach leaves to wilt in the residual heat.
9. Serve with the quinoa for a filing main meal or enjoy on its own.

Top tip: Extra virgin olive oil (EVOO) is a rich source of heart-healthy polyphenols and antioxidants. Choose cold-pressed if possible.

Edamame and lentil khichadi

Serves 6

1 cup brown rice
2 cups split yellow lentils (toor dal), pre-soaked
9-12 cups water
2 tsp turmeric powder
1 tsp asafoetida *hing* (optional)

2 chopped carrots, diced
1 cup green beans, diced
½ cup frozen peas
½ cup frozen edamame beans
1-2 tsp salt (to taste)
1 tsp olive oil (optional)
2 tsp cumin seeds
3-4 dry red chillies

1. Soak the brown rice and yellow lentils for 3-4 hours combined in room temperature water. Ensure they are covered by at least 5 cm (2 inches) while soaking.
2. Rinse thoroughly.
3. Bring to the boil with 9-12 cups water.
4. Add the turmeric and asafoetida once boiling, then turn down the heat and simmer for 30 minutes.
5. At this point, add in the carrots, beans, peas and edamame beans and stir mixture thoroughly. Lentils absorb a huge amount of water so ensure the mixture is quite liquid.
6. Simmer for an additional 30 minutes or longer. It should be soft and almost mushy when fully cooked. Add salt to taste.
7. Finally, heat the oil in a pan (or omit if oil-free) for the 'tadka'– that is, the seasoning for the khichadi. Add in the cumin seeds, turmeric and asafoetida and break the red chillies into the pan depending on spice preference. Be careful not to burn and stir for a minute.
8. Add to the khichadi mixture and stir thoroughly then turn off the heat and allow to rest for 5 minutes with the lid on the pot.
9. Serve a bowl of khichadi with a corn or lentil papad/poppadum and a dollop of soya yoghurt.
10. Store any leftovers in the fridge in an airtight container and enjoy within 3 days.

Top tip: Lentils may be small but they're nutritional powerhouses, packed with plant protein, fibre and iron. They're also great for the soil and are the top 'climate friendly' protein according to the Environmental Working Group.

Indian red lentil dal and rice

Serves 6-8

Brown rice
3 cups brown rice
6 cups water

1. Thoroughly rinse the brown rice in a sieve.
2. Add to a pan of boiling water on the stove, bring to the boil and then lower the heat to simmer.
3. Cook for around 20 minutes with the lid on, on a low heat, checking occasionally.
4. Eat immediately or cool and then refrigerate (eat within one day).

Indian red lentil dal
1 tbsp cumin seeds
1 tbsp cumin powder
1 tsp garam masala
1 tsp turmeric powder (or 2.5 cm (1 inch) fresh root, grated)
½ tsp red chilli powder
1 large yellow onion, diced
4 cloves garlic, diced
1 red chilli, diced (optional)

2.5 cm (1 inch) fresh ginger, grated

1 tbsp tomato paste

2 cups split red lentils, rinsed and drained

4 cups vegetable broth

2 cups water

4 tomatoes, diced (can omit to make pantry-friendly)

1 tsp salt (optional – to taste)

¼ tsp black pepper

4 handfuls spinach leaves or kale, chopped

1 bunch coriander, chopped including stems

1 lemon, juiced

1. Soak the red lentils in slightly warm water for a few hours to improve their digestibility. Lentils don't require soaking so this is an optional step. Give them a good rinse and set aside.

2. Heat a large pan and dry-roast the cumin seeds, cumin, powder, garam masala, turmeric powder and red chilli powder until they are fragrant. Do this on a low heat for a couple of minutes and be very careful not to let them burn - they should not be smoking!

3. Add a splash of water (or olive oil if you're not cooking oil-free) and the onion and sauté for a few minutes.

4. Add the chilli, garlic and ginger and another tiny splash of water if needed to deglaze the pan.

5. Add the tomato paste and stir.

6. Add the drained lentils and mix.

7. Add the vegetable broth and water and bring to the boil, then reduce to a simmer.

8. After 20 minutes of simmering, add in the diced tomatoes, salt and black pepper.

9. Continue to cook for another 15 minutes or until the lentils are fully cooked.

10. Turn the heat off and add in the spinach and coriander including the coriander stems (full of flavour). They will wilt in the residual heat if you put the lid on. Reserve some of the coriander for garnish.

11. Serve with brown or red rice and an extra squeeze of lemon juice.

Top tip: Cumin has many benefits for health as do most herbs and spices. Cumin seeds and powder can help with digestion, weight management, blood sugar and cholesterol control. The healthiest, longest-living societies around the world (Blue Zones) eat legumes (beans, peas, lentils) every day and often more than once a day.

Green pea minestrone soup

Serves 6

3 litres water
2 low-salt vegan stock cubes (optional)
1 tbsp dried basil
1 large onion, finely chopped
3-4 cloves garlic, crushed or diced finely
2 green chillies, slit lengthways
1 400-g can chopped tomatoes (double the fresh quantity to avoid cans)
4 fresh large tomatoes, diced
2 potatoes, diced into small cubes
2 carrots, diced
1 large handful green beans, diced
1 head broccoli, diced including stalks

1 cup frozen or fresh peas

1 400 g can butter, cannellini or haricot beans

1 courgette, diced

1 cup wholewheat pasta (or gluten-free brown rice pasta if gluten-free)

½ tsp freshly ground black pepper

Salt (optional)

Red chilli flakes (optional for sprinkling)

1 handful fresh basil leaves, chopped

1. In a large pan, add the boiling water, then the optional stock cubes, dried basil, onion, garlic, chillies and both the canned and fresh tomatoes and bring to the boil. Keep chopping the vegetables and adding as you go along.

2. Add the potatoes and carrots next as they take longer to cook. Keep the pan covered and on medium heat.

3. After approximately 10 minutes, add the beans and broccoli.

4. After another 10 minutes add the peas, butter beans and courgette, and the pasta last. Add some more hot water if needed.

5. Bring to the boil and then cover and simmer for 10-12 minutes until the pasta is al dente and the potatoes are cooked.

6. Season to taste with salt and pepper and add the basil as a garnish. Sprinkle on red chilli flakes if you like the heat.

7. Serve hot with seeded rye or gluten-free bread.

8. Leftovers make great next-day lunches.

Top tip: Peas are legumes, a group that includes beans, lentils and peanuts too. What do the 'Blue Zones' - the places on Earth where people live the longest - have in common? The consumption of legumes. The long-living populations in these areas eat at least four times as many beans as we do, on average. Try to eat 2-3 portions of legumes a day. A portion is only a handful or 80 g and is easily achieved.

Red lentil ragù with wholewheat spaghetti

Serves 4

75-100 g dry spaghetti (wholewheat or spelt or gluten-free option)
1 cup split red lentils
1 tsp olive oil (swap for water/vegetable stock for oil-free)
1 red onion, diced
1 red chilli, chopped finely
4 cloves garlic, crushed or diced finely
3 carrots, chopped finely
6-8 chestnut mushrooms, chopped finely
1 red bell pepper, diced
4 tsp mixed Italian herbs (thyme, oregano, basil)
1 tsp onion powder (optional)
½ tsp black pepper
1 400-g can diced tomatoes
1 tbsp tomato paste
1 cup vegetable broth
1 tsp salt (optional)
To serve: fresh basil and nutritional yeast

1. Wash the lentils thoroughly and drain. Add to pot with 4 cups water. Simmer on a medium heat for around 15 minutes until just cooked, stirring once in a while. (You can also swap this step for pre-cooked red lentils to save time.)

2. Prepare the spaghetti or pasta according to the instructions on the packet. Drain and set aside. If you are gluten-free, use a gluten-free alternative such as brown rice pasta.

3. Add the oil (or water/vegetable stock) to a pan, along with the chopped onion, and sauté for 2-3 minutes before adding the chilli and garlic. After another 2-3 minutes, add the carrots, mushrooms and red bell pepper and mix together.

4. Add the mixed herbs, onion powder and black pepper and coat well.

5. Add the tomatoes, tomato paste and vegetable stock and bring to the boil. Once boiling, turn down and simmer for 15 minutes. Season with salt and pepper to taste.

6. Add in the cooked lentils, and a splash of water if the consistency is too thick. Taste and adjust herbs and spices at this point if needed.

7. To serve, add some sprigs of fresh basil and some nutritional yeast. While best with spaghetti, this also tastes fantastic on its own or on top of potatoes. Serve with a green salad of rocket leaves, cucumber and lemon with balsamic vinegar.

Top tips: Sunbathe your mushrooms. When exposed to UV light, mushrooms generate their own vitamin D. This nutrient is essential for our immune system and helps us absorb calcium for strong bones and teeth. Mushrooms also contain beta-glucans which activate the immune system, reducing cancer risk including of breast cancer. Choose red onions over white onions as they contain more antioxidants and flavonoids, which are anti-inflammatory and anti-cancer.

Pinto bean chilli with red rice quinoa

Serves 4-6

Red rice quinoa recipe
1 cup red rice (soaking for a few hours (then rinsing and
    draining) significantly reduces cooking time)
1 cup quinoa
4 cups water

1. Thoroughly rinse the red rice in a sieve.
2. Add to a pot of boiling water on the stove, bring to the boil
    and then lower the heat to simmer.
3. Cook for around 30-40 minutes with the lid on, on a low heat,
    checking occasionally if more water is needed.
4. Eat immediately. (If you have leftovers, cool and refrigerate;
    eat within one day.)

Pinto bean chilli
1 tsp extra virgin olive oil (or water)
1 medium onion, chopped
4 cloves garlic, crushed and or diced
1 hot red chilli, finely diced
1 bell pepper, chopped
1 400-g can diced tomatoes
300 g tomato passata
1 tsp ground cumin
½ tsp chilli powder
1 tsp ground cinnamon
1 tsp oregano
1 bay leaf
1 tsp hot smoked paprika

2 400-g cans pinto beans (or 3 cups cooked pinto beans), rinsed and drained

1 400-g can jackfruit (separate into pieces with your fingers or chop)

1 cup vegetable broth

2 tsp raw cacao powder

1 tsp garlic powder

¼ tsp freshly ground black pepper

1 tsp salt (optional)

To serve (optional): red rice quinoa and fresh coriander leaves

1. In a large saucepan, sauté the onion in olive oil (or water, if oil-free) until softened, then add the garlic, red chilli and bell pepper.
2. Add the canned tomatoes, passata, beans, ground cumin, chilli powder, cinnamon, oregano, bay leaf and paprika and bring to the boil for 1 minute.
3. Reduce to a simmer and add in the pinto beans and jackfruit.
4. Add the vegetable broth if the mixture looks a little thick as it will reduce as it cooks.
5. Add in the cacao powder, garlic powder, pepper and salt. Keep on a low simmer for 30 minutes until tender, checking occasionally and stirring.
6. Check the seasoning. If it's bitter, add 1 tbsp sweetener such as maple syrup.
8. Serve with red rice and fresh coriander leaves. This dish keeps well in the fridge for a few days.

Top tips:

- Adding herbs and spices (in this recipe, basil, cinnamon, oregano, pepper and cumin) to any dish increases flavour several fold while increasing the antioxidant and phytonutrient content which are beneficial to health. Crushing or chopping garlic releases the enzyme allinase that helps in the formation of allicin, a healthy organic sulphur compound that reduces inflammation and has anti-cancer properties. Leave garlic for 10 minutes before cooking or freezing after crushing to allow for the maximum benefit.

Baked sweet potato, guacamole and black bean salad

Serves 2

2 large, sweet potatoes with skins, washed and scrubbed
For the guacamole
    2 ripe avocados
    1 lime, juiced
    2 cloves garlic, finely minced
    ¼ tsp ground cumin
    Pinch salt (optional)
For the black bean salad
    1 400-g can black beans, rinsed and drained
    ½ medium red onion, diced
    1 clove garlic, finely minced
    1 small jalapeño pepper, finely diced (optional)
    1 lime, juiced
    1 tsp apple cider vinegar
    ¼ tsp hot smoked paprika (optional)
    ¼ tsp ground cumin
    1 red bell pepper, finely diced
    1 tomato, finely diced
    1 handful coriander leaves, chopped

1. Preheat a fan oven to 200ºC.
2. Prick sweet potatoes with a knife in a few places to shorten the baking time and prevent them from bursting, then put them in the oven and bake for 1 hour.
3. To prepare the guacamole, mash the avocado with the back of a fork and mix with the remaining ingredients.
4. To prepare the black bean salad, mix all of the ingredients together and refrigerate. This is best done for around at least 4 hours before serving as the flavours really come together.
5. Serve the baked sweet potato with the guacamole and black bean salad. Another topping could include paprika hummus (page 365).

Top tips:

- Start all main meals with a salad (even if it just a cup of dark green leaves and some beetroot or cherry tomatoes).

- Make salad a main meal, especially in the summer, and make it colourful and plentiful.

Tangy tomato sweet potato chickpea curry

Serves 2

400 g cooked chickpeas (rinse and drain)
2 medium-sized sweet potatoes, washed with skins on, diced into cubes
1 tbsp coriander powder
1-1½ tsp chilli powder
½ tsp turmeric powder
¼ tsp pepper powder

1 stick cinnamon or ½-1 tsp cinnamon powder
¼ tsp brown sugar or jaggery
Salt to taste
4 cm (1½ inches) ginger, grated
3 medium tomatoes, chopped
4 small red onions (or 1 large)
250 ml boiling water
2-3 handfuls spinach or kale at the end to wilt in for extra greens
To serve: small handful freshly chopped coriander leaves

1. In a heated pan, dry-roast without burning all the spices, until you get the aroma of the roasted spices.
2. Add the chopped onions to the spice mix, cook for a 2-3 minutes on high heat.
3. Add the ginger and a splash of hot water and cook on medium heat for about 5 minutes until the onions caramelise slightly.
4. Add the chopped tomatoes and tomato paste and the sugar and salt and cook for 2-3 minutes, mixing thoroughly.
5. Add the canned tomatoes, diced sweet potatoes and hot water.
6. Mix and cover and cook on medium heat for about 5 minutes.
7. Add the chickpeas, mix them in and bring to the boil, then cover and cook for 10-15 minutes on low heat to allow the tomatoes to thicken and coat the chickpeas.
8. Add the coriander and turn the heat off.
9. Add the spinach to boost your greens if you wish. Enjoy hot or cold, with brown rice, wholemeal flatbread or a salad.

Top tip: Sweet potatoes are a great source of fibre and are very satiating, with a low glycaemic load. Their deep orange colour is a sign of their rich antioxidant content.

Almond butter noodles with vegetables and tofu

Serves 4

300 g uncooked brown rice/wholewheat noodles
1 x 400-g pack calcium-set tofu
2 tbsp low-sodium soya sauce, or tamari if gluten-free
1 small red onion, diced
3 cloves garlic, crushed and finely diced
1 large red chilli, finely diced
Pinch of salt (optional)
2.5 cm (1 inch) ginger, grated
2 carrots, finely sliced
1 yellow (or green) courgette, finely sliced
1 red bell pepper, thinly sliced
2 cups curly kale, roughly chopped
2 spring onions, finely diced
4 tbsp sesame seeds, lightly toasted in a dry pan
Dressing:
  ½ cup almond butter, unsalted
  1 tsp garlic powder
  1 tbsp sriracha
  1 tsp maple syrup (optional but helps bring out the flavour)
  3 tbsp low-sodium soya sauce
  ½ lime, juiced
  Water to thin as desired

1. Drain the tofu and pat dry. Slice into cubes and toss with the
    soya sauce. Refrigerate for a few hours if possible then bake in
    a preheated oven for 20 minutes at 200ºC until firm.

2. Prepare the noodles according to the packet instructions and rinse under cold water immediately so they don't stick.
3. Blend the dressing ingredients and set aside.
4. In a hot pan with a little water, sauté the onion, garlic and chilli with a pinch of salt.
5. Add the ginger and carrots and sauté for a few minutes, adding a little hot water if needed to deglaze the pan.
6. Partially cover and add the courgette followed by the red bell pepper 2-3 minutes later.
5. Once the courgette is tender but not too soft, add the kale and baked tofu. Stir thoroughly.
6. Add the noodles and drizzle the dressing on top, then turn off the heat and toss until noodles are well coated, being careful not to break the noodles too much.
7. Serve hot with the toasted sesame seeds and sliced spring onion to garnish.

Top tip: You can get all the calcium you need from plants. Just one serving of this meal provides over 603 mg of calcium (86% of the daily requirement as the UK RDA for adults is 700 mg).

Stir-fried baked tofu, mushrooms and broccoli with red peppers

Serves 4

1 400-g block calcium-set extra-firm tofu, drained
2 cups mixed mushrooms, such as maitake, shiitake, oyster, button, and/or cremini, cleaned and sliced into pieces
2 red peppers, chopped

1 broccoli, chopped including the florets and stalk

4 spring onions, chopped finely

5-cm (2-inch) piece ginger, chopped finely

1 red chilli, diced

3 tbsp tamari, divided

3 tbsp rice vinegar

3 tbsp Shaoxing wine (Chinese rice wine) or mirin

1 tbsp sesame oil (optional)

To serve: brown rice or soba (buckwheat) noodles, sesame seeds

1. Chop the block of tofu into ½ inch pieces and bake in a pre-heated oven at 180 degrees Celsius for 20 minutes.
2. Stir rice vinegar, wine and soya sauce in a bowl.
3. Heat the oil in a large wide pan or wok over medium high heat (or add a tablespoon of water if oil-free). Add broccoli and cook for a few minutes.
4. Add the mushrooms, spring onions, red pepper and ginger and cook, until mushrooms and spring onions are lightly browned, and the red pepper is tender for about 5 to 7 minutes.
5. Add the baked tofu and the vinegar, wine and tamari mixture to the pan. Mix until all ingredients are coated
6. Remove from heat. Taste and season with extra soya sauce if desired.

To serve: Enjoy the stir-fry with brown rice or soba noodles. Garnish with sesame seeds.

Top tip: Broccoli is rich in sulforaphane, a powerful anti-cancer, anti-ageing and anti-inflammatory compound. Load up on cruciferous vegetables such as arugula, cauliflower and cabbage to reap its benefits.

Side dishes

Balsamic-drenched soya aubergine

Serves 4

3 medium-sized aubergines (eggplants)
1 tbsp cumin powder
1 tsp turmeric powder
1 pinch pepper
1 tsp red chilli powder
3 tbsp balsamic vinegar
2-3 tbsp low salt soya or tamari sauce

1. Slice aubergines into 5-7.5-cm (2–3-inch) slender long slices. Dry roast all spices in a heated pan until you get aroma.
2. Add the sliced aubergine. Mix through and add a couple of tablespoons of water, cover and cook for 10 minutes in low heat.
3. Add the soya sauce and balsamic vinegar and mix thoroughly, increase heat until slightly caramelised for a couple of minutes, mix through and cover and cook until cooked through for another 10 minutes.
4. Increase heat for a minute or two until you see a glazed appearance.
5. Enjoy in a wrap or as a side dish or in top of quinoa or rice with a side salad.

Top tips: Aubergines or eggplants belong to the family, Solanaceae, as do tomatoes, potatoes, bell and chilli peppers. These are absolutely safe and packed with nutrients. There is a theory that links inflammation with tomatoes, aubergine and potatoes (nightshades), which is not borne out scientifically, so one should be very careful before excluding these nutritious vegetables from the diet. Remember, the greater the variety of plants you eat, the better your gut health and better your overall health.

Cucumber or sweetcorn mint raita

Serves 4

1 small can (250 g) sweet corn OR ½ large -1 small cucumber, grated
250 ml soya or plant yoghurt
4 tbsp soya or plant milk
1 tbsp garden mint sauce or 1 tbsp finely chopped fresh mint
½ tsp fresh cumin powder

1. Whip the soya yoghurt to a smooth consistency with the soya milk, mint sauce and cumin powder.
2. Add the sweet corn or grated cucumber and a pinch of salt if you wish.

Top tip: Sweetcorn is a complex starchy carbohydrate that is full of fibre. Cucumbers consist of about 95% water and are a good source of electrolytes while mint is very cooling and benefits your digestion.

Beetroot rocket salad

Serves 4

2 large handfuls rocket leaves
3 cooked beetroots, chopped
1 handful crushed walnuts and/or seeds
1 large handful mung bean or broccoli sprouts (optional)
1 tsp seaweed flakes (optional)
1 large glug balsamic vinegar

1. This is as easy as it gets: toss all the ingredients together and serve!

Top tips:

- Studies have shown that eating nitrate-rich foods like beetroot and leafy greens, such as rocket, can improve brain function, reduce blood pressure and improve exercise intensity and duration by increased nitric oxide production which helps dilate blood vessels.[5]

- Beetroot and leafy greens may also help change the structure of the brain which becomes more rigid as we age. The neuroplasticity of the brain can improve with learning new skills like dancing as well as with aerobic exercise and by eating nitrate-rich foods.

- Beetroot is rich in minerals and vitamins with 100 g providing 27% of the daily requirement for folate (vitamin B9) and nearly 3 g of fibre.

Paprika hummus

Serves 4

1 400-g can chickpeas, drained and rinsed but set the aquafaba
  aside
1 400-g can cannellini beans, drained and discard the aquafaba
  (see Top tips)
4 cloves raw garlic
½ tsp black pepper
½ tsp salt
½ tsp cumin powder
2 lemons, juiced
2 tbsp tahini
½ tsp paprika for dressing
1-2 tbsp premium-quality extra virgin olive oil (optional)

1. Drain water from cannellini beans and rinse.
2. Save the water from the chickpea BPA free can (aquafaba) and use as much of it as you need to blend to a smooth consistency with all the other ingredients in a good quality blender.
3. Use most of the aquafaba water if you prefer a runnier hummus. Add as you go along to reach desired consistency.

Top tips:
- Aquafaba is the viscous water in which legume seeds such as chickpeas have been cooked. Aquafaba can be used as an egg replacement as it mimics egg whites in cooking, e.g. in meringues and marshmallows.
- Eating legumes (chickpeas and cannellini beans in this recipe) every day is great for short-term and long-term health as they are full of fibre, protein, minerals and vitamins.

Snacks, drinks and desserts

Green smoothie

Serves 2

2 medium-sized frozen bananas (break bananas into thirds to freeze - easier to blend)
½ cucumber
Thumb-sized piece ginger
1 handful baby spinach leaves, washed
1 stem fresh mint including leaves
½-¾ cup fortified soya milk (or other plant-based milk)
1 tbsp ground flax or hemp seeds

1. Mix all of the ingredients in a strong blender.
2. Add more milk depending on desired consistency.
3. Top with extra hemp seeds, a sprig of mint or some fruit.

Top tip: Sip and chew your smoothie very slowly over 30 minutes at least, to activate the salivary enzymes and digestion, which is really important for gut and overall health. Then rinse your mouth afterwards with water to protect the enamel of your teeth.

Sunshine turmeric shot

Serves 4

2 oranges, juiced (or any other fresh juice)
1 lemon, juiced
2 tsp turmeric powder

¼ tsp pepper powder

1 tsp fresh finely grated ginger or ginger powder

1. Stir through, makes about 4 shots.
2. Add a cup of water.
3. Consume a shot daily. You can have it with just water if you prefer.

Top tips:

- Curcumin is the bright golden-yellow pigment in turmeric powder that has been studied the most. This phytochemical is considered to have anti-inflammatory, anti-cancer and antioxidant properties and is widely used in Ayurvedic medicine. Large trials are lacking but several studies have indicated support for the anti-cancer effects of curcumin, which may have a beneficial role in lung disease, Alzheimer's disease, arthritis, and ulcerative colitis skin conditions. Fresh or dried turmeric can be added to lentil dal, stews and soups and even to plant milk lattes.

- Piperine, a compound in black pepper, helps to increase the bioavailability of turmeric. Even just a little pinch of pepper ($\frac{1}{20}$ of a teaspoon) can significantly boost absorption.

Ginger turmeric tea

Serves 2

2.5 cm (1 inch) fresh turmeric root, sliced thinly (or ¾ tsp turmeric powder)

2.5 cm (1 inch) fresh ginger root, sliced thinly

3 cups filtered water

¼ tsp ground black pepper
½ tsp ground cinnamon
1 tsp maple syrup or sweetener of choice (optional)
1 lemon, sliced into rounds

1. Add turmeric, ginger and water to a small saucepan and bring to the boil. Reduce to a simmering heat and add in the black pepper and cinnamon. Simmer for 5 minutes.
2. Sieve the mixture. Let cool for a few minutes before adding in sliced lemons so as not to destroy the vitamin C. If it is too spicy for you, dilute with a little hot water and squeeze of lemon. Add in your sweetener of choice if desired.

Top tips:

*   Include fresh or dried ginger in your diet regularly as studies have shown it can make a difference to period pain and flow.

*   Ginger also helps with nausea so is a great aid in pregnancy.

Cacao, date and almond balls

Makes 12 energy balls

8 medium medjool dates, be careful to remove the pits
1 cup raw almonds
3 tbsp raw cacao powder
2 tbsp almond butter (or peanut butter)
1 tbsp chia seeds (optional)
1 pinch sea salt

Note: If using other dates, soak in water beforehand then drain to make them easier to process. You may need one or two more dates.

1.   Pulse the almonds in a food processor until broken into smaller pieces.
2.   Add remaining ingredients and blitz until well combined. It should come together easily in your hands when rolling. If it's too dry, add a dollop of almond butter and mix again. If it's too wet add a bit more cacao powder.
3.   Store in the fridge for 5 days or so and enjoy as a naturally sweet treat. These can also be frozen for up to a month.

Top tip: Dates are a great addition to dishes for sweetness and come packed with fibre.

Apricot, coconut and tahini energy balls

Makes 20 balls

1 cup dried apricots
½ medjool dates
4 tbsp tahini
1 cup desiccated coconut
½ cup raw cashews
1 tbsp water
1 tbsp chia seeds
1 tsp vanilla extract
1 pinch sea salt
1 dash cinnamon

1. Add the dates and apricots to the food processor and pulse for a minute until finely chopped.
2. Add coconut, cashews, water, chia seeds, vanilla extract, salt and cinnamon. Process for a couple of minutes or until well combined
3. Add 4 tbsp tahini and combine well. It should be perfect but if it is too dry, add a little extra tahini. If too wet, add in some more coconut.
4. Take tablespoon amounts of the mixture and roll into balls in your hands.
5. Chill in the fridge for at least an hour before serving.

Top tip: Dried apricots, tahini and chia seeds are good sources of calcium. This is the perfect snack for breastfeeding too, as calcium requirements increase at this time.

Banana, oat and walnut cookies

Makes 8 medium-sized cookies

1 medium mashed banana (overripe and spotty)
¼ cup peanut butter (or nut butter of choice OR sunflower seed butter if nut free and 1 tbsp maple syrup as it tends to be more bitter)
1 cup rolled oats
3 tbsp walnuts, crumbled into pieces
¼ tsp salt
½ tsp ground cinnamon
1 tbsp chia seeds
½ tsp vanilla extract
1 tbsp maple syrup (optional)

2 tbsp freeze-dried raspberries OR desiccated coconut OR dark chocolate chips

1. Preheat your fan oven to 170ºC.
2. Mash the banana thoroughly then add the peanut butter (or substitute) until it forms a paste.
3. Add the rolled oats, walnuts, salt, cinnamon, chia seeds, vanilla extract, maple syrup and freeze-dried raspberries/ desiccated coconut or dark chocolate chips.
4. Mix thoroughly until well combined.
5. Form into balls and pat down flat on a baking tray lined with parchment paper or a silicone baking mat.
6. Bake for 20 minutes (check on them after 15 minutes as oven temperatures can vary).
7. Enjoy with a cup of herbal tea.

Top tip: Pure maple syrup has a lower glycaemic index than refined sugar, meaning it raises blood sugar less quickly. However, it should still be consumed sparingly.

34

It is never too late
What we eat is bigger than just personal health

What's on our plates does matter

Our healthcare system struggles to cope on a daily basis with the burden of chronic disease, the majority of which could be addressed by lifestyle changes including healthier, plant-predominant dietary patterns. Major nutrition and dietetic organisations around the world, including the British Dietetic Association, all state that a plant-based diet can meet nutritional requirements at all stages of life, from birth to old age. It is one of the healthiest choices you can make, whether you have PCOS or not.

Planetary health

We are all connected. Planetary health is a fairly new field that recognises the health of the planet as a system that needs our urgent attention. Human health and the health of our planet are inextricably linked and our civilisation depends on human health, flourishing natural systems and the wise stewardship of natural resources (The Rockefeller Foundation-Lancet Commission on Planetary Health).

With natural systems being degraded to an unprecedented extent in human history, both our health and that of our planet are in peril.[1] The global food system is a major driver of the climate crisis and the emissions from animal agriculture are greater than those from all forms of transportation combined.

The time is now

An urgent transition to a plant-based food system is essential for the health of humans, non-human animals and the future of our planet. There is a desperate need to improve access to healthy plant-based foods and make them affordable to all and to demand that governments stop subsidising meat and dairy. Regardless of the distance from the farm to your plate, even the most sustainably produced animal foods generate more greenhouse gas emissions than any plant foods.[1] Plant-based diets are best for the environment and human health. A shift to a plant-forward planetary health diet, as outlined by The EAT-Lancet Commission in 2019, along with targets for sustainable food production can prevent as many as 11 million premature adult deaths per year and drive the transition toward a sustainable global food system by 2050. Millions more will avoid going hungry. Food can be a powerful driver of change.[2]

Killing animals is killing us too

Animal agriculture and the food we eat are inextricably linked to zoonotic diseases. Three in four emerging infectious diseases now come from animals, from transmission from the wildlife trade and factory farms. Whether its swine flu in pigs, avian flu in birds or SARS-CoV originating in civets, the underlying theme is the same. Our exploitation of animals and our destruction of their wild habitats have brought us into closer contact than ever before, thereby increasing the risk of zoonotic disease transmission.

Factory farming has been described as a 'perfect storm environment' for infectious diseases, with poultry farms a 'ticking time bomb'. We need to protect vulnerable slaughterhouse workers, who are predominantly from low-income communities and have suffered the brunt of COVID-19 outbreaks due to the nature of their dangerous work. Studies have found that slaughterhouse work is connected to higher rates of post-traumatic stress disorder (PTSD) and higher incidents of domestic violence and alcohol and drug abuse.[2]

The frequent and widespread use of antibiotics on farm animals and fish has also contributed to a huge rise in the number of antibiotic-resistant infections which endanger human lives. The United Nations has already warned that an extra 10 million people may die by 2050 as a result of antibiotic resistance which is completely preventable.[3]

The COVID-19 pandemic, one of the worst we have seen in generations, has already further strained all health resources. It has been particularly disastrous for those of lower socioeconomic means and communities of colour. It's now not a question of whether there will be another pandemic, but when.

Many drops make an ocean

We often feel we cannot make a difference at an individual level. Most of us agree that climate change is real but there is a gap between our thinking and our actions. We know something needs to be done to avert the climate crisis, but we are unsure of what we can do to help. While we need to demand system change, those of us who are able to do so can make a positive difference every time we decide what we choose to eat. Choosing plants over animal products is that difference; choosing beans over beef.

Be the change

Many people genuinely want to change but do not know how to or are confused or scared. You may be put off by healthcare professionals who may disapprove of your decision to adopt a plant-based diet as they are not aware of the science themselves. Remember, most doctors are not given any significant nutrition education in medical school. It is little wonder that people are confused, especially as most health professionals get their nutrition knowledge from the same social media and newspapers that the general public read, rather than peer-reviewed medical nutrition journals.

Plant-based options are growing

Our diets should be centred around whole plant foods that promote health, such as whole grains, legumes, fruit, vegetables, nuts and seeds. There is no need to miss out if you have cravings either, as innovation in food technology has led to tasty plant-based meat, dairy, egg and seafood alternatives without the immense environmental impact or slaughter.

Planetary health, human health and animal justice

The most wonderful thing about eating mostly or only plants is that not only is a plant-based diet optimal for humans, but also the healthiest for the planet and the kindest diet for the fellow beings with whom we share our beautiful home. There is now consensus that to sustain both human and planetary health, a global transition to a plant-based food system is necessary.

A starting point

Once you have identified your 'why', there are plenty of reliable resources to guide you. Our guide in this book on how to transition to a plant-based diet (see Chapter 24) as well as our simple, flavourful plant-based recipes, can help you navigate the change, feeling empowered rather than overwhelmed.

Conclusion
Our hopes and future outlook

We hope that you have found within these pages the answers you have been searching for. Rather than seeing it as a burden, PCOS can be a catalyst to make the nutrition and lifestyle changes that will transform your life. We have seen the power of this for ourselves, our patients and our loved ones. You can regain your health and live the life you truly deserve.

While the future looks exciting for Lifestyle Medicine and plant-based nutrition, there is still a long way to go. You already know that PCOS is the most common endocrine condition in women, affecting at least one in 10 women and AFAB people of reproductive age, and yet it receives far less attention than it deserves. At the heart of our work, and of this book, is our emphasis on knowing your body better. This means empowering you to better navigate this complex condition as an individual and as a patient. However, it also means raising informed awareness of PCOS to drive greater research funding and public policy attention. By engaging with this book, you are already taking one step forward. You are demystifying this condition for yourself and the people you know and love.

Finally, this isn't just a book about PCOS. The nutrition and lifestyle approaches we have detailed are not limited to this condition alone. These are the building blocks for living a long and healthy life. Do take the time to continue to notice the intimate connections between your mind and body and how each of these influences the other.

We wish you all the luck on your journey to a full and wonderful life, *Living PCOS Free.*

Dr Nitu Bajekal with **Rohini Bajekal**

Resources

Useful websites

1. Dr Nitu Bajekal MD ObGyn: nitubajekal.com/pcos/
2. Rohini Bajekal, Nutritionist: rohinibajekal.com
3. Brenda Davis, Registered Dietitian: brendadavisrd.com
4. ESHRE International evidence-based guideline for the assessment and management of polycystic ovary syndrome (PCOS): www.monash.edu/__data/assets/pdf_file/0004/1412644/PCOS_Evidence-Based-Guidelines_20181009.pdf
5. NICE, National Institute for Health and Care Excellence, England Guidance (providing advice and information services for health, public health and social care professionals): https://cks.nice.org.uk/topics/polycystic-ovary-syndrome/
6. Up To Date – Evidence-based clinical resource for medical and patient information: www.uptodate.com/contents/polycystic-ovary-syndrome-pcos-beyond-the-basics
7. The Royal College of Obstetrics and Gynaecology (RCOG, UK): www.rcog.org.uk/en/patients/patient-leaflets/polycystic-ovary-syndrome-pcos-what-it-means-for-your-long-term-health/
8. NHS,UK (National Health Service): www.nhs.uk/conditions/polycystic-ovary-syndrome-pcos/
9. Plant Based Health Professionals (Organisation educating health professionals, members of the public and policy

makers): www.plantbasedhealthprofessionals.com/wp-content/uploads/PCOS-factsheet-210709.pdf

10. ACLM (American College of Lifestyle Medicine): www.lifestylemedicine.org/Scientific-Evidence
11. Dylan Cutler, PhD, Online Holistic Health Educator: http://phruitfuldish.com
12. Centers for Disease Control and Prevention (CDC), USA: www.cdc.gov/diabetes/basics/pcos.html
13. Mayo Clinic, USA: www.mayoclinic.org/diseases-conditions/pcos/symptoms-causes/syc-20353439
14. BDA (British Dietetic Association): www.bda.uk.com/resource/polycystic-ovary-syndrome-pcos-diet.html
15. WHO (World Health Organization): www.who.int/news-room/fact-sheets/detail/physical-activity
16. PCRM (Physicians Committee for Responsible Medicine) – non-profit organisation: www.pcrm.org/news/exam-room-podcast/best-diet-pcos
17. Harvard School of Public Health, USA: www.hsph.harvard.edu/nutritionsource/healthy-eating-plate

Support groups and other helpful organisations

1. Verity UK – PCOS charity: verity-pcos.org.uk
2. Cysters – charity removing cultural barriers in BAME communities surrounding reproductive health including PCOS: cysters.org
3. PCOS Awareness Organisation – non-profit organisation dedicated to the advocacy of PCOS: pcosaa.org
4. PCOS Challenge – a global non-profit PCOS support organisation: pcoschallenge.org
5. Daisy Network – A charity for women with POI (premature ovarian insufficiency): daisynetwork.org

Resources

6. The Eve Appeal – charity funding research and raising awareness of the five gynaecological cancers. eveappeal.org.uk
7. BAATN – The Black, African and Asian Therapy Network: baatn.org.uk
8. Black Minds Matter – connecting Black individuals and families with free mental health services: blackmindsmatteruk.com
9. BEAT – UK eating disorder charity: beateatingdisorders.org.uk
10. Mind – mental health charity: mind.org.uk
11. OCD UK – charity run by and for people with OCD: ocdaction.org.uk
12. UK SMART Recovery – charity that provides help and support for those with any form of addiction: smartrecovery.org.uk
13. Papyrus – UK suicide prevention: papyrus-uk.org
14. Made in Hackney – local community food kitchen offering in-person and online classes: madeinhackney.org

Recipe blogs we love

1. Vegan Richa by Richa Hingle (veganricha.com)
2. Rainbow Plant Life by Nisha Vora (rainbowplantlife.com)
3. WoonHeng (woonheng.com)
4. The Korean Vegan (thekoreanvegan.com)
5. Sweet Potato Soul (sweetpotatosoul.com)
6. The Vegan Nigerian (thevegannigerian.com)
7. Minimalist Baker (minimalistbaker.com)
8. Pick Up Limes (pickuplimes.com)
9. Deliciously Ella (deliciouslyella.com)
10. Love and Lemons (loveandlemons.com)

Glossary

Acanthosis nigricans: a type of skin change characterised by darkened patches of skin that may have a thicker, velvety texture. The development of acanthosis nigricans in those with PCOS is often related to insulin resistance and/or excess weight.

Adenomyosis: is where the lining of the womb pushes into the muscle layer of the womb, also known as uterine or internal endometriosis.

AGEs: advanced glycation end-products. These harmful compounds are formed when protein or fat combine with sugar in the bloodstream. This process is called glycation.

Amenorrhoea: absence of menstrual periods in women of reproductive age.

Androgen: any hormone made by the body that causes characteristics such as excess hair growth. Testosterone is one of the androgens.

Anorexia nervosa (AN): an eating disorder resulting in low body weight due to restriction of food intake or persistent behaviour which interferes with weight gain.

Anovulation: when an egg (ovum) doesn't release from the ovary during the menstrual cycle.

Anti-Müllerian hormone (AMH): a hormone produced by granulosa cells of pre-antral and antral follicles in the ovary and used sometimes to predict ovarian reserve and function.

Antioxidant: any substance that inhibits oxidation – for example, vitamin C or E that remove potentially damaging oxidising agents in a living organism.

Assigned female at birth (AFAB): when a person's gender identity is different from the female sex they were assigned at birth.

Atypical eating disorders: closely resemble anorexia nervosa, bulimia nervosa, and/or binge eating, but do not meet the precise diagnostic criteria.

Binge eating disorder (BED): recurrent episodes of binge eating in the absence of compensatory behaviours. Episodes are marked by feelings of lack of control.

BIPOC: Black, Indigenous, and people of colour.

Bisphenol A (BPA): an industrial chemical that has been used to make certain plastics and resins since the 1950s.

Blood pressure (BP): is recorded as two numbers. The first (top) number is 'systolic blood pressure', which measures how much pressure your blood exerts on the artery walls when the heart beats. The second (bottom) number is 'diastolic blood pressure', which is the amount of pressure exerted on your artery walls while your heart is resting between beats. An ideal blood pressure is considered to be between 90/60 mm Hg and 120/80 mm Hg. High blood pressure is considered to be 140/90 mm Hg or higher. Low blood pressure is considered to be 90/60 mm Hg or lower.

Blue Zones: geographic areas in which people have low rates of chronic disease and live longer than anywhere else.

Body mass index (BMI): a measure based on a person's weight and height to estimate if a person is underweight, at a healthy weight, overweight, or obese. A BMI of 18.5-24.9 is considered a healthy weight, 25-29.9 is considered overweight and 30 or higher is considered obese. It is an imperfect measure, but since women with PCOS may be at risk for excess weight and complications related to excess weight, health providers look to the BMI as an added way to monitor weight status.

Bulimia nervosa (BN): recurrent episodes of extreme overeating over a short time period (binge eating) followed by compensatory behaviour such as self-induced vomiting, laxative abuse or excessive exercise.

Carnitine: substance made in the muscle and liver tissue and found in certain foods, such as meat, poultry, fish and some dairy products. It is used by many cells in the body to make energy from fatty acids.

Cholesterol: a waxy fatty substance. It is a sterol, a type of lipid found in most body tissues. Cholesterol and its derivatives are needed to make hormones and vitamin D, for example.

Circadian rhythm: biological changes that occur over an approximately 24-hour cycle as part of the body's internal clock. They are dependent in large part on environmental cues, like light and darkness, to help the brain regulate biological processes, such as sleep/wake cycles and the release of hormones.

Clinical: concerned with or based on actual observation and treatment of disease in patients rather than experimentation or theory.

Cognitive behavioural therapy (CBT): a talking therapy that can help you manage your problems by changing the way you think and behave.

Colposcopy: a method of viewing the cervix, vulva or vagina under magnification with an instrument called a colposcope.

Combined oral contraceptive pill (COCP): often just called 'the pill', it contains artificial versions of oestrogen and progesterone, which are produced naturally in the ovaries. If taken correctly, it is a very effective form of contraception.

C-reactive protein (CRP): a plasma protein that rises in the blood when there is inflammation or infection. It can be identified by a simple blood test.

Dementia: a general term for the impaired ability to remember, think, or make decisions that interferes with doing everyday activities. Alzheimer's disease is the most common type of dementia (CDC).

Disordered eating: a variety of abnormal eating behaviours and body image concerns that, by themselves, do not warrant diagnosis of an eating disorder. Some of the most common types of disordered eating are dieting and restrictive eating.

Dysmenorrhoea: discomfort and pain during the menstrual period.

Endocrine system: the series of glands that produce hormones that work their effects on distant organs, controlling important functions such as reproduction, through a complex messenger system with feedback loops.

Endometrial hyperplasia: a condition in which the lining of the uterus grows too thick.

EVOO: extra virgin olive oil – the highest grade of virgin olive oil derived by cold mechanical extraction from olives without the use of solvents or refining methods.

Excess weight: excess body fat.

Fasting blood glucose: a test to determine how much glucose (sugar) is in a blood sample after an overnight fast.

FODMAPs: common short-chain, fermentable carbohydrates that are widespread throughout a number of food groups, including wheat. Research has shown that ingesting FODMAPs can provoke gastrointestinal symptoms in susceptible individuals. A diet low in FODMAPs is clinically recommended for the management of irritable bowel syndrome (IBS).

Follicle-stimulating hormone (FSH): a hormone made by the pituitary gland in the brain that helps an egg to mature.

Free sugars: include all monosaccharides and disaccharides added to foods by the manufacturer, cook or consumer, plus sugars naturally present in honey, syrups and unsweetened fruit juices. Within this definition, lactose (milk sugar) when naturally present in milk and milk products and sugars contained within the cellular structure of foods (particularly fruit and vegetables) are excluded.

Gestational diabetes mellitus: Diabetes that begins during pregnancy.

Glycaemic index (GI): a rating system for foods containing carbohydrates, showing how quickly or slowly each food affects your blood sugar (glucose) level when that food is eaten on its own.

Glycaemic load (GL): a measure that considers the amount of carbohydrate in a portion of food together with how quickly it raises blood glucose levels.

HbA1c (glycated haemoglobin): your average blood glucose (sugar) levels for the last two to three months.

Heart disease: includes conditions that narrow or block blood vessels (coronary heart disease). This can lead to a heart attack, angina and some strokes. Heart disease also covers conditions that affect your heart's muscle or valves or cause abnormal rhythms (arrhythmias) (British Heart Foundation).

Homocysteine: an amino acid. Vitamins B12, B6 and B9 (folate) break down homocysteine to create other chemicals your body needs.

Hormones: chemical messengers that are released directly into the blood, which carries them to distant organs and tissues of the body to exert their functions.

Insulin-like growth factor-1 (IGF-1): a hormone that, along with growth hormone (GH), helps promote normal bone and tissue growth and development.

Infertility: the inability to get pregnant after 12 months or more of regular unprotected sexual intercourse.

Insulin resistance: when cells in your body are unable to respond to insulin and therefore cannot take up glucose. This is the main cause of type 2 diabetes but occurs in a number of related conditions, including PCOS.

Irritable bowel syndrome (IBS): a common condition that affects the digestive system. It causes symptoms like stomach cramps, bloating, diarrhoea and constipation.

Laparoscopy: a surgical procedure in which a thin, lighted telescope called a laparoscope is inserted through a small incision (cut) in the abdomen. The laparoscope is used to view the pelvic organs.

Lean PCOS: a term for those living with PCOS who are classed as being in the healthy body weight range.

Lifestyle Medicine: according to the American College of Lifestyle Medicine (ACLM), the leading medical professional organisation providing standardised education for Lifestyle Medicine education: 'Lifestyle Medicine is the use of a whole food, plant-predominant dietary lifestyle, regular physical activity, restorative sleep, stress management, avoidance of risky substances and positive social connection as a primary therapeutic modality for treatment and reversal of chronic disease.'

Luteinising hormone (LH): a hormone made in the pituitary gland that helps an egg to be released from the ovary.

Macronutrients: the nutrients that provide most of the energy, or fuel, the human body needs to function properly. Macronutrients include proteins, carbohydrates and fats. These nutrients provide the calories (energy) in your diet.

Metabolic syndrome: a combination of problems that can lead to type 2 diabetes and heart disease. These problems include high blood pressure, having excess weight or having too much fat around your waist, higher-than-normal blood sugar level, lower-than-normal levels of 'good' cholesterol, and high levels of fats in the blood (triglycerides).

Micronutrients: these include vitamins and minerals, as well as compounds like phytonutrients (plant nutrients) that play a vital part in optimal health. Micronutrients are only needed in tiny amounts. Eating a varied diet, rich in colourful fruit and vegetables, is the best way to get all the necessary micronutrients.

Minimally processed: unprocessed or minimally processed foods are whole foods in which the vitamins and nutrients are still intact. The food is in its natural (or nearly natural) state. These foods may be minimally altered by removal of inedible parts.

Neu5Gc: common sialic acid type of sugar in mammals. Dietary sources that are rich in Neu5Gc include red meats such as beef, pork, lamb and, to a much lesser extent, cow's milk products.

Obesity: a state characterised by excessive body fat.

Obsessive-compulsive disorder (OCD): a common, chronic and long-lasting disorder in which a person has uncontrollable, recurring thoughts (obsessions) and/or behaviours (compulsions) that they feel the urge to repeat over and over.

Oligomenorrhoea: the medical term for infrequent menstrual periods (fewer than six to eight per year).

Overweight and Obesity: above a weight considered in the healthy range, with likely excessive fat accumulation that may impair health. There are pitfalls in management (See BMI). For adults, WHO defines overweight as a BMI $\geq$ 25 and obesity as a BMI$\geq$ 30.

Ovulation: the release of an egg (ovum) from the ovary into the fallopian tube around 13-15 days before the start of a period (usually mid-cycle).

Ovulation induction: the process of using medications to stimulate ovulation (release of an egg) in women who have irregular or absent ovulation (anovulation). Letrozole and Clomiphene are both medications used for ovulation induction.

Oxidative stress: an imbalance between free radicals and antioxidants in your body.

PCO/PCOM – Polycystic ovary (PCO) or polycystic ovary morphology (PCOM): defined under the Rotterdam criteria (see page 40) as a follicle number per ovary of 12 or more (usually $\geq$ 20) and/or an ovarian volume of more than 10 cc in at least one ovary.

PCOS/Polycystic ovary syndrome/Polycystic ovarian syndrome /PCOD: terms used interchangeably for an endocrine (hormone) disorder affecting ovarian function.

Physical activity: any bodily movement produced by skeletal muscles that requires energy expenditure.

Phytonutrients: a broad name for a wide variety of compounds produced by plants and found in fruit, vegetables, beans, grains, and other plants. Examples are antioxidants and isoflavones.

Phyto-oestrogens: plant oestrogens, including isoflavones and lignans. They are found in several different types of food, including soya, grains, beans and some fruit and vegetables.

Polyphenols: compounds naturally found in plants that have anti-oxidant and anti-inflammatory properties.

Prediabetes: a condition in which blood sugar is high, but not high enough to be diagnosed as type 2 diabetes.

Premature ovarian insufficiency (POI) (previously known as **premature ovarian failure** or **premature menopause**): a condition that causes the ovaries to stop working before the age of 40.

Premenstrual syndrome (PMS): the name for the symptoms women can experience in the weeks before their period. These include mood swings, tender breasts, food cravings, fatigue, irritability and depression.

Probiotic: foods that contain beneficial live bacteria while **prebiotic foods** feed the good bacteria that already live in your gut.

Prolactin: a hormone made by the pituitary gland, a small gland at the base of the brain. It causes the breasts to grow and make milk during pregnancy and after birth.

Reproductive age: from the start of your first period until menopause is reached around age 51.

Sex hormone-binding globulin (SHBG): a protein produced by the liver that attaches itself to sex hormones, including testosterone, controlling how much of these hormones is delivered to the body's tissues. A blood SHBG test tells us if there is too much or too little testosterone available for use by the body.

Structured exercise: any activity requiring physical effort, carried out to sustain or improve health and fitness.

Subfertility: generally describes any form of reduced fertility with prolonged time of unwanted non-conception.

Ultra-processed/Highly processed: foods with many added ingredients, such as sugar, salt, fat and artificial colours or preservatives and made mostly from substances extracted from foods, such as fats, starches, added sugars and hydrogenated fats.

Vagina: a tube-like structure surrounded by muscles that leads from the uterus to the outside of the body.

Vulva: the external female genital area.

WHO – World Health Organization: a part of the United Nations that deals with major health issues around the world.

Womb or Endometrial cancer: cancer that affects the womb (uterus) and usually starts in the lining of the womb (endometrium).

Popular diet patterns

Plant-based: a diet consisting completely of plants, or mainly of plants.

Veganism: an ethical lifestyle that excludes all animal-derived food from the diet, including meat, poultry, fish, eggs, dairy and honey.

Vegetarianism: a diet pattern that excludes meat, poultry and fish but sometimes includes eggs and dairy.

Whole food plant-based: a diet pattern that consists entirely of whole or minimally processed fruit, vegetables, whole grains, legumes, nuts, seeds, herbs and spices. It excludes all animal products, including red meat, poultry, fish, eggs and dairy products. This diet pattern minimises the consumption of added salt, oil and sugar.

Types of research study mentioned in this book

Cohort study: a type of longitudinal study that typically follows a group of people (cohort) over time to understand the causes of a disease or condition. Cohort studies can be prospective (forward-looking) or retrospective (backward-looking).

Longitudinal study: participants (subjects) are followed over time with continuous or repeated monitoring of risk factors or health outcomes, or both.

Meta-analysis: a statistical technique for combining data from multiple studies on a particular topic. Meta-analyses can be performed when there are multiple scientific studies addressing the same question, with each individual study reporting measurements that are expected to have some degree of error.

Observational study: a study in which researchers do not intervene; they simply observe study subjects to determine whether there's a correlation between an exposure and disease risk within a given population. Researchers measure activities, events, or processes as precisely and completely as possible without personal interpretation, so the outcome is not affected.

Randomised control trial (RCT): a study design that randomly assigns participants into an experimental group (who receive the variable being tested in a study) or a control group (who do not receive the variable being tested). As the study is conducted, the only expected difference between the control and experimental groups in a RCT is the outcome variable being studied.

Systematic review: a type of review that summarises the results of available carefully designed healthcare studies (controlled trials) and provides a high level of evidence on the effectiveness of healthcare interventions.

References

Introduction

1. Conway G, Dewailly D, Diamanti-Kandarakis E, Escobar-Morreale HF, Franks S, Gambineri A, et al. The polycystic ovary syndrome: a position statement from the European Society of Endocrinology. *European Journal of Endocrinology* 2014; 171(4): P1-P29. doi: 10.1530/EJE-14-0253.
2. Pasquali R, Diamanti-Kandarakis E, Gambineri A. Management of endocrine disease: Secondary polycystic ovary syndrome: theoretical and practical aspects. *European Journal of Endocrinology* 2016;175(4): R157-R169. doi: 10.1530/EJE-16-0374.
3. Deswal R, Narwal V, Dang A, Pundir C. The Prevalence of Polycystic Ovary Syndrome: A Brief Systematic Review. *Journal of Human Reproductive Sciences* 2020; 13(4): 261-271. doi: 10.4103/jhrs.JHRS_95_18
4. Bozdag G, Mumusoglu S, Zengin D, Karabulut E, Yildiz BO. The prevalence and phenotypic features of polycystic ovary syndrome: a systematic review and meta-analysis. *Human Reproduction* 2016; 31(12): 2841-2855. doi: 10.1093/humrep/dew218.
5. March WA, Moore VM, Willson KJ, Phillips DIW, Norman RJ, Davies MJ. The prevalence of polycystic ovary syndrome in a community sample assessed under contrasting diagnostic criteria. *Human Reproduction* 2010; 25(2): 544-551. doi: 10.1093/humrep/dep399
6. Monash University MA. PCOS Evidence-Based guidelines [Internet]. 2018 [cited 2021 Nov 4]. www.monash.edu/__data/assets/pdf_file/0004/1412644/PCOS_Evidence-Based-Guidelines_20181009.pdf
7. Royal College of Obstetricians and Gynaecologists. Long-Term Consequences of Polycystic ovary syndrome. 2014 [cited 2021 Nov 4]. www.rcog.org.uk/globalassets/documents/guidelines/gtg_33.pdf
7a. Subramanian A, Anand A, Adderley NJ, Okoth K, Toulis KA, Gokhale K, Sainsbury C, O'Reilly MW, Arlt W, Nirantharakumar K. Increased COVID-19 infections in women with polycystic ovary syndrome: a population-based study. *Eur J Endocrinol.* 2021 May;184(5):637-645. doi: 10.1530/EJE-20-1163. PMID: 33635829; PMCID: PMC8052516.)
7b. Riestenberg, C., Jagasia, A., Markovic, D., Buyalos, R. P., & Azziz, R. (2022). Health Care-Related Economic Burden of Polycystic Ovary Syndrome in the United States: Pregnancy-Related and Long-Term Health Consequences. *The*

Journal of Clinical Endocrinology and Metabolism, 107(2), 575–585. https://doi.org/10.1210/clinem/dgab613

8. Azziz R, Dumesic DA, Goodarzi MO. Polycystic ovary syndrome: an ancient disorder? *Fertility and Sterility* 2011; 95(5): 1544-1548. doi: 10.1016/j.fertnstert.2010.09.032.

9. Hirschberg AL. Female hyperandrogenism and elite sport. *Endocrine Connections* 2020; 9(4): R81-R82. doi: 10.1530/EC-19-0537

10. National Institute for Health and Care Excellence (NICE). Polycystic Ovary Syndrome Causes [Internet]. 2018 [cited 2021 Nov 4]. https://cks.nice.org.uk/topics/polycystic-ovary-syndrome/background-information/causes/

11. Zhu J, Pujol-Gualdo N, Wittemans LBL, Lindgren CM, Laisk T, Hirschhorn JN, Chan YM. Evidence From Men for Ovary-independent Effects of Genetic Risk Factors for Polycystic Ovary Syndrome. *J Clin Endocrinol Metab.* 2021 Nov 19:dgab838. doi: 10.1210/clinem/dgab838. Epub ahead of print. PMID: 34969092.

12. Merkin SS, Azziz R, Seeman T, Calderon-Margalit R, Daviglus M, Kiefe C, et al. Socioeconomic Status and Polycystic Ovary Syndrome. *Journal of Women's Health* 2011; 20(3): 413–419. doi:10.1089/jwh.2010.2303

13. Cockerham WC, Hamby BW, Oates GR. The Social Determinants of Chronic Disease. *American Journal of Preventive Medicine* 2017; 52(1): S5–S12. doi: 10.1016/j.amepre.2016.09.010

Chapter 1: Periods: a vital sign – Know your body

1. American Academy of Pediatrics Committee on Adolescence; American College of Obstetricians and Gynecologists Committee on Adolescent Health Care, Diaz A Laufer MR, Breech LL . Menstruation in Girls and Adolescents: Using the Menstrual Cycle as a Vital Sign. *Pediatrics* 2006; 118(5): 2245-2250. doi: 10.1542/peds.2006-2481.

2. ACOG. Using the menstrual cycle as a vital sign. 2015 [cited 2021 Nov 4]. www.acog.org/clinical/clinical-guidance/committee-opinion/articles/2015/12/menstruation-in-girls-and-adolescents-using-the-menstrual-cycle-as-a-vital-sign

3. Rees M. The age of menarche. *ORGYN* 1995; (4): 2-4. PMID: 12319855

4. Intimina. Women and their bodies: 25% of women can't correctly identify vagina. 10 November 2020 [cited 2021 Nov 4]. www.intimina.com/blog/women-and-their-bodies/

Chapter 2: Demystifying PCOS – understanding the condition

1. Monash University MA. PCOS Evidence-Based guidelines [Internet]. 2018 [cited 2021 Nov 4]. Available from: www.monash.edu/__data/assets/pdf_file/0004/1412644/PCOS_Evidence-Based-Guidelines_20181009.pdf

2. Conway G, Dewailly D, Diamanti-Kandarakis E, Escobar-Morreale HF, Franks S, Gambineri A, et al. The polycystic ovary syndrome: a position statement from

the European Society of Endocrinology. *European Journal of Endocrinology* 2014; 171(4): P1-29. doi: 10.1530/EJE-14-0253

3. National Institute for Health and Care Excellence (NICE). PCOS prevalence [Internet]. 2018 [cited 2021 Nov 5]. Available from: https://cks.nice.org.uk/topics/polycystic-ovary-syndrome/background-information/prevalence/

4. Royal College of Obstetricians and Gynaecologists. Long-Term Consequences of Polycystic ovary syndrome. 2014 [cited 2021 Nov 4]; Available from: www.rcog.org.uk/globalassets/documents/guidelines/gtg_33.pdf

5. Bozdag G, Mumusoglu S, Zengin D, Karabulut E, Yildiz BO. The prevalence and phenotypic features of polycystic ovary syndrome: a systematic review and meta-analysis. *Human Reproduction* 2016; 31(12): 2841-2855. doi: 10.1093/humrep/dew218

6. March WA, Moore VM, Willson KJ, Phillips DIW, Norman RJ, Davies MJ. The prevalence of polycystic ovary syndrome in a community sample assessed under contrasting diagnostic criteria. *Human Reproduction* 2010; 25(2): 544-551. doi: 10.1093/humrep/dep399

7. Ding T, Hardiman PJ, Petersen I, Wang F-F, Qu F, Baio G. The prevalence of polycystic ovary syndrome in reproductive-aged women of different ethnicity: a systematic review and meta-analysis. *Oncotarget* 2017; 8(56): 96351-96358. doi: 10.18632/oncotarget.19180

8. Legro RS, Driscoll D, Strauss JF, Fox J, Dunaif A. Evidence for a genetic basis for hyperandrogenemia in polycystic ovary syndrome. *Proceedings of the National Academy of Sciences* 1998; 95(25): 14956-14960. doi: 10.1073/pnas.95.25.14956

9. Álvarez-Blasco F, Botella-Carretero JI, San Millán JL, Escobar-Morreale HF. Prevalence and Characteristics of the Polycystic Ovary Syndrome in Overweight and Obese Women. *Archives of Internal Medicine* 2006; 166(19): 2081-2086. doi: 10.1001/archinte.166.19.2081

10. Davis S, Knight S, White V, Claridge C, Davis BJ, Bell R. Preliminary indication of a high prevalence of polycystic ovary syndrome in indigenous Australian women. *Gynecol Endocrinol* 2002; 16(6): 443–446. PMID: 12626030

11. Azziz R. Epidemiology, phenotype, and genetics of the polycystic ovary syndrome in adults [Internet]. *UpToDate* 2021 [cited 2021 Nov 5]. Available from: www.uptodate.com/contents/epidemiology-phenotype-and-genetics-of-the-polycystic-ovary-syndrome-in-adults

12. Sam S. Obesity and Polycystic Ovary Syndrome. *Obesity Management* 2007; 3(2): 69-73. doi: 10.1089/obe.2007.0019

13. Azziz R. Polycystic Ovary Syndrome Is a Family Affair. *Journal of Clinical Endocrinology & Metabolism* 2008; 93(5): 1579-1581. doi.org/10.1210/jc.2008-0477

14. Baillargeon J-P, Carpentier AC. Brothers of women with polycystic ovary syndrome are characterised by impaired glucose tolerance, reduced insulin sensitivity and related metabolic defects. *Diabetologia* 2007; 50(12): 2424-2432. doi: 10.1007/s00125-007-0831-9.

15. di Guardo F, Cerana MC, D'urso G, Genovese F, Palumbo M. Male PCOS equivalent and nutritional restriction: Are we stepping forward? *Medical Hypotheses* 2019; 126: 1-3. doi: 10.1016/j.mehy.2019.03.003.

16. Witchel SF, Oberfield S, Rosenfield RL, Codner E, Bonny A, Ibáñez L, et al. The Diagnosis of Polycystic Ovary Syndrome during Adolescence. *Hormone Research in Paediatrics* 2015; 83(6). doi: 10.1159/000375530.

17. National Institute for Health and Care Excellence (NICE). Polycystic Ovary Syndrome Causes [Internet]. 2018 [cited 2021 Nov 4]. Available from: https://cks.nice.org.uk/topics/polycystic-ovary-syndrome/background-information/causes/
18. Yau TT, Ng NY, Cheung L, Ma RC. Polycystic ovary syndrome: a common reproductive syndrome with long-term metabolic consequences. *Hong Kong Medical Journal* 2017; 23(6): 622-634. doi: 10.12809/hkmj176308.

Chapter 3: PCOS: what to look out for – Signs and symptoms

1. Gibson-Helm M, Teede H, Dunaif A, Dokras A. Delayed diagnosis and a lack of information associated with dissatisfaction in women with polycystic ovary syndrome. *Journal of Clinical Endocrinology & Metabolism* 2017; 102(2): 604-612. doi: 10.1210/jc.2016-2963.
2. Conway G, Dewailly D, Diamanti-Kandarakis E, Escobar-Morreale HF, Franks S, Gambineri A, et al. The polycystic ovary syndrome: a position statement from the European Society of Endocrinology. *European Journal of Endocrinology* 2014; 171(4): P1-P29. doi: 10.1530/EJE-14-0253.
3. Azziz R, Carmina E, Dewailly D, Diamanti-Kandarakis E, Escobar-Morreale HF, Futterweit W, et al. The Androgen Excess and PCOS Society criteria for the polycystic ovary syndrome: the complete task force report. *Fertility and Sterility* 2009; 91(2): 456-488. doi: 10.1016/j.fertnstert.2008.06.035.
4. Witchel SF, Oberfield S, Rosenfield RL, Codner E, Bonny A, Ibáñez L, et al. The Diagnosis of Polycystic Ovary Syndrome during Adolescence. *Hormone Research in Paediatrics* 2015; 83(6). doi: 10.1159/000375530.
5. Baillargeon J-P, Carpentier AC. Brothers of women with polycystic ovary syndrome are characterised by impaired glucose tolerance, reduced insulin sensitivity and related metabolic defects. *Diabetologia* 2007; 50(12): 2424-2432. doi: 10.1007/s00125-007-0831-9.
6. di Guardo F, Cerana MC, D'urso G, Genovese F, Palumbo M. Male PCOS equivalent and nutritional restriction: Are we stepping forward? *Medical Hypotheses* 2019; 126: 1-3. doi: 10.1016/j.mehy.2019.03.003.
7. Vink JM, Sadrzadeh S, Lambalk CB, Boomsma DI. Heritability of Polycystic Ovary Syndrome in a Dutch Twin-Family Study. *Journal of Clinical Endocrinology & Metabolism* 2006; 91(6): 2100-2104. doi: 10.1210/jc.2005-1494.
8. Legro RS, Driscoll D, Strauss JF, Fox J, Dunaif A. Evidence for a genetic basis for hyperandrogenemia in polycystic ovary syndrome. *Proceedings of the National Academy of Sciences USA* 1998; 95(25): 14956-14960. doi: 10.1073/pnas.95.25.14956
9. Bray GA. The epidemic of obesity and changes in food intake: the Fluoride Hypothesis. *Physiology & Behavior* 2004; 82(1): 115-121. doi: 10.1016/j.physbeh.2004.04.033.

Chapter 4: Solving the PCOS puzzle – Diagnosis of PCOS

1. Copp T, Hersch J, Muscat DM, McCaffery KJ, Doust J, Dokras A, et al. The benefits and harms of receiving a polycystic ovary syndrome diagnosis: a qualitative study of women's experiences. *Human Reproduction Open* 2019; 2019(4): hoz026. doi: 10.1093/hropen/hoz026.
2. The Rotterdam ESHRE/ASRM-sponsored PCOS consensus workshop group. Revised 2003 consensus on diagnostic criteria and long-term health risks related to polycystic ovary syndrome (PCOS). Human Reproduction [Internet]. 2004 Jan 1 [cited 2021 Nov 6];19(1). Available from: https://academic.oup.com/humrep/article/19/1/41/690226
3. Monash University MA. PCOS Evidence-Based guidelines [Internet]. 2018 [cited 2021 Nov 4]. Available from: www.monash.edu/__data/assets/pdf_file/0004/1412644/PCOS_Evidence-Based-Guidelines_20181009.pdf
3a. Yue CY, Lu LK, Li M, Zhang QL, Ying CM. (2018). Threshold value of anti-Mullerian hormone for the diagnosis of polycystic ovary syndrome in Chinese women. *PloS one* 2018; 13(8): e0203129. doi.org/10.1371/journal.pone.0203129).
4. Álvarez-Blasco F, Botella-Carretero JI, San Millán JL, Escobar-Morreale HF. Prevalence and Characteristics of the Polycystic Ovary Syndrome in Overweight and Obese Women. *Archives of Internal Medicine* 2006; 166(19): 2081-2086. doi: 10.1001/archinte.166.19.2081
5. Witchel SF, Oberfield S, Rosenfield RL, Codner E, Bonny A, Ibáñez L, et al. The Diagnosis of Polycystic Ovary Syndrome during Adolescence. *Hormone Research in Paediatrics* 2015; 83(6). doi: 10.1159/000375530
6. Conway G, Dewailly D, Diamanti-Kandarakis E, Escobar-Morreale HF, Franks S, Gambineri A, et al. The polycystic ovary syndrome: a position statement from the European Society of Endocrinology. *European Journal of Endocrinology* 2014; 171(4): P1-P29. doi: 10.1530/EJE-14-0253.

Chapter 5: The missing link – Insulin resistance in PCOS

1. Marshall JC, Dunaif A. Should all women with PCOS be treated for insulin resistance? *Fertility and Sterility* 2012; 97(1): 18-22. doi: 10.1016/j.fertnstert.2011.11.036.
2. Rosenfield RL, Ehrmann DA. The Pathogenesis of Polycystic Ovary Syndrome (PCOS): The Hypothesis of PCOS as Functional Ovarian Hyperandrogenism Revisited. *Endocrine Reviews* 2016; 37(5): 467-520. doi: 10.1210/er.2015-1104.
3. Prapas N, Karkanaki A, Prapas I, Kalogiannidis I, Katsikis I, Panidis D. Genetics of Polycystic Ovary Syndrome. *Hippokratia* 2009; 13(4): 216-223. PMID: 20011085
4. Diamanti-Kandarakis E, Dunaif A. Insulin Resistance and the Polycystic Ovary Syndrome Revisited: An Update on Mechanisms and Implications. *Endocrine Reviews* 2012; 33(6): 981-1030. doi: 10.1210/er.2011-1034
5. de Luca C, Olefsky JM. Inflammation and insulin resistance. *FEBS letters* 2008; 582(1): 97–105. doi.org/10.1016/j.febslet.2007.11.057

6. Sharma S, Tripathi P. Gut microbiome and type 2 diabetes: where we are and where to go? *Journal of Nutritional Biochemistry* 2019; 63: 101–108. doi.org/10.1016/j.jnutbio.2018.10.003

7. Hall J. Endocrine-disrupting chemicals. *Up To Date* [Internet]. [cited 2021 Nov 6]; Available from: www.uptodate.com/contents/endocrine-disrupting-chemicals

8. Barrett E, Sobolewski M. Polycystic Ovary Syndrome: Do Endocrine-Disrupting Chemicals Play a Role? *Seminars in Reproductive Medicine* 2014; 32(03): 166-176. doi: 10.1055/s-0034-1371088.

9. Monash University MA. PCOS Evidence-Based guidelines [Internet]. 2018 [cited 2021 Nov 4]. Available from: www.monash.edu/__data/assets/pdf_file/0004/1412644/PCOS_Evidence-Based-Guidelines_20181009.pdf

10. Qu X, Donnelly R. Sex Hormone-Binding Globulin (SHBG) as an Early Biomarker and Therapeutic Target in Polycystic Ovary Syndrome. *International Journal of Molecular Sciences* 2020; 21(21): 8191. doi: 10.3390/ijms21218191.

11. Tymchuk CN, Tessler SB, Barnard RJ. Changes in Sex Hormone-Binding Globulin, Insulin, and Serum Lipids in Postmenopausal Women on a Low-Fat, High-Fiber Diet Combined With Exercise. *Nutrition and Cancer* 2000; 38(2): 158-162. doi: 10.1207/S15327914NC382_3.

12. Tuso P, Ismail MH, Ha BP, Bartolotto C. Nutritional Update for Physicians: Plant-Based Diets. *Permanente Journal* 2013; 17(2): 61-66. doi: 10.7812/TPP/12-085.

13. Erickson ML, Jenkins NT, McCully KK. Exercise after You Eat: Hitting the Postprandial Glucose Target. *Frontiers in Endocrinology* 2017; 8: 228. doi: 10.3389/fendo.2017.00228

14. Kim CH, Chon SJ, Lee SH. Effects of lifestyle modification in polycystic ovary syndrome compared to metformin only or metformin addition: A systematic review and meta-analysis. *Scientific Reports* 2020; 10(1): 7802. doi: 10.1038/s41598-020-64776-w.

15. Royal College of Obstetricians and Gynaecologists. Long-Term Consequences of Polycystic ovary syndrome. 2014 [cited 2021 Nov 4]; Available from: www.rcog.org.uk/globalassets/documents/guidelines/gtg_33.pdf

16. Wakeman M, Archer DT. Metformin and Micronutrient Status in Type 2 Diabetes: Does Polypharmacy Involving Acid-Suppressing Medications Affect Vitamin B12 Levels? *Diabetes, Metabolic Syndrome and Obesity: Targets and Therapy* 2020; 13: 2093-2108. doi: 10.2147/DMSO.S237454.

17. Aroda VR, Edelstein SL, Goldberg RB, Knowler WC, Marcovina SM, Orchard TJ, et al. Long-term Metformin Use and Vitamin B12 Deficiency in the Diabetes Prevention Program Outcomes Study. *Journal of Clinical Endocrinology & Metabolism* 2016; 101(4): 1754-1761. doi: 10.1210/jc.2015-3754.

Chapter 6: Androgen excess – Hyperandrogenism

1. Tymchuk CN, Tessler SB, Barnard RJ. Changes in Sex Hormone-Binding Globulin, Insulin, and Serum Lipids in Postmenopausal Women on a Low-Fat, High-Fiber Diet Combined With Exercise. *Nutrition and Cancer* 2000; 38(2): 158-162. doi: 10.1207/S15327914NC382_3.

2. Dolfing JG, Stassen CM, van Haard PMM, Wolffenbuttel BHR, Schweitzer DH. Comparison of MRI-assessed body fat content between lean women with

polycystic ovary syndrome (PCOS) and matched controls: less visceral fat with PCOS. *Human Reproduction* 2011; 26(6): 1495-1500. doi.org/10.1093/humrep/der070

3. Ehrmann DA, Liljenquist DR, Kasza K, Azziz R, Legro RS, Ghazzi MN. Prevalence and Predictors of the Metabolic Syndrome in Women with Polycystic Ovary Syndrome. *Journal of Clinical Endocrinology & Metabolism* 2006; 91(1): 48-53. doi: 10.1210/jc.2005-1329.

4. National Institute for Health and Care Excellence (NICE). Polycystic Ovary Syndrome Causes [Internet]. 2018 [cited 2021 Nov 4]. Available from: https://cks.nice.org.uk/topics/polycystic-ovary-syndrome/background-information/causes/

5. McMacken M, Shah S. A plant-based diet for the prevention and treatment of type 2 diabetes. *Journal of Geriartric Cardiology* 2017; 14(5): 342-354. doi: 10.11909/j.issn.1671-5411.2017.05.009

Chapter 7: One size does not fit all – Body weight and PCOS

1. Tanas R, Bernasconi S, Marsella M, Corsello G. What's the name? Weight stigma and the battle against obesity. *Italian Journal of Pediatrics* 2020; 46(1): 60. doi.org/10.1186/s13052-020-00821-8

2. Ee C, Smith C, Moran L, MacMillan F, Costello M, Baylock B, Teede H. "The whole package deal": experiences of overweight/obese women living with polycystic ovary syndrome. *BMC Women's Health* 2020; 20: 221. doi.org/10.1186/s12905-020-01090-7

3. Azziz R, Barbieri RL, Martin KA. Epidemiology, phenotype, and genetics of the polycystic ovary syndrome in adults. *UpToDate* 2021. [cited 2021 Nov 5] Available from: www.uptodate.com/contents/epidemiology-phenotype-and-genetics-of-the-polycystic-ovary-syndrome-in-adults?topicRef=7436&source=see_link

4. Geller G, Watkins PA. Addressing Medical Students' Negative Bias Toward Patients With Obesity Through Ethics Education. *AMA Journal of Ethics* 2018; 20(10): E948-E959. doi: 10.1001/amajethics.2018.948.

5. Phelan SM, Burgess DJ, Yeazel MW, Hellerstedt WL, Griffin JM, Ryn M. Impact of weight bias and stigma on quality of care and outcomes for patients with obesity. *Obesity Reviews* 2015; 16(4): 319-326. doi: 10.1111/obr.12266.

6. Phelan SM, Dovidio JF, Puhl RM, Burgess DJ, Nelson DB, Yeazel MW, et al. Implicit and explicit weight bias in a national sample of 4,732 medical students: The medical student CHANGES study. *Obesity* 2014; 22(4): 1201-1208. doi: 10.1002/oby.20687

7. Volger S, Vetter ML, Dougherty M, Panigrahi E, Egner R, Webb V, et al. Patients' Preferred Terms for Describing Their Excess Weight: Discussing Obesity in Clinical Practice. *Obesity* 2012; 20(1): 147-150. doi: 10.1038/oby.2011.217

8. HSPH. Measuring Obesity From Calipers to CAT Scans, Ten Ways to Tell Whether a Body Is Fat or Lean. *Obesity Prevention Source* [cited 2021 Nov 6]. Available from: www.hsph.harvard.edu/obesity-prevention-source/obesity-definition/how-to-measure-body-fatness/

References

9. Brennan KM, Kroener LL, Chazenbalk GD, Dumesic DA. Polycystic Ovary Syndrome: Impact of Lipotoxicity on Metabolic and Reproductive Health. *Obstetrical & Gynecological Survey* 2019; 74(4): 223-231. doi: 10.1097/OGX.0000000000000661.

10. Dolfing JG, Stassen CM, van Haard PMM, Wolffenbuttel BHR, Schweitzer DH. Comparison of MRI-assessed body fat content between lean women with polycystic ovary syndrome (PCOS) and matched controls: less visceral fat with PCOS. *Human Reproduction* 2011; 26(6): 1495-1500. doi.org/10.1093/humrep/der070

11. Rosenberg S. The Relationship Between PCOS and Obesity: Which Comes First? *Science Journal of the Lander College of Arts and Sciences* 2019; 13(1). Available from: https://touroscholar.touro.edu/ sjlcas/vol13/iss1/5

12. Monash University MA. *International evidence-based guideline for the assessment and management of polycystic ovary syndrome.* Monash Univeristy, Melbourne Australia, 2018 [cited 2021 Nov 4]. Available from: www.monash.edu/__data/assets/pdf_file/0004/1412644/PCOS_Evidence-Based-Guidelines_20181009.pdf

13. Brennan L, Teede H, Skouteris H, Linardon J, Hill B, Moran L. Lifestyle and Behavioral Management of Polycystic Ovary Syndrome. *Journal of Women's Health* 2017; 26(8): 836-848. doi: 10.1089/jwh.2016.5792

14. Carmina E, Campagna AM, Lobo RA. A 20-Year Follow-up of Young Women with Polycystic Ovary Syndrome. Obstetrics & Gynecology. 2012; 119(2, Part 1): 263-269. doi: 10.1097/AOG.0b013e31823f7135

15. Gibson-Helm M, Teede H, Dunaif A, Dokras A. Delayed diagnosis and a lack of information associated with dissatisfaction in women with polycystic ovary syndrome. *Journal of Clinical Endocrinology & Metabolism* 2017; 102(2): 604-612. doi: 10.1210/jc.2016-2963.

16. Azziz R. Polycystic Ovary Syndrome Is a Family Affair. *Journal of Clinical Endocrinology & Metabolism* 2008; 93(5): 1579-1581. doi.org/10.1210/jc.2008-0477

17. Brady C, Mousa SS, Mousa SA. Polycystic ovary syndrome and its impact on women's quality of life: More than just an endocrine disorder. *Drug, Healthcare and Patient Safety* 2009; 1: 9-15. doi: 10.2147/dhps.s4388.

18. Afshin A, Sur PJ, Fay KA, Cornaby L, Ferrara G, Salama JS, et al. Health effects of dietary risks in 195 countries, 1990–2017: a systematic analysis for the Global Burden of Disease Study 2017. *Lancet* 2019; 393(10184): 1958-1972. doi.org/10.1016/S0140-6736(19)30041-8

19. Mazidi M, Katsiki N, Mikhailidis DP, Sattar N, Banach M. Lower carbohydrate diets and all-cause and cause-specific mortality: a population-based cohort study and pooling of prospective studies. *European Heart Journal* 2019; 40(34): 2870-2879. doi.org/10.1093/eurheartj/ehz174

20. Seidelmann SB, Claggett B, Cheng S, Henglin M, Shah A, Steffen LM, et al. Dietary carbohydrate intake and mortality: a prospective cohort study and meta-analysis. *Lancet Public Health* 2018; 3(9): e419-e428. doi: 10.1016/S2468-2667(18)30135-X

21. Lim SS, Hutchison SK, van Ryswyk E, Norman RJ, Teede HJ, Moran LJ. Lifestyle changes in women with polycystic ovary syndrome. *Cochrane Database of Systematic Reviews* 2019; 3(3): CD007506. doi: 10.1002/14651858.CD007506.pub4.

22. Lim SS, Davies MJ, Norman RJ, Moran LJ. Overweight, obesity and central obesity in women with polycystic ovary syndrome: a systematic review and meta-analysis. *Human Reproduction Update* 2012; 18(6): 618-637. doi: 10.1093/humupd/dms030.

23. Pasquali R, Gambineri A, Cavazza C, Ibarra Gasparini D, Ciampaglia W, Cognigni GE, et al. Heterogeneity in the responsiveness to long-term lifestyle intervention and predictability in obese women with polycystic ovary syndrome. *European Journal of Endocrinology* 2011; 164(1): 53-60. https://eje.bioscientifica.com/view/journals/eje/164/1/53.xml

24. Holbrey S, Coulson NS. A qualitative investigation of the impact of peer to peer online support for women living with Polycystic Ovary Syndrome. *BMC Women's Health* 2013; 13(1): 51. www.biomedcentral.com/1472-6874/13/51

25. Lee R, Joy Mathew C, Jose MT, Elshaikh AO, Shah L, Cancarevic I. A Review of the Impact of Bariatric Surgery in Women with Polycystic Ovary Syndrome. *Cureus* 2020; 12(10): e10811. doi: 10.7759/cureus.10811

26. Escobar-Morreale HF, Botella-Carretero JI, Álvarez-Blasco F, Sancho J, San Millán JL. The polycystic ovary syndrome associated with morbid obesity may resolve after weight loss induced by bariatric surgery. *Journal of Clinical Endocrinology & Metabolism* 2005; 90(12): 6364-6369. doi: 10.1210/jc.2005-1490.

Chapter 8: Not just teenage angst – Adolescent PCOS

1. Rosenfield RL, Ehrmann DA. The Pathogenesis of Polycystic Ovary Syndrome (PCOS): The Hypothesis of PCOS as Functional Ovarian Hyperandrogenism Revisited. *Endocrine Reviews* 2016; 37(5): 467-520. doi: 10.1210/er.2015-1104.

2. Abbott DH, Barnett DK, Bruns CM, Dumesic DA. Androgen excess fetal programming of female reproduction: a developmental aetiology for polycystic ovary syndrome? *Human Reproduction Update* 2005; 11(4): 357-374. doi: 10.1093/humupd/dmi013

3. Witchel SF, Oberfield SE, Peña AS. Polycystic Ovary Syndrome: Pathophysiology, Presentation, and Treatment With Emphasis on Adolescent Girls. *Journal of the Endocrine Society* 2019; 3(8): 1545-1573. doi: 10.1210/js.2019-00078.

4. Paschou SA, Ioannidis D, Vassilatou E, Mizamtsidi M, Panagou M, Lilis D, et al. Birth Weight and Polycystic Ovary Syndrome in Adult Life: Is There a Causal Link? *PLoS One* 2015; 10(3): e0122050. doi: 10.1371/journal.pone.0122050

5. Monash University MA. PCOS Evidence-Based guidelines [Internet]. 2018 [cited 2021 Nov 4]. Available from: www.monash.edu/__data/assets/pdf_file/0004/1412644/PCOS_Evidence-Based-Guidelines_20181009.pdf

6. Golden NH, Schneider M, Wood C. Preventing Obesity and Eating Disorders in Adolescents. *Pediatrics* 2016; 138(3): e20161649. doi: 10.1542/peds.2016-1649.

7. Skovlund CW, Mørch LS, Kessing LV, Lidegaard Ø. Association of Hormonal Contraception With Depression. *JAMA Psychiatry* 2016; 73(11): 1154-1162. doi: 10.1001/jamapsychiatry.2016.2387.

8. McKetta S, Keyes KM. Oral contraceptive use and depression among adolescents. *Annals of Epidemiology* 2019; 29: 46-51. doi: 10.1016/j.annepidem.2018.10.002.

Chapter 9: It's not fair – How PCOS affects people of colour

1. Ding T, Hardiman PJ, Petersen I, Wang F-F, Qu F, Baio G. The prevalence of polycystic ovary syndrome in reproductive-aged women of different ethnicity: a systematic review and meta-analysis. *Oncotarget* 2017; 8(56): 96351-96358. doi: 10.18632/oncotarget.19180.
2. Li R, Yu G, Yang D, Li S, Lu S, Wu X, et al. Prevalence and predictors of metabolic abnormalities in Chinese women with PCOS: a cross- sectional study. *BMC Endocrine Disorders* 2014; 14(1): 76. doi.org/10.1186/1472-6823-14-76
3. Ganie M, Vasudevan V, Wani I, Baba M, Arif T, Rashid A. Epidemiology, pathogenesis, genetics & management of polycystic ovary syndrome in India. *Indian Journal of Medical Research* 2019; 150(4): 333-344. doi: 10.4103/ijmr.IJMR_1937_17
4. Goodarzi MO, Quiñones MJ, Azziz R, Rotter JI, Hsueh WA, Yang H. Polycystic ovary syndrome in Mexican-Americans: prevalence and association with the severity of insulin resistance. *Fertility and Sterility* 2005; 84(3): 766-769. doi: 10.1016/j.fertnstert.2005.03.051.
5. Kauffman RP, Baker VM, Dimarino P, Gimpel T, Castracane VD. Polycystic ovarian syndrome and insulin resistance in white and Mexican American women: A comparison of two distinct populations. *American Journal of Obstetrics and Gynecology* 2002; 187(5): 1362-1369. doi: 10.1067/mob.2002.126650.
6. Boyle JA, Cunningham J, O'Dea K, Dunbar T, Norman RJ. Prevalence of polycystic ovary syndrome in a sample of Indigenous women in Darwin, Australia. *Medical Journal of Australia* 2012; 196(1): 62-66. doi: 10.5694/mja11.10553
7. Davis S, Knight S, White V, Claridge C, Davis BJ, Bell R. Preliminary indication of a high prevalence of polycystic ovary syndrome in indigenous Australian women. *Gynecol Endocrinol* 2002; 16(6): 443-446. https://pubmed.ncbi.nlm.nih.gov/12626030/
8. Diamanti-Kandarakis E, Kouli CR, Bergiele AT, Filandra FA, Tsianateli TC, Spina GG, et al. A Survey of the Polycystic Ovary Syndrome in the Greek Island of Lesbos: Hormonal and Metabolic Profile. *Journal of Clinical Endocrinology & Metabolism* 1999; 84(11): 4006-4011. doi: 10.1210/jcem.84.11.6148.
9. Royal College of Obstetricians and Gynaecologists. Long-Term Consequences of Polycystic ovary syndrome. 2014 [cited 2021 Nov 4]; Available from: www.rcog.org.uk/globalassets/documents/guidelines/gtg_33.pdf
10. Wijeyaratne CN, Balen AH, Barth JH, Belchetz PE. Clinical manifestations and insulin resistance (IR) in polycystic ovary syndrome (PCOS) among South Asians and Caucasians: is there a difference? *Clinical Endocrinology* 2002; 57(3): 343-350. doi: 10.1046/j.1365-2265.2002.01603.x.
11. Engmann L, Jin S, Sun F, Legro RS, Polotsky AJ, Hansen KR, et al. Racial and ethnic differences in the polycystic ovary syndrome metabolic phenotype. *American Journal of Obstetrics and Gynecology* 2017; 216(5): 493.e1-493.e13. doi: 10.1016/j.ajog.2017.01.003.

12. Monash University MA. PCOS Evidence-Based guidelines [Internet]. 2018 [cited 2021 Nov 4]. Available from: www.monash.edu/__data/assets/pdf_file/0004/1412644/PCOS_Evidence-Based-Guidelines_20181009.pdf

13. Lo JC, Feigenbaum SL, Yang J, Pressman AR, Selby J v., Go AS. Epidemiology and Adverse Cardiovascular Risk Profile of Diagnosed Polycystic Ovary Syndrome. *Journal of Clinical Endocrinology & Metabolism* 2006; 91(4): 1357-1363. doi: 10.1210/jc.2005-2430.

14. Boyd R. The World's Leading Medical Journals Don't Write About Racism. That's a Problem. 2021 Apr [cited 2021 Nov 6]; Available from: https://time.com/5956643/medical-journals-health-racism/

15. Byrd W. An American Health Dilemma: A Medical History of African Americans and the Problem of Race: Beginnings to 1900 [Internet]. 2000 [cited 2021 Nov 6]. Available from: www.taylorfrancis.com/books/mono/10.4324/9780203904107/american-health-dilemma-michael-byrd-linda-clayton

16. MBRRACE- UK. Saving Lives, Improving Mothers' Care. 2021 [cited 2021 Nov 6]; Available from: www.npeu.ox.ac.uk/assets/downloads/mbrrace-uk/reports/MBRRACE-UK_Maternal_Report_June_2021_-_FINAL_v10.pdf

17. Knight. Driving policy change to prevent maternal deaths. 2019 [cited 2021 Nov 6]; Available from: www.ox.ac.uk/research/research-impact/driving-policy-change-prevent-maternal-deaths

18. Kar P. Partha Kar: Covid-19 and ethnicity—why are all our angels white? *BMJ* 2020; 369: m1804. doi: 10.1136/bmj.m1804.

19. Hoffman KM, Trawalter S, Axt JR, Oliver MN. Racial bias in pain assessment and treatment recommendations, and false beliefs about biological differences between blacks and whites. *Proceedings of the National Academy of Sciences* 2016; 113(16): 4296-4301. doi.org/10.1073/pnas.1516047113

20. Carlin E, Kramer B. Hair, Hormones, and Haunting: Race as a Ghost Variable in Polycystic Ovary Syndrome. *Science, Technology, & Human Values* 2020; 45(5): 779-803. doi.org/10.1177/0162243920908647

Chapter 10: You are in the driving seat – Lifestyle Medicine

1. WHO. WHO reveals leading causes of death and disability worldwide: 2000-2019. 2020 Dec [cited 2021 Nov 6]; Available from: www.who.int/news/item/09-12-2020-who-reveals-leading-causes-of-death-and-disability-worldwide-2000-2019

2. British Heart Foundation. Women and Heart Disease. [cited 2021 Nov 6]; Available from: www.bhf.org.uk/informationsupport/heart-matters-magazine/medical/women-and-heart-disease

3. Office for National Statistics UK. Leading causes of death, UK: 2001 to 2018. [cited 2021 Nov 6]; Available from: www.ons.gov.uk/peoplepopulationandcommunity/healthandsocialcare/causesofdeath/articles/leadingcausesofdeathuk/2001to2018

4. ACLM. What is Lifestyle Medicine. [cited 2021 Nov 6]; Available from: 3. https://lifestylemedicine.org/What-is-Lifestyle-Medicine

5. GBD 2019 Diseases and Injuries Collaborators: Vos T, Lim SS, Abbafati C, Abbas KM, Abbasi M, Abbasifard M, et al. Global burden of 369 diseases and injuries in 204 countries and territories, 1990–2019: a systematic analysis for the Global Burden of Disease Study 2019. *Lancet* 2020; 396(10258): 1204-1222. doi: 10.1016/S0140-6736(20)30925-9.

6. NHS. Fruit and vegetable intake [Internet]. 2018 [cited 2021 Nov 6]. Available from: http://healthsurvey.hscic.gov.uk/data-visualisation/data-visualisation/explore-the-trends/fruit-vegetables.aspx

7. ACLM. Scientific Evidence. [cited 2021 Nov 6]; Available from: www.lifestylemedicine.org/Scientific-Evidence#Diabetes

8. Hurtado-Barroso S, Trius-Soler M, Lamuela-Raventós RM, Zamora-Ros R. Vegetable and Fruit Consumption and Prognosis Among Cancer Survivors: A Systematic Review and Meta-Analysis of Cohort Studies. *Advances in Nutrition* 2020; 11(6): 1569-1582. doi: 10.1093/advances/nmaa082.

Chapter 11: The domino effect – The six pillars of lifestyle in PCOS

1. National Institute for Health and Care Excellence (NICE). Polycystic Ovary Syndrome Causes [Internet]. 2018 [cited 2021 Nov 4]. Available from: https://cks.nice.org.uk/topics/polycystic-ovary-syndrome/background-information/causes/

2. Royal College of Obstetricians and Gynaecologists. Long-Term Consequences of Polycystic Ovary Syndrome. 2014 [cited 2021 Nov 4]; Available from: www.rcog.org.uk/globalassets/documents/guidelines/gtg_33.pdf

3. Monash University MA. PCOS Evidence-Based guidelines [Internet]. 2018 [cited 2021 Nov 4]. Available from: www.monash.edu/__data/assets/pdf_file/0004/1412644/PCOS_Evidence-Based-Guidelines_20181009.pdf

4. Lim SS, Hutchison SK, van Ryswyk E, Norman RJ, Teede HJ, Moran LJ. Lifestyle changes in women with polycystic ovary syndrome. *Cochrane Database of Systematic Reviews* 2019; 3(3): CD007506. doi: 10.1002/14651858.CD007506.pub4.

5. Moran LJ, Noakes M, Clifton PM, Tomlinson L, Norman RJ. Dietary Composition in Restoring Reproductive and Metabolic Physiology in Overweight Women with Polycystic Ovary Syndrome. *Journal of Clinical Endocrinology & Metabolism* 2003; 88(2): 812-819. doi: 10.1210/jc.2002-020815

6. Gibson-Helm M, Teede H, Dunaif A, Dokras A. Delayed diagnosis and a lack of information associated with dissatisfaction in women with polycystic ovary syndrome. *Journal of Clinical Endocrinology & Metabolism* 2017; 102(2): 604-612. doi: 10.1210/jc.2016-2963.

7. Uusitupa M, Khan TA, Viguiliouk E, Kahleova H, Rivellese AA, Hermansen K, et al. Prevention of Type 2 Diabetes by Lifestyle Changes: A Systematic Review and Meta-Analysis. *Nutrients* 2019; 11(11): 2611. doi: 10.3390/nu11112611

8. ACLM. Scientific Evidence. [cited 2021 Nov 6]; Available from: www.lifestylemedicine.org/Scientific-Evidence#Diabetes

References

9. Loef M, Walach H. The combined effects of healthy lifestyle behaviors on all-cause mortality: A systematic review and meta-analysis. *Preventive Medicine* 2012; 55(3): 163-170. doi: 10.1016/j.ypmed.2012.06.017.

10. Vos T, Lim SS, Abbafati C, Abbas KM, Abbasi M, Abbasifard M, et al. Global burden of 369 diseases and injuries in 204 countries and territories, 1990-2019: a systematic analysis for the Global Burden of Disease Study 2019. *Lancet* 2020; 396(10258): 1204-1222. doi: 10.1016/S0140-6736(20)30925-9.

11. Afshin A, Sur PJ, Fay KA, Cornaby L, Ferrara G, Salama JS, et al. Health effects of dietary risks in 195 countries, 1990-2017: a systematic analysis for the Global Burden of Disease Study 2017. *Lancet* 2019; 393(10184): 1958-1972. doi: 10.1016/S0140-6736(19)30041-8

11a. 2021 Global Nutrition Report: The state of global nutrition. Bristol, UK: Development Initiatives. Nutrition Accountability Framework. Available from: https://globalnutritionreport.org/ [cited 7 February 2022]

12. Hupin D, Roche F, Gremeaux V, Chatard J-C, Oriol M, Gaspoz J-M, et al. Even a low-dose of moderate-to-vigorous physical activity reduces mortality by 22% in adults aged ≥60 years: a systematic review and meta-analysis. *British Journal of Sports Medicine* 2015; 49(19): 1262-1267. doi: 10.1136/bjsports-2014-094306

13. Guthold, R, Stevens GA, Riley LM, Bull FC. Worldwide trends in insufficient physical activity from 2001 to 2016: a pooled analysis of 358 population-based surveys with 1·9 million participants. *The Lancet. Global Health* 2018; 6(10): e1077–e1086. doi.org/10.1016/S2214-109X(18)30357-7

14. Gov.UK. Physical Activity: Ethnicity - Facts and Figures. 2020 [cited 2021 Nov 6]; Available from: www.ethnicity-facts-figures.service.gov.uk/health/diet-and-exercise/physical-activity/latest

15. Patten RK, Boyle RA, Moholdt T, Kiel I, Hopkins WG, Harrison CL, Stepto NK. Exercise Interventions in Polycystic Ovary Syndrome: A Systematic Review and Meta-Analysis. *Frontiers in Physiology* 2020; 11: 606. doi: 10.3389/fphys.2020.00606

16. dos Santos IK, Ashe MC, Cobucci RN, Soares GM, de Oliveira Maranhão TM, Dantas PMS. The effect of exercise as an intervention for women with polycystic ovary syndrome. *Medicine* 2020; 99(16): e19644. doi: 10.1097/MD.0000000000019644.

17. Stepto NK, Patten RK, Tassone EC, Misso ML, Brennan L, Boyle J, et al. Exercise Recommendations for Women with Polycystic Ovary Syndrome: Is the Evidence Enough? *Sports Medicine* 2019; 49(8): 1143-1157. doi: 10.1007/s40279-019-01133-6.

18. Benham JL, Yamamoto JM, Friedenreich CM, Rabi DM, Sigal RJ. Role of exercise training in polycystic ovary syndrome: a systematic review and meta-analysis. *Clinical Obesity* 2018; 8(4): 275-284. doi: 10.1111/cob.12258

19. NHS UK. Physical activity guidelines for adults aged 19 to 64 [Internet]. 2021 [cited 2021 Nov 6]. Available from: www.nhs.uk/live-well/exercise/

20. CDC USA. How much physical activity do adults need? 2020 [cited 2021 Nov 6]; Available from: www.cdc.gov/physicalactivity/basics/adults/index.htm

21. National Institute for Health and Care Excellence (NICE). Insomnia [Internet]. 2021 [cited 2021 Nov 7]. Available from: https://cks.nice.org.uk/topics/insomnia/references/

22. Haugland BSM, Hysing M, Baste V, Wergeland GJ, Rapee RM, Hoffart A, et al. Sleep Duration and Insomnia in Adolescents Seeking Treatment for Anxiety in

Primary Health Care. *Frontiers in Psychology* 2021; 12: 638879. doi: 10.3389/fpsyg.2021.638879

23. Wang Y-H, Wang J, Chen S-H, Li J-Q, Lu Q-D, Vitiello M v., et al. Association of Longitudinal Patterns of Habitual Sleep Duration With Risk of Cardiovascular Events and All-Cause Mortality. *JAMA Network Open* 2020 May 22;3(5): e205246. doi: 10.1001/jamanetworkopen.2020.5246.

24. Jehan S, Zizi F, Pani-Perumal SR, et al. Shift Work and Sleep: Medical Implications and Management. *Sleep Med Disord* 2017; 1(2): 00008. PMID: 29517053

25. Szkiela M, Kusideł E, Makowiec-D'browska T, Kaleta D. Night Shift Work—A Risk Factor for Breast Cancer. *International Journal of Environmental Research and Public Health* 2020; 17(2): 659. doi: 10.3390/ijerph17020659.

26. Pace-Schott EF, Germain A, Milad MR. Effects of sleep on memory for conditioned fear and fear extinction. *Psychological Bulletin* 2015; 141(4): 835-857. doi.org/10.1037/bul0000014

27. Léger D, Poursain B, Neubauer D, Uchiyama M. An international survey of sleeping problems in the general population. *Current Medical Research and Opinion* 2008; 24(1): 307-317. doi: 10.1185/030079907x253771

28. Jehan S, Auguste E, Hussain M, et al. Sleep and premenstrual Syndrome. *J Sleep Med Disord* 2016; 3(5): 1061. PMID: 28239684

29. St-Onge M-P, Mikic A, Pietrolungo CE. Effects of Diet on Sleep Quality. *Advances in Nutrition* 2016; 7(5): 938-949. doi: 10.3945/an.116.012336.

30. Castro-Diehl C, Wood AC, Redline S, Reid M, Johnson DA, Maras JE, et al. Mediterranean diet pattern and sleep duration and insomnia symptoms in the Multi-Ethnic Study of Atherosclerosis. *Sleep* 2018; 41(11): zsy158. doi: 10.1093/sleep/zsy158.

31. Mitchell MD, Gehrman P, Perlis M, Umscheid CA. Comparative effectiveness of cognitive behavioral therapy for insomnia: a systematic review. *BMC Family Practice* 2012; 13(1): 40. doi.org/10.1186/1471-2296-13-40

32. Mental health Foundation UK. Stress and Coping. 2021 [cited 2021 Nov 7]; Available from: www.mentalhealth.org.uk/news/ stressed-nation-74-uk-overwhelmed-or-unable-cope-some-point-past-year

33. Keles B, McCrae N, Grealish A. A systematic review: the influence of social media on depression, anxiety and psychological distress in adolescents. *International Journal of Adolescence and Youth* 2020; 25(1): 79-93. doi: 10.1080/02673843.2019.1590851

34. Seabrook EM, Kern ML, Rickard NS. Social Networking Sites, Depression, and Anxiety: A Systematic Review. *JMIR Mental Health* 2016; 3(4): e50. doi: 10.2196/mental.5842.

35. Patel A, Sharma PSVN, Narayan P, Binu V, Dinesh N, Pai P. Prevalence and predictors of infertility-specific stress in women diagnosed with primary infertility: A clinic-based study. *Journal of Human Reproductive Sciences* 2016; 9(1): 28-34. doi: 10.4103/0974-1208.178630.

36. Papalou O, Diamanti-Kandarakis E. The role of stress in PCOS. *Expert Review of Endocrinology & Metabolism* 2017; 12(1): 87-95. doi: 10.1080/17446651.2017.1266250.

37. Basu BR, Chowdhury O, Saha S. Possible link between stress-related factors and altered body composition in women with polycystic ovarian syndrome. Journal

of Human Reproductive Sciences 2018; 11(1): 10-18.
doi: 10.4103/jhrs.JHRS_78_17

38. Legro RS. Obesity and PCOS: Implications for Diagnosis and Treatment. *Seminars in Reproductive Medicine* 2012; 30(06): 496-506.
doi: 10.1055/s-0032-1328878.

39. Furuyashiki A, Tabuchi K, Norikoshi K, Kobayashi T, Oriyama S. A comparative study of the physiological and psychological effects of forest bathing (Shinrin-yoku) on working age people with and without depressive tendencies. *Environmental Health and Preventive Medicine* 2019; 24(1): 46.
doi: 10.1186/s12199-019-0800-1.

40. Kotera Y, Richardson M, Sheffield D. Effects of Shinrin-Yoku (Forest Bathing) and Nature Therapy on Mental Health: a Systematic Review and Meta-analysis. *International Journal of Mental Health and Addiction* 2020; 28 July.
doi.org/10.1007/s11469-020-00363-4

41. Li Y, Lv M-R, Wei Y-J, Sun L, Zhang J-X, Zhang H-G, Li B. Dietary patterns and depression risk: A meta-analysis. *Psychiatry Research* 2017; 253: 373-382.
doi: 10.1016/j.psychres.2017.04.020.

42. Vajdi M, Farhangi MA. A systematic review of the association between dietary patterns and health-related quality of life. *Health and Quality of Life Outcomes* 2020; 18(1): 337. doi: 10.1186/s12955-020-01581-z.

43. Nucci D, Fatigoni C, Amerio A, Odone A, Gianfredi V. Red and Processed Meat Consumption and Risk of Depression: A Systematic Review and Meta-Analysis. *International Journal of Environmental Research and Public Health* 2020; 17(18): 6686. doi: 10.3390/ijerph17186686.

44. Adjibade M, Julia C, Allès B, Touvier M, Lemogne C, Srour B, et al. Prospective association between ultra-processed food consumption and incident depressive symptoms in the French NutriNet-Santé cohort. *BMC Medicine* 2019; 17(1): 78.
doi: 10.1186/s12916-019-1312-y.

45. Alcohol Change UK. Alcohol in the UK. 2021 [cited 2021 Nov 7]; Available from: https://alcoholchange.org.uk/alcohol-facts/fact-sheets/alcohol-statistics

46. WHO. Alcohol Facts. 2018 [cited 2021 Nov 7]; Available from: www.who.int/news-room/fact-sheets/detail/alcohol

47. American Cancer Society. Known and Probable Human Carcinogens. 2021 [cited 2021 Nov 7]; Available from: www.cancer.org/cancer/cancer-causes/general-info/known-and-probable-human-carcinogens.html

48. Cancer Research UK. How does Smoking Cause Cancer . 2021 Mar [cited 2021 Nov 7]; Available from: www.cancerresearchuk.org/about-cancer/causes-of-cancer/smoking-and-cancer/how-does-smoking-cause-cancer

49. Pau CT, Keefe CC, Welt CK. Cigarette smoking, nicotine levels and increased risk for metabolic syndrome in women with polycystic ovary syndrome. *Gynecological Endocrinology* 2013; 29(6): 551-555.
doi: 10.3109/09513590.2013.788634

50. National Institute for Health and Care Excellence (NICE). Management of PCOS in Adults [Internet]. 2018 [cited 2021 Nov 7]. Available from: https://cks.nice.org.uk/topics/polycystic-ovary-syndrome/management/management-adults/

51. de Angelis C, Nardone A, Garifalos F, Pivonello C, Sansone A, Conforti A, et al. Smoke, alcohol and drug addiction and female fertility. *Reproductive Biology and Endocrinology* 2020; 18(1): 21. doi: 10.1186/s12958-020-0567-7.

52. Gill J. The effects of moderate alcohol consumption on female hormone levels and reproductive function. *Alcohol and Alcoholism* 2000; 35(5): 417-423. doi: 10.1093/alcalc/35.5.417.

53. Chavarro JE, Rich-Edwards JW, Rosner BA, Willett WC. Caffeinated and Alcoholic Beverage Intake in Relation to Ovulatory Disorder Infertility. *Epidemiology* 2009; 20(3): 374-381. doi: 10.1097/EDE.0b013e31819d68cc.

54. Cancer Research UK. Breast Cancer Statistics UK. 2018 [cited 2021 Nov 7]; Available from: www.cancerresearchuk.org/health-professional/cancer-statistics/statistics-by-cancer-type/breast-cancer

55. Park B, Kim J-H, Lee ES, Jung S-Y, Lee SY, Kang H-S, et al. Role of aldehyde dehydrogenases, alcohol dehydrogenase 1B genotype, alcohol consumption, and their combination in breast cancer in East-Asian women. *Scientific Reports* 2020; 10(1): 6564. doi: 10.1038/s41598-020-62361-9.

56. Wise LA, Palmer JR, Harlow BL, et al. Risk of uterine leiomyomata in relation to tobacco, alcohol and caffeine consumption in the Black Women's Health Study. *Human Reproduction* 2004; 19(8): 1746-1754. doi: 10.1093/humrep/deh309.

57. Royal College of Obstetricians and Gynaecologists (RCOG UK). RCOG statement on new research on drinking during pregnancy. 2017 [cited 2021 Nov 7]; Available from: www.rcog.org.uk/en/news/rcog-statement-on-new-research-on-drinking-during-pregnancy/

58. AGE UK. Loneliness and Isolation. 2018 [cited 2021 Nov 7]; Available from: www.ageuk.org.uk/our-impact/policy-research/loneliness-research-and-resources/loneliness-isolation-understanding-the-difference-why-it-matters/

59. Health Resources and Services Administration. The Loneliness Epidemic . 2019 [cited 2021 Nov 7]; Available from: www.hrsa.gov/enews/past-issues/2019/january-17/loneliness-epidemic

60. Harvard University. Loneliness and Cigarette Smoking. 2018 [cited 2021 Nov 7]; Available from: https://sitn.hms.harvard.edu/flash/2018/loneliness-an-epidemic/

61. Xia N, Li H. Loneliness, Social Isolation, and Cardiovascular Health. *Antioxidants & Redox Signaling* 2018; 28(9): 837-851. doi: 10.1089/ars.2017.7312.

62. Williams S, Sheffield D, Knibb RC. 'Everything's from the inside out with PCOS': Exploring women's experiences of living with polycystic ovary syndrome and co-morbidities through SkypeTM interviews. *Health Psychology Open* 2015; 2(2): 2055102915603051. doi: 10.1177/2055102915603051.

63. Lu P, Oh J, Leahy KE, Chopik WJ. Friendship Importance Around the World: Links to Cultural Factors, Health, and Well-Being. *Frontiers in Psychology* 2021; 11: 570839. doi: 10.3389/fpsyg.2020.570839.

Chapter 12: Full of beans – The benefits of plant-based nutrition for PCOS

1. Lally P, van Jaarsveld CHM, Potts HWW, Wardle J. How are habits formed: Modelling habit formation in the real world. *European Journal of Social Psychology* 2010; 40(6): 998-1009. doi.org/10.1002/ejsp.674

2. Hall KD, Kahan S. Maintenance of Lost Weight and Long-Term Management of Obesity. *Medical Clinics of North America* 2018; 102(1): 183-197. doi: 10.1016/j.mcna.2017.08.012.

3. Anderson JW, Konz EC, Frederich RC, Wood CL. Long-term weight-loss maintenance: a meta-analysis of US studies. *American Journal of Clinical Nutrition* 2001; 74(5): 579-584. doi: 10.1093/ajcn/74.5.579.

4. Cao V, Makarem N, Maguire M, Samayoa I, Xi H, Liang C, et al. History of Weight Cycling Is Prospectively Associated With Shorter and Poorer-Quality Sleep and Higher Sleep Apnea Risk in Diverse US Women. *Journal of Cardiovascular Nursing* 2021; 36(6): 573-581.

5. Tomiyama AJ, Mann T, Vinas D, Hunger JM, DeJager J, Taylor SE. Low Calorie Dieting Increases Cortisol. *Psychosomatic Medicine* 2010; 72(4): 357-364. doi: 10.1097/PSY.0b013e3181d9523c.

6. National Insitute of Mental Health USA. Eating Disorders: About More Than Food. 2021 [cited 2021 Nov 7]; Available from: www.nimh.nih.gov/health/publications/eating-disorders

7. Katz DL, Meller S. Can We Say What Diet Is Best for Health? *Annual Review of Public Health* 2014; 35(1): 83-103. doi.org/10.1146/annurev-publhealth-032013-182351

8. ACLM. Scientific Evidence. [cited 2021 Nov 6]; Available from: www.lifestylemedicine.org/Scientific-Evidence#Diabetes

8a. Jenkins D, et al. The effect of a plant-based low-carbohydrate ("Eco-Atkins") diet on body-weight and blood lipid concentrations in hyperlipidemic subjects. *Arch Intern Med* 2009; 169: 1046-1054.

9. Seidelmann SB, Claggett B, Cheng S, Henglin M, Shah A, Steffen LM, et al. Dietary carbohydrate intake and mortality: a prospective cohort study and meta-analysis. *Lancet Public Health* 2018; 3(9): E419-E428. doi.org/10.1016/S2468-2667(18)30135-X

10. Vos T, Lim SS, Abbafati C, Abbas KM, Abbasi M, Abbasifard M, et al. Global burden of 369 diseases and injuries in 204 countries and territories, 1990–2019: a systematic analysis for the Global Burden of Disease Study 2019. *Lancet* 2020; 396(10258): 1204-1222. doi.org/10.1016/S0140-6736(20)30925-9

11. Afshin A, Sur PJ, Fay KA, Cornaby L, Ferrara G, Salama JS, et al. Health effects of dietary risks in 195 countries, 1990–2017: a systematic analysis for the Global Burden of Disease Study 2017. *Lancet* 2019; 393(10184): 1958-1972. doi: 10.1016/S0140-6736(19)30041-8.

12. Kelly J, Karlsen M, Steinke G. Type 2 Diabetes Remission and Lifestyle Medicine: A Position Statement From the American College of Lifestyle Medicine. *American Journal of Lifestyle Medicine* 2020; 14(4): 406-419. doi: 10.1177/1559827620930962.

13. Barnett A. The Nature of Crops: Why Do We Eat So Few of the Edible Plants. 2015 [cited 2021 Nov 7]; Available from: www.newscientist.com/article/mg22730301-400-the-nature-of-crops-why-do-we-eat-so-few-of-the-edible-plants/

14. Buettner D, Skemp S. Blue Zones. *American Journal of Lifestyle Medicine* 2016; 10(5): 318-321. doi: 10.1177/1559827616637066.

15. Kim H, Caulfield LE, Garcia-Larsen V, Steffen LM, Coresh J, Rebholz CM. Plant-Based Diets Are Associated With a Lower Risk of Incident Cardiovascular Disease, Cardiovascular Disease Mortality, and All-Cause Mortality in a General

References

Population of Middle-Aged Adults. *Journal of the American Heart Association* 2019 Aug 20; 8(16): e012865. doi: 10.1161/JAHA.119.012865.

16. Plant-based or vegan diet may be best for keeping type 2 diabetes in check. Science News 30 October 2018 www.sciencedaily.com/releases/2018/10/181030184510.htm Source: Anastasios Toumpanakis, Triece Turnbull, Isaura Alba-Barba. Effectiveness of plant-based diets in promoting well-being in the management of type 2 diabetes: a systematic review. *BMJ Open Diabetes Research & Care* 2018; 6 (1): e000534. doi: 10.1136/bmjdrc-2018-000534

17. Kassam S. Plant-based diets for the prevention and treatment of type 2 diabetes. 2020 [cited 2021 Nov 7]; Available from: https://plantbasedhealthprofessionals.com/plant-based-diets-for-the-prevention-and-treatment-of-type-2-diabetes

18. Rigi S, Mousavi SM, Benisi-Kohansal S, Azadbakht L, Esmaillzadeh A. The association between plant-based dietary patterns and risk of breast cancer: a case–control study. *Scientific Reports* 2021; 11(1): 3391. doi: 10.1038/s41598-021-82659-6.

19. McMacken M. A plant-based diet for the prevention and treatment of type 2 diabetes. Journal of Geriartric Cardiology [Internet]. 2017 May [cited 2021 Nov 6]; Available from: www.ncbi.nlm.nih.gov/pmc/articles/PMC5466941/

20. Kim H, Rebholz CM, Hegde S, LaFiura C, Raghavan M, Lloyd JF, et al. Plant-based diets, pescatarian diets and COVID-19 severity: a population-based case–control study in six countries. *BMJ Nutrition, Prevention & Health* 2021 Jun; 4(1). doi:10.1136/bmjnph-2021-000272

21. CDC USA. Leading Causes of Death. 2021 Oct [cited 2021 Nov 7]; Available from: www.cdc.gov/nchs/fastats/leading-causes-of-death.htm

22. Tan BL, Norhaizan ME, Liew W-P-P. Nutrients and Oxidative Stress: Friend or Foe? *Oxidative Medicine and Cellular Longevity* 2018; 2018: 9719584. doi: 10.1155/2018/9719584.

23. Nurses Health Study. 2016 [cited 2021 Nov 7]; Available from: https://nurseshealthstudy.org/

24. Fung TT, van Dam RM, Hankinson SE, et al. Low-Carbohydrate Diets and All-Cause and Cause-Specific Mortality: two cohort studies. *Annals of Internal Medicine* 2010; 153(5): 289-298. doi: 10.7326/0003-4819-153-5-201009070-00003.

25. AlEssa HB, Cohen R, Malik VS, Adebamowo SN, Rimm EB, Manson JE, et al. Carbohydrate quality and quantity and risk of coronary heart disease among US women and men. *American Journal of Clinical Nutrition* 2018; 107(2): 257-267. doi: 10.1093/ajcn/nqx060.

26. Ho FK, Gray SR, Welsh P, Petermann-Rocha F, Foster H, Waddell H, et al. Associations of fat and carbohydrate intake with cardiovascular disease and mortality: prospective cohort study of UK Biobank participants. *Br Med J* 2020; 368: m688. doi: 10.1136/bmj.m688.

27. Moran LJ, Noakes M, Clifton PM, Tomlinson L, Norman RJ. Dietary Composition in Restoring Reproductive and Metabolic Physiology in Overweight Women with Polycystic Ovary Syndrome. *Journal of Clinical Endocrinology & Metabolism* 2003; 88(2): 812-819. doi: 10.1210/jc.2002-020815.

28. Larsson SC, Wallin A, Wolk A. Dietary Approaches to Stop Hypertension Diet and Incidence of Stroke. *Stroke* 2016; 47(4): 986-990. doi: 10.1161/STROKEAHA.116.012675

References

29. Asemi Z, Esmaillzadeh A. DASH Diet, Insulin Resistance, and Serum hs-CRP in Polycystic Ovary Syndrome: A Randomized Controlled Clinical Trial. *Hormone and Metabolic Research* 2014; 47(03): 232-238. doi: 10.1055/s-0034-1376990

30. Moran LJ, Hutchison SK, Norman RJ, Teede HJ. Lifestyle changes in women with Polycystic Ovary Syndrome. *Cochrane Database of Systematic Reviews* 2011; 16(2): CD007506. doi: 10.1002/14651858.CD007506.pub2.

31. Wright N, Wilson L, Smith M, Duncan B, McHugh P. The BROAD study: A randomised controlled trial using a whole food plant-based diet in the community for obesity, ischaemic heart disease or diabetes. *Nutrition & Diabetes* 2017; 7(3): e256. doi: 10.1038/nutd.2017.3.

32. Karamali M, Kashanian M, Alaeinasab S, Asemi Z. The effect of dietary soy intake on weight loss, glycaemic control, lipid profiles and biomarkers of inflammation and oxidative stress in women with polycystic ovary syndrome: a randomised clinical trial. *Journal of Human Nutrition and Dietetics* 2018; 31(4): 533-543. doi: 10.1111/jhn.12545.

33. Turner-McGrievy GM, Davidson CR, Wingard EE, Billings DL. Low glycemic index vegan or low-calorie weight loss diets for women with polycystic ovary syndrome: a randomized controlled feasibility study. *Nutrition Research* 2014; 34(6): 552-558. doi: 10.1016/j.nutres.2014.04.011.

34. Faghfoori Z, Fazelian S, Shadnoush M, Goodarzi R. Nutritional management in women with polycystic ovary syndrome: A review study. *Diabetes & Metabolic Syndrome: Clinical Research & Reviews* 2017; 11(S1): S429-S432. doi: 10.1016/j.dsx.2017.03.030.

35. Barnard ND, Scialli AR, Hurlock D, Bertron P. Diet and sex-hormone binding globulin, dysmenorrhea, and premenstrual symptoms. *Obstetrics & Gynecology* 2000; 95(2): 245-250. doi: 10.1016/s0029-7844(99)00525-6.

36. Tantalaki E, Piperi C, Livadas S, Kollias A, Adamopoulos C, Koulouri A, et al. Impact of dietary modification of advanced glycation end products (AGEs) on the hormonal and metabolic profile of women with polycystic ovary syndrome (PCOS). *Hormones* 2014; 13(1): 65-73. doi: 10.1007/BF03401321.

37. Kudesia R, Alexander M, Gulati M, Kennard A, Tollefson M. Dietary Approaches to Women's Sexual and Reproductive Health. *American Journal of Lifestyle Medicine* 2021; 15(4): 414-424. doi: 10.1177/15598276211007113.

38. Yang Y, Zhao L-G, Wu Q-J, Ma X, Xiang Y-B. Association Between Dietary Fiber and Lower Risk of All-Cause Mortality: A Meta-Analysis of Cohort Studies. *American Journal of Epidemiology* 2015; 181(2): 83-91. doi: 10.1093/aje/kwu257.

39. Eslamian G, Baghestani A-R, Eghtesad S, Hekmatdoost A. Dietary carbohydrate composition is associated with polycystic ovary syndrome: a case-control study. *Journal of Human Nutrition and Dietetics* 2017; 30(1): 90-97. doi: 10.1111/jhn.12388

40. Merhi Z. Advanced glycation end products and their relevance in female reproduction. *Human Reproduction* 2014; 29(1): 134-145. doi: 10.1093/humrep/det383

41. Gibson R, Eriksen R, Chambers E, Gao H, Aresu M, Heard A, et al. Intakes and Food Sources of Dietary Fibre and Their Associations with Measures of Body Composition and Inflammation in UK Adults: Cross-Sectional Analysis of the Airwave Health Monitoring Study. *Nutrients* 2019; 11(8): 1839. doi: 10.3390/nu11081839.

42. British Dietetic Association. Fibre Food Fact Sheet. 2021 Apr [cited 2021 Nov 7]; Available from: www.bda.uk.com/resource/fibre.html

43. Leach JD. Evolutionary perspective on dietary intake of fibre and colorectal cancer. *European Journal of Clinical Nutrition* 2007; 61(1): 140-142. doi.org/10.1038/sj.ejcn.1602486

44. Monteiro CA, Moubarac J-C, Levy RB, Canella DS, Louzada ML da C, Cannon G. Household availability of ultra-processed foods and obesity in nineteen European countries. *Public Health Nutrition* 2018; 21(1): 18-26. doi: 10.1017/S1368980017001379

45. McDonald P. Colorectal quotations. *Journal of the Royal Society of Medicine* 2005; 98(2): 77-78. doi: 10.1258/jrsm.98.2.77

46. Zhang B, Shen S, Bi Y, Zhu D. Gut Microbiota as a Potential Target for Treatment of Polycystic Ovary Syndrome. *Diabetes* 2018; 67(Supplement 1).

47. Gorbach SL, Goldin BR. Diet and the excretion and enterohepatic cycling of estrogens. *Preventive Medicine* 1987l; 16(4): 525-531. doi: 10.1016/0091-7435(87)90067-3.

48. Madigan M, Karhu E. The role of plant-based nutrition in cancer prevention. *Journal of Unexplored Medical Data* 2018; 3(11): 9. doi: 10.20517/2572-8180.2018.05

49. Nybacka Å, Hellström PM, Hirschberg AL. Increased fibre and reduced trans fatty acid intake are primary predictors of metabolic improvement in overweight polycystic ovary syndrome-Substudy of randomized trial between diet, exercise and diet plus exercise for weight control. *Clinical Endocrinology* 2017; 87(6): 680-688. doi: 10.1111/cen.13427.

50. Szabo Z, Koczka V, Marosvolgyi T, Szabo E, Frank E, Polyak E, et al. Possible Biochemical Processes Underlying the Positive Health Effects of Plant-Based Diets—A Narrative Review. *Nutrients* 2021; 13(8): 2593. doi: 10.3390/nu13082593

51. Song M, Fung TT, Hu FB, Willett WC, Longo VD, Chan AT, et al. Association of Animal and Plant Protein Intake With All-Cause and Cause-Specific Mortality. *JAMA Internal Medicine* 2016; 176(10): 1453-1463. doi: 10.1001/jamainternmed.2016.4182.

52. Carmina E, Legro RS, Stamets K, Lowell J, Lobo RA. Difference in body weight between American and Italian women with polycystic ovary syndrome: influence of the diet. *Human Reproduction* 2003; 18(11): 2289-2293. doi: 10.1093/humrep/deg440.

53. Merhi Z, Kandaraki EA, Diamanti-Kandarakis E. Implications and Future Perspectives of AGEs in PCOS Pathophysiology. *Trends in Endocrinology & Metabolism* 2019; 30(3): 150-162. doi: 10.1016/j.tem.2019.01.005

54. Garg D, Merhi Z. Advanced Glycation End Products: Link between Diet and Ovulatory Dysfunction in PCOS? *Nutrients* 2015; 7(12): 10129-10144. doi: 10.3390/nu7125524

55. Liao Y, Huang R, Sun Y, Yue J, Zheng J, Wang L, et al. An inverse association between serum soluble receptor of advanced glycation end products and hyperandrogenism and potential implication in polycystic ovary syndrome patients. *Reproductive Biology and Endocrinology* 2017; 15(1): 9. doi.org/10.1186/s12958-017-0227-8

56. Uribarri J, Woodruff S, Goodman S, Cai W, Chen X, Pyzik R, et al. Advanced Glycation End Products in Foods and a Practical Guide to Their Reduction in

the Diet. *Journal of the American Dietetic Association* 2010; 110(6): 911-916.e12. doi: 10.1016/j.jada.2010.03.018

57. Scheijen JLJM, Clevers E, Engelen L, Dagnelie PC, Brouns F, Stehouwer CDA, et al. Analysis of advanced glycation endproducts in selected food items by ultra-performance liquid chromatography tandem mass spectrometry: Presentation of a dietary AGE database. *Food Chemistry* 2016; 190: 1145-1150. doi: 10.1016/j.foodchem.2015.06.049.

Chapter 13: You cannot meditate away a broken leg – Lifestyle Medicine complements conventional medicine

1. Gaynes R. The Discovery of Penicillin—New Insights After More Than 75 Years of Clinical Use. Emerging Infectious Diseases. 2017 May;23(5): 849-853. doi: 10.3201/eid2305.161556

2. Loudon I. Ignaz Phillip Semmelweis' studies of death in childbirth. Journal of the Royal Society of Medicine. 2013 Nov 24;106(11): 461-463. doi: 10.1177/0141076813507844

3. Callaway E, Ledford H, Viglione G, Watson T, Witze A. COVID and 2020: An extraordinary year for science. *Nature* 2020; 588(7839): 550-552. doi: 10.1038/d41586-020-03437-4. www.nature.com/immersive/d41586-020-03437-4/index.html

4. Schindler AE. Non-Contraceptive Benefits of Oral Hormonal Contraceptives. *International Journal of Endocrinology and Metabolism* 2012; 11(1): 41-47. doi: 10.5812/ijem.4158

5. Collaborative Group on Epidemiological Studies on Endometrial Cancer. Endometrial cancer and oral contraceptives: an individual participant meta-analysis of 27 276 women with endometrial cancer from 36 epidemiological studies. *Lancet Oncology* 2015; 16(9): 1061-1070. doi: 10.1016/S1470-2045(15)00212-0.

6. Cancer Research UK. Does the Contraceptive Pill Increase cancer Risk? 24 March 2021 [cited 2021 Nov 7]; Available from: www.cancerresearchuk.org/about-cancer/causes-of-cancer/hormones-and-cancer/does-the-contraceptive-pill-increase-cancer-risk

7. Barbieri R, Ehrmann DA. Patient education: Polycystic Ovary Syndrome (PCOS) (Beyond the Basics). Up To Date [Internet]. 12 May 2021 [cited 2021 Nov 7]; Available from: www.uptodate.com/contents/polycystic-ovary-syndrome-pcos-beyond-the-basics

Chapter 14: When your periods go missing – Periods in PCOS

1. Shufelt C, Torbati T, Dutra E. Hypothalamic Amenorrhea and the Long-Term Health Consequences. *Seminars in Reproductive Medicine* 2017; 35(3): 256-262. doi: 10.1055/s-0037-1603581
2. Rosenfield RL, Ehrmann DA. The Pathogenesis of Polycystic Ovary Syndrome (PCOS): The Hypothesis of PCOS as Functional Ovarian Hyperandrogenism Revisited. *Endocrine Reviews* 2016; 37(5): 467-529. doi: 10.1210/er.2015-1104
3. Monash University MA. PCOS Evidence-Based guidelines [Internet]. 2018 [cited 2021 Nov 4]. Available from: www.monash.edu/__data/assets/pdf_file/0004/1412644/PCOS_Evidence-Based-Guidelines_20181009.pdf
4. Magnay JL, O'Brien S, Gerlinger C, Seitz C. A systematic review of methods to measure menstrual blood loss. *BMC Women's Health* 2018; 18(1): 142. doi: 10.1186/s12905-018-0627-8
5. Schoep ME, Adang EMM, Maas JWM, de Bie B, Aarts JWM, Nieboer TE. Productivity loss due to menstruation-related symptoms: a nationwide cross-sectional survey among 32 748 women. *BMJ Open* 2019; 9(6): e026186. doi: 10.1136/bmjopen-2018-026186.
6. Jeong JY, Kim MK, Lee I, Yun J, Won Y bin, Yun BH, et al. Polycystic ovarian morphology is associated with primary dysmenorrhea in young Korean women. *Obstetrics & Gynecology Science* 2019; 62(5): 329-334. doi: 10.5468/ogs.2019.62.5.329
7. Hager M, Wenzl R, Riesenhuber S, Marschalek J, Kuessel L, Mayrhofer D, et al. The Prevalence of Incidental Endometriosis in Women Undergoing Laparoscopic Ovarian Drilling for Clomiphene-Resistant Polycystic Ovary Syndrome: A Retrospective Cohort Study and Meta-Analysis. *Journal of Clinical Medicine* 2019; 8(8): 1210. doi: 10.3390/jcm8081210
8. Barnard ND, Scialli AR, Hurlock D, Bertron P. Diet and sex-hormone binding globulin, dysmenorrhea, and premenstrual symptoms. *Obstetrics & Gynecology* 2000; 95(2): 245-250. doi: 10.1016/s0029-7844(99)00525-6
9. Kiddy DS, Hamilton-Fairley D, Bush A, Short F, Anyaoku V, Reed MJ, Franks Sl. Improvement in endocrine and ovarian function during dietary treatment of obese women with polycystic ovary syndrome. *Clinical Endocrinology* 1992; 36(1): 105-111. doi: 10.1111/j.1365-2265.1992.tb02909.x
10. Huber-Buchholz M-M, Carey DGP, Norman RJ. Restoration of Reproductive Potential by Lifestyle Modification in Obese Polycystic Ovary Syndrome: Role of Insulin Sensitivity and Luteinizing Hormone1. *Journal of Clinical Endocrinology & Metabolism* 1999; 84(4): 1470-1474. doi: 10.1210/jcem.84.4.5596.
11. Sakkas H, Bozidis P, Touzios C, Kolios D, Athanasiou G, Athanasopoulou E, et al. Nutritional Status and the Influence of the Vegan Diet on the Gut Microbiota and Human Health. *Medicina* 2020; 56(2): 88. doi: 10.3390/medicina56020088
12. Hooda J, Shah A, Zhang L. Heme, an Essential Nutrient from Dietary Proteins, Critically Impacts Diverse Physiological and Pathological Processes. *Nutrients* 2014; 6(3): 1080-1102. doi: 10.3390/nu6031080
13. Kaluza J, Wolk A, Larsson SC. Heme Iron Intake and Risk of Stroke. Stroke: a prospective study of men. *Stroke* 2013; 44(2): 334-339. doi: 10.1161/STROKEAHA.112.679662.

14. Karamali M, Kashanian M, Alaeinasab S, Asemi Z. The effect of dietary soy intake on weight loss, glycaemic control, lipid profiles and biomarkers of inflammation and oxidative stress in women with polycystic ovary syndrome: a randomised clinical trial. *Journal of Human Nutrition and Dietetics* 2018; 31(4): 533-543. doi: 10.1111/jhn.12545.

15. Chen CX, Barrett B, Kwekkeboom KL. Efficacy of Oral Ginger (Zingiber officinale) for Dysmenorrhea: A Systematic Review and Meta-Analysis. *Evidence-Based Complementary and Alternative Medicine* 2016; 2016: 6295737. doi.org/10.1155/2016/6295737

16. Rad HA, Basirat Z, Bakouei F, Moghadamnia AA, Khafri S, Farhadi Kotenaei ZF, et al. Effect of Ginger and Novafen on menstrual pain: A cross-over trial. *Taiwanese Journal of Obstetrics and Gynecology* 2018; 57(6): 806-809. doi: 10.1016/j.tjog.2018.10.006.

17. Kashefi F, Khajehei M, Alavinia M, Golmakani E, Asili J. Effect of Ginger (Zingiber officinale) on Heavy Menstrual Bleeding: A Placebo-Controlled, Randomized Clinical Trial. *Phytotherapy Research* 2015; 29(1): 114-119. doi: 10.1002/ptr.5235

Chapter 15: Getting pregnant – Fertility, preconception and pregnancy in PCOS

1. Monash University MA. PCOS Evidence-Based Guidelines [Internet]. 2018 [cited 2021 Nov 4]. Available from: www.monash.edu/__data/assets/pdf_file/0004/1412644/PCOS_Evidence-Based-Guidelines_20181009.pdf

2. Balen AH, Morley LC, Misso M, Franks S, Legro RS, Wijeyaratne CN, et al. The management of anovulatory infertility in women with polycystic ovary syndrome: an analysis of the evidence to support the development of global WHO guidance. *Human Reproduction Update* 2016; 22(6): 687-708. doi: 10.1093/humupd/dmw025.

3. Datta J, Palmer MJ, Tanton C, Gibson LJ, Jones KG, Macdowall W, et al. Prevalence of infertility and help seeking among 15 000 women and men. *Human Reproduction* 2016; 31(9): 2108-2118. doi: 10.1093/humrep/dew123.

4. Singla R, Gupta Y, Khemani M, Aggarwal S. Thyroid disorders and polycystic ovary syndrome: An emerging relationship. *Indian Journal of Endocrinology and Metabolism* 2015; 19(1): 25-29. doi: 10.4103/2230-8210.146860

5. Ulrich J, Goerges J, Keck C, Müller-Wieland D, Diederich S, Janssen OE. Impact of Autoimmune Thyroiditis on Reproductive and Metabolic Parameters in Patients with Polycystic Ovary Syndrome. *Experimental and Clinical Endocrinology & Diabetes* 2018; 126(04): 198-204. doi: 10.1055/s-0043-110480

6. Kim CH, Chon SJ, Lee SH. Effects of lifestyle modification in polycystic ovary syndrome compared to metformin only or metformin addition: A systematic review and meta-analysis. *Scientific Reports* 2020; 10(1): 7802. doi: 10.1038/s41598-020-64776-w

7. Palomba S, Falbo A, Orio F, Zullo F. Effect of preconceptional metformin on abortion risk in polycystic ovary syndrome: a systematic review and meta-analysis of randomized controlled trials. *Fertility and Sterility* 2009; 92(5): 1646-1658. doi: 10.1016/j.fertnstert.2008.08.087

References

8. Vanky E, Stridsklev S, Heimstad R, Romundstad P, Skogøy K, Kleggetveit O, et al. Metformin versus Placebo from First Trimester to Delivery in Polycystic Ovary Syndrome: A Randomized, Controlled Multicenter Study. *Journal of Clinical Endocrinology & Metabolism* 2010; 95(12): E448-E455. doi: 10.1210/jc.2010-0853

9. Barbieri R. Metformin for treatment of PCOS. *Up To Date* [Internet]. 2021 [cited 2021 Nov 8]; Available from: www.uptodate.com/contents/metformin-for-treatment-of-the-polycystic-ovary-syndrome

10. Hutchison JC, Truong TT, Salamonsen LA, Gardner DK, Evans J. Advanced glycation end products present in the obese uterine environment compromise preimplantation embryo development. *Reproductive BioMedicine Online* 2020; 41(5): 757-766. doi: 10.1016/j.rbmo.2020.07.026.

11. Rausch ME, Legro RS, Barnhart HX, Schlaff WD, Carr BR, Diamond MP, et al. Predictors of Pregnancy in Women with Polycystic Ovary Syndrome. *Journal of Clinical Endocrinology & Metabolism* 2009; 94(9): 3458-3466. doi: 10.1210/jc.2009-0545.

12. Balen AH, Rutherford AJ. Managing anovulatory infertility and polycystic ovary syndrome. *BMJ* 2007; 335(7621): 663-666. doi: 10.1136/bmj.39335.462303.80

13. Melo AS, Ferriani RA, Navarro PA. Treatment of infertility in women with polycystic ovary syndrome: approach to clinical practice. *Clinics* 2015; 70(11): 765-769. doi: 10.6061/clinics/2015(11)09.

14. Wu J, Chen D, Liu N. Effectiveness of acupuncture in polycystic ovary syndrome. *Medicine* 2020; 99(22): e20441. doi: 10.1097/MD.0000000000020441.

15. Vulpoi C, Lecomte C, Guilloteau D, Lecomte P. Ageing and reproduction: is polycystic ovary syndrome an exception? *Annales d'Endocrinologie* 2007; 68(1): 45-50. doi: 10.1016/j.ando.2006.12.005.

16. Li J, Liu X, Hu L, Zhang F, Wang F, Kong H, et al. A Slower Age-Related Decline in Treatment Outcomes After the First Ovarian Stimulation for in vitro Fertilization in Women with Polycystic Ovary Syndrome. *Frontiers in Endocrinology* 2019; 10: 834. doi.org/10.3389/fendo.2019.00834

17. Weghofer A, Munne S, Chen S, Barad D, Gleicher N. Lack of association between polycystic ovary syndrome and embryonic aneuploidy. *Fertility and Sterility* 2007; 88(4): 900-905. doi: 10.1016/j.fertnstert.2006.12.018

18. Royal College of Obstetricians and Gynaecologists (RCOG UK). RCOG statement on new research on drinking during pregnancy. 2017 [cited 2021 Nov 7]; Available from: www.rcog.org.uk/en/news/rcog-statement-on-new-research-on-drinking-during-pregnancy/

19. Royal College of Obstetricians and Gynaecologists (RCOG UK). Alcohol and Pregnancy. 2018 Jan [cited 2021 Nov 8]; Available from: www.rcog.org.uk/en/patients/patient-leaflets/alcohol-and-pregnancy/

20. Royal College of Obstetricians and Gynaecologists (RCOG UK). Healthy eating and vitamin supplements in pregnancy. 2014 Oct [cited 2021 Nov 8]; Available from: www.rcog.org.uk/globalassets/documents/patients/patient-information-leaflets/pregnancy/pi-healthy-eating-and-vitamin-supplements-in-pregnancy.pdf

21. Royal College of Obstetricians and Gynaecologists (RCOG UK). New research suggests caffeine raises stillbirth risk in pregnancy. 2020 Nov [cited 2021 Nov 8]; Available from: www.rcog.org.uk/en/news/new-research-suggests-caffeine-raises-stillbirth-risk-in-pregnancy/

References

22. Heazell AEP, Timms K, Scott RE, Rockliffe L, Budd J, Li M, et al. Associations between consumption of coffee and caffeinated soft drinks and late stillbirth—Findings from the Midland and North of England stillbirth case-control study. *European Journal of Obstetrics & Gynecology and Reproductive Biology* 2021; 256: 471-477. doi: 10.1016/j.ejogrb.2020.10.012

23. Pasquali R, Gambineri A, Cavazza C, Ibarra Gasparini D, Ciampaglia W, Cognigni GE, et al. Heterogeneity in the responsiveness to long-term lifestyle intervention and predictability in obese women with polycystic ovary syndrome. *European Journal of Endocrinology* 2011; 164(1): 53-60. doi: 10.1530/EJE-10-0692

24. Katib A. Mechanisms linking obesity with male infertility. *Central European Journal of Urology* 2015; 68(1): 79-85. doi: 10.5173/ceju.2015.01.435

25. McDiarmid MA, Gardiner PM, Jack BW. The clinical content of preconception care: environmental exposures. *American Journal of Obstetrics and Gynecology* 2008; 199(6 Suppl 2): S357-361. doi: 10.1016/j.ajog.2008.10.044

26. Sackey JB-MD. The preconception office visit [Internet]. UpToDate. [cited 2021 Nov 12]. Available from: www.uptodate.com/contents/the-preconception-office-visit

27. Royal College of Obstetricians and Gynaecologists (RCOG UK). Healthy eating and vitamin supplements in pregnancy [Internet]. 2014 [cited 2021 Nov 12]. Available from: www.rcog.org.uk/globalassets/documents/patients/patient-information-leaflets/pregnancy/pi-healthy-eating-and-vitamin-supplements-in-pregnancy.pdf

28. Tsarna E, Reedijk M, Birks LE, Guxens M, Ballester F, Ha M, et al. Associations of Maternal Cell-Phone Use During Pregnancy With Pregnancy Duration and Fetal Growth in 4 Birth Cohorts. *American Journal of Epidemiology* 2019; 188(7): 1270-1280. doi: 10.1093/aje/kwz092

29. Higgins JA, Carpenter E, Everett BG, Greene MZ, Haider S, Hendrick CE. Sexual Minority Women and Contraceptive Use: Complex Pathways Between Sexual Orientation and Health Outcomes. *American Journal of Public Health* 2019; 109(12): 1680-1686. doi: 10.2105/AJPH.2019.305211

30. Palomba S, Falbo A, Chiossi G, Orio F, Tolino A, Colao A, et al. Low-Grade Chronic Inflammation in Pregnant Women With Polycystic Ovary Syndrome: A Prospective Controlled Clinical Study. *Journal of Clinical Endocrinology & Metabolism* 2014; 99(8): 2942-2951. doi: 10.1210/jc.2014-1214

31. Qin JZ, Pang LH, Li MJ, Fan XJ, Huang RD, Chen HY. Obstetric complications in women with polycystic ovary syndrome: a systematic review and meta-analysis. *Reproductive Biology and Endocrinology* 2013; 11(1): 56. doi: 10.1186/1477-7827-11-56.

32. National Institute for Health and Care Excellence (NICE). Management of PCOS in Adults [Internet]. 2018 [cited 2021 Nov 7]. Available from: https://cks.nice.org.uk/topics/polycystic-ovary-syndrome/management/management-adults/

33. National Institute for Health and Care Excellence (NICE). Fertility: Assessment and treatment of people with fertility problems [Internet]. 2013 [cited 2021 Nov 8]. Available from: www.nice.org.uk/guidance/cg156/evidence/full-guideline-pdf-188539453

34. Barbieri R. Polycystic Ovary Syndrome. *Up To Date* [Internet]. 2021 [cited 2021 Nov 7]; Available from: www.uptodate.com/contents/polycystic-ovary-syndrome-pcos-beyond-the-basics

35. British Dietetic Association. Vegetarian, vegan and plant-based diet: Food Fact Sheet. 2021 Apr [cited 2021 Nov 8]; Available from: www.bda.uk.com/resource/vegetarian-vegan-plant-based-diet.html
36. American Dietetic Association. Position of the American Dietetic Association: Vegetarian Diets. Journal of the American Dietetic Association. 2009 Jul;109(7).
37. Melina V, Craig W, Levin S. Position of the Academy of Nutrition and Dietetics: Vegetarian Diets. *Journal of the Academy of Nutrition and Dietetics* 2016; 116(12): 1970-1980. doi: 10.1016/j.jand.2016.09.025
38. Joham AE, Ranasinha S, Zoungas S, Moran L, Teede HJ. Gestational Diabetes and Type 2 Diabetes in Reproductive-Aged Women With Polycystic Ovary Syndrome. Journal of Clinical Endocrinology & Metabolism 2014; 99(3): E447-E452. doi: 10.1210/jc.2013-2007
38a. Alur-Gupta S, et al. Postpartum complications increased in women with polycystic ovary syndrome. *Am J Obstet Gynecol* 2021; 224(3): 280.e1-280.e13. doi: 10.1016/j.ajog.2020.08.048.
38b. Tay CT, et al Perinatal Mental Health in Women with Polycystic Ovary Syndrome: A Cross-Sectional Analysis of an Australian Population-Based Cohort. *J Clin Med* 2019; 8(12): 2070. doi: 10.3390/jcm8122070.
38c. Koric A, et al Polycystic ovary syndrome and postpartum depression symptoms: a population-based cohort study. *Am J Obstet Gynecol* 2021; 224(6): 591.e1-591.e12. doi: 10.1016/j.ajog.2020.12.1215.
39. Royal College of Obstetricians and Gynaecologists. Long-Term Consequences of Polycystic ovary syndrome. 2014 [cited 2021 Nov 4]; Available from: www.rcog.org.uk/globalassets/documents/guidelines/gtg_33.pdf
40. Durnwald C, Nathan DM, Werner EF, Barss VA. Gestational diabetes mellitus: Glycemic control and maternal prognosis. *UpToDate* 2021 Sep. Available from: www.uptodate.com/contents/gestational-diabetes-mellitus-glycemic-control-and-maternal-prognosis
41. Lo JC, Yang J, Gunderson EP, Hararah MK, Gonzalez JR, Ferrara A. Risk of Type 2 Diabetes Mellitus following Gestational Diabetes Pregnancy in Women with Polycystic Ovary Syndrome. *Journal of Diabetes Research* 2017; 2017: 5250162. doi: 10.1155/2017/5250162
42. Perak AM, Lancki N, Kuang A, Labarthe DR, Allen NB, Shah SH, et al. Associations of Maternal Cardiovascular Health in Pregnancy With Offspring Cardiovascular Health in Early Adolescence. *JAMA* 2021; 325(7): 658-668. doi: 10.1001/jama.2021.0247
43. ACLM. Scientific Evidence. [cited 2021 Nov 6]; Available from: www.lifestylemedicine.org/Scientific-Evidence#Diabetes
44. McMacken M. A plant-based diet for the prevention and treatment of type 2 diabetes. Journal of Geriartric Cardiology [Internet]. 2017 May [cited 2021 Nov 6]; Available from: www.ncbi.nlm.nih.gov/pmc/articles/PMC5466941/

Chapter 16: Spot the symptom – Acne

1. Graber E. Acne vulgaris: Overview of management [Internet]. UpToDate. [cited 2021 Nov 12]. Available from: www.uptodate.com/contents/acne-vulgaris-overview-of-management

References

2. Thiboutot DZA. Pathogenesis, clinical manifestations, and diagnosis of acne vulgaris [Internet]. UpToDate. [cited 2021 Nov 12]. Available from: www.uptodate.com/contents/pathogenesis-clinical-manifestations-and-diagnosis-of-acne-vulgaris

3. Reszko ABD. Postadolescent acne in women [Internet]. UpToDate. [cited 2021 Nov 12]. Available from: www.uptodate.com/contents/postadolescent-acne-in-women

4. Spencer EH, Ferdowsian HR, Barnard ND. Diet and acne: a review of the evidence. *International Journal of Dermatology* 2009; 48(4): 339-347. doi: 10.1111/j.1365-4632.2009.04002.x.

5. Gainder S, Sharma B. Update on Management of Polycystic Ovarian Syndrome for Dermatologists. *Indian Dermatology Online Journal* 2019; 10(2): 97–105. doi: 10.4103/idoj.IDOJ_249_17

6. Özdemir S, Özdemir M, Gorkemli H, Kiyici A, Bodur S. Specific dermatologic features of the polycystic ovary syndrome and its association with biochemical markers of the metabolic syndrome and hyperandrogenism. *Acta Obstetricia et Gynecologica Scandinavica* 2010; 89(2): 199–204. doi: 10.3109/00016340903353284

7. Degitz K, Placzek M, Borelli C, Plewig G. Pathophysiology of acne. *J Dtsch Dermatol Ges* 2007; 5(4): 316-323. doi: 10.1111/j.1610-0387.2007.06274.x.

8. Smith RN, Mann NJ, Braue A, Mäkeläinen H, Varigos GA. A low-glycemic-load diet improves symptoms in acne vulgaris patients: a randomized controlled trial. *American Journal of Clinical Nutrition* 2007; 86(1): 107-115. doi: 10.1093/ajcn/86.1.107

9. Rausch ME, Legro RS, Barnhart HX, Schlaff WD, Carr BR, Diamond MP, et al. Predictors of Pregnancy in Women with Polycystic Ovary Syndrome. *Journal of Clinical Endocrinology & Metabolism* 2009; 94(9): 3458-3466. doi: 10.1210/jc.2009-0545

10. Lee YB, Byun EJ, Kim HS. Potential Role of the Microbiome in Acne: A Comprehensive Review. *Journal of Clinical Medicine* 2019; 8(7): 987. doi: 10.3390/jcm8070987

11. O'Neill CA, Monteleone G, McLaughlin JT, Paus R. The gut-skin axis in health and disease: A paradigm with therapeutic implications. *BioEssays* 2016; 38(11): 1167-1176. doi: 10.1002/bies.201600008

12. Bowe WP, Logan AC. Acne vulgaris, probiotics and the gut-brain-skin axis - back to the future? *Gut Pathogens* 2011; 3: 1. doi: 10.1186/1757-4749-3-1

13. Kumar S, Mahajan BB, Kamra N. Future perspective of probiotics in dermatology: an old wine in new bottle. *Dermatology Online Journal* 2014; 20(9): 13030/qt8br333fc. PMID: 25244173

14. Solway J, McBride M, Haq F, Abdul W, Miller R. Diet and Dermatology: The Role of a Whole-food, Plant-based Diet in Preventing and Reversing Skin Aging-A Review. *Journal of Clinical and Aesthetic Dermatology* 2020; 13(5): 38-43. PMC7380694

15. Messina M. Soy and Health Update: Evaluation of the Clinical and Epidemiologic Literature. *Nutrients* 2016; 8(12): 754. doi: 10.3390/nu8120754

16. Adebamowo CA, Spiegelman D, Danby FW, Frazier AL, Willett WC, Holmes MD. High school dietary dairy intake and teenage acne. *Journal of the American Academy of Dermatology* 2005; 52(2): 207-214. doi: 10.1016/j.jaad.2004.08.007

17. Solway J, McBride M, Haq F, Abdul W, Miller R. Diet and Dermatology: The Role of a Whole-food, Plant-based Diet in Preventing and Reversing Skin Aging-A Review. *Journal of Clinical and Aesthetic Dermatology* 2020; 13(5): 38-43. PMID: 32802255
18. Burris J, Rietkerk W, Woolf K. Acne: The Role of Medical Nutrition Therapy. *Journal of the Academy of Nutrition and Dietetics* 2013; 113(3): 416-430. doi: 10.1016/j.jand.2012.11.016
19. Capitanio B, Sinagra JL, Ottaviani M, Bordignon V, Amantea A, Picardo M. Acne and smoking. *Dermato-Endocrinology* 2009; 1(3): 129-135. doi: 10.4161/derm.1.3.9638
20. Elsaie ML. Hormonal treatment of acne vulgaris: an update. *Clinical, Cosmetic and Investigational Dermatology* 2016; 9: 241-248. doi: 10.2147/CCID.S114830
21. Albuquerque RGR, Rocha MAD, Bagatin E, Tufik S, Andersen ML. Could adult female acne be associated with modern life? *Archives of Dermatological Research* 2014; 306(8): 683-688. doi: 10.1007/s00403-014-1482-6.
22. Hayashi N, Imori M, Yanagisawa M, Seto Y, Nagata O, Kawashima M. Make-up improves the quality of life of acne patients without aggravating acne eruptions during treatments. *European Journal of Dermatology* 2005; 15(4): 284-287. PMID: 16048760
23. Conrado AB, Ierodiakonou D, Gowland MH, Boyle RJ, Turner PJ. Food anaphylaxis in the United Kingdom: analysis of national data, 1998-2018. *BMJ* 2021; 372: n251. doi.org/10.1136/bmj.n251

Chapter 17: Treating the root cause – Excessive facial and body hair growth

1. The Rotterdam ESHRE/ASRM-sponsored PCOS consensus workshop group. Revised 2003 consensus on diagnostic criteria and long-term health risks related to polycystic ovary syndrome (PCOS). *Human Reproduction* 2004; 19(1): 41-47. doi.org/10.1093/humrep/deh098
2. Hadjiconstantinou M, Mani H, Patel N, Levy M, Davies M, Khunti K, et al. Understanding and supporting women with polycystic ovary syndrome: a qualitative study in an ethnically diverse UK sample. *Endocrine Connections* 2017; 6(5): 323-330. doi: 10.1530/EC-17-0053
3. Kitzinger C, Willmott J. 'The thief of womanhood': women's experience of polycystic ovarian syndrome. *Social Science & Medicine* 2002; 54(3): 349-361. doi.org/10.1016/S0277-9536(01)00034-X
4. Barbieri R, Ehrmann D. Treatment of polycystic ovary syndrome in adults [Internet]. *UpToDate* [cited 2021 Nov 12]. Available from: www.uptodate.com/contents/treatment-of-polycystic-ovary-syndrome-in-adults
5. Zhao Y, Qiao J. Ethnic differences in the phenotypic expression of polycystic ovary syndrome. *Steroids* 2013; 78(8): 755-760. doi: 10.1016/j.steroids.2013.04.006
6. Grant P, Ramasamy S. An Update on Plant Derived Anti-Androgens. *International Journal of Endocrinology and Metabolism* 2012; 10(2): 497–502.

7. Grant P. Spearmint herbal tea has significant anti-androgen effects in polycystic ovarian syndrome. a randomized controlled trial. *Phytotherapy Research* 2010; 24(2): 186–188.
8. Matheson E, Bain J. Hirsutism in Women. *American Family Physician* 2019; 100(3): 168-175.
9. Martin KA, Chang RJ, Ehrmann DA, Ibanez L, Lobo RA, Rosenfield RL, et al. Evaluation and Treatment of Hirsutism in Premenopausal Women: An Endocrine Society Clinical Practice Guideline. *Journal of Clinical Endocrinology & Metabolism* 2008; 93(4): 1105-1120. doi: 10.1210/jc.2007-2437.
10. Ramos-e-Silva M, de Castro MCR, Carneiro JR LV. Hair removal. *Clinics in Dermatology* 2001; 19(4): 437-444. doi: 10.1016/s0738-081x(01)00200-0.

Chapter 18: It's not all down the drain – Female-pattern hair loss

1. Carmina E, Azziz R, Bergfeld W, Escobar-Morreale HF, Futterweit W, Huddleston H, et al. Female Pattern Hair Loss and Androgen Excess: A Report From the Multidisciplinary Androgen Excess and PCOS Committee. *Journal of Clinical Endocrinology & Metabolism* 2019; 104(7): 2875-2891. doi: 10.1210/jc.2018-02548
2. Gainder S, Sharma B. Update on Management of Polycystic Ovarian Syndrome for Dermatologists. *Indian Dermatology Online Journal* 2019; 10(2): 97–105. doi: 10.4103/idoj.IDOJ_249_17
3. Herskovitz I, Tosti A. Female Pattern Hair Loss. *International Journal of Endocrinology and Metabolism* 2013; 11(4): e9860. doi: 10.5812/ijem.9860
4. British Association of Dermatologists' (BAD). Female Pattern Hair Loss (Androgenetic Alopecia) [Internet]. 2019 [cited 2021 Nov 12]. Available from: www.bad.org.uk/shared/get-file.ashx?id=3830&itemtype=document
5. McMichael A. Female pattern hair loss (androgenetic alopecia in women): Pathogenesis, clinical features, and diagnosis. *UpToDate* Available from: www.uptodate.com/contents/female-pattern-hair-loss-androgenetic-alopecia-in-females-pathogenesis-clinical-features-and-diagnosis
6. Quinn M, Shinkai K, Pasch L, Kuzmich L, Cedars M, Huddleston H. Prevalence of androgenic alopecia in patients with polycystic ovary syndrome and characterization of associated clinical and biochemical features. *Fertility and Sterility* 2014; 101(4): 1129-1134. doi: 10.1016/j.fertnstert.2014.01.003
7. Cela E, Robertson C, Rush K, Kousta E, White D, Wilson H, et al. Prevalence of polycystic ovaries in women with androgenic alopecia. *European Journal of Endocrinology* 2003; 149(5): 439-442. doi: 10.1530/eje.0.1490439

8. Lizneva D, Gavrilova-Jordan L, Walker W, Azziz R. Androgen excess: Investigations and management. *Best Practice & Research Clinical Obstetrics & Gynaecology* 2016; 37: 98-118. doi: 10.1016/j.bpobgyn.2016.05.003

9. Tosti A, Piraccini BM, Sisti A, Duque-Estrada B. Hair loss in women. *Minerva Ginecologica* 2009; 61(5): 61(5): 445-452. PMID: 19749676

10. Guo EL, Katta R. Diet and hair loss: effects of nutrient deficiency and supplement use. *Dermatology Practical & Conceptual* 2017; 7(1): 1-10. doi: 10.5826/dpc.0701a01

11. McMichael A. Female pattern hair loss (androgenetic alopecia in women): Pathogenesis, clinical features, and diagnosis [Internet]. UpToDate. [cited 2021 Nov 12]. Available from: www.uptodate.com/contents/female-pattern-hair-loss-androgenetic-alopecia-in-women-pathogenesis-clinical-features-and-diagnosis

Chapter 19: Making your peace with PCOS – Anxiety, depression, sexual problems and mood disorders

1. Chaudhari AP, Mazumdar K, Mehta PD. Anxiety, Depression, and Quality of Life in Women with Polycystic Ovarian Syndrome. *Indian Journal of Psychological Medicine* 2018; 40(3): 239-246. doi: 10.4103/IJPSYM.IJPSYM_561_17

2. Zhuang J, Wang X, Xu L, Wu T, Kang D. Antidepressants for polycystic ovary syndrome. *Cochrane Database of Systematic Reviews* 2013; 2013(5): CD008575. doi: 10.1002/14651858.CD008575.pub2.

3. Williams J, Nieuwsma J. Screening for depression in adults. *UpToDate* [cited 2021 Nov 12]. Available from: www.uptodate.com/contents/screening-for-depression-in-adults

4. Brutocao C, Zaiem F, Alsawas M, Morrow AS, Murad MH, Javed A. Psychiatric disorders in women with polycystic ovary syndrome: a systematic review and meta-analysis. *Endocrine* 2018; 62(2): 318-325. doi: 10.1007/s12020-018-1692-3.

5. National Institute for Health and Care Excellence (NICE). Management of PCOS in Adults [Internet]. 2018 [cited 2021 Nov 7]. Available from: https://cks.nice.org.uk/topics/polycystic-ovary-syndrome/management/management-adults/

6. Royal College of Obstetricians and Gynaecologists. Long-Term Consequences of Polycystic ovary syndrome. 2014 [cited 2021 Nov 4]; Available from: www.rcog.org.uk/globalassets/documents/guidelines/gtg_33.pdf

7. Monash University MA. PCOS Evidence-Based guidelines [Internet]. 2018 [cited 2021 Nov 4]. Available from: www.monash.edu/__data/assets/pdf_file/0004/1412644/PCOS_Evidence-Based-Guidelines_20181009.pdf

8. Berni TR, Morgan CL, Berni ER, Rees DA. Polycystic Ovary Syndrome Is Associated With Adverse Mental Health and Neurodevelopmental Outcomes. *Journal of Clinical Endocrinology & Metabolism* 2018; 103(6): 2116-2125. doi: 10.1210/jc.2017-02667.

9. Eftekhar T, Sohrabvand F, Zabandan N, Shariat M, Haghollahi F, Ghahghaei-Nezamabadi A. Sexual dysfunction in patients with polycystic ovary syndrome and its affected domains. *Iranian Journal of Reproductive Medicine* 2014; 12(8): 539-546. PMID: 25408703; PMCID: PMC4233312

10. Fliegner M, Richter-Appelt H, Krupp K, Brunner F. Sexual Function and Socio-Sexual Difficulties in Women with Polycystic Ovary Syndrome (PCOS). *Geburtshilfe und Frauenheilkunde* 2019; 79(05): 498-509. doi: 10.1055/a-0828-7901

11. Greenwood EA, Pasch LA, Cedars MI, Legro RS, Huddleston HG. Association between depression, symptom experience, and quality of life in polycystic ovary syndrome. *American Journal of Obstetrics and Gynecology* 2018; 219(3): 279. e1-279.e7. doi: 10.1016/j.ajog.2018.06.017

12. Shifren J. Overview of sexual dysfunction in women: Epidemiology, risk factors, and evaluation. *UpToDate* [cited 2021 Nov 12]. Available from: www.uptodate.com/contents/overview-of-sexual-dysfunction-in-women-epidemiology-risk-factors-and-evaluation

13. Jones GL, Hall JM, Balen AH, Ledger WL. Health-related quality of life measurement in women with polycystic ovary syndrome: a systematic review. *Human Reproduction Update* 2007; 14(1): 15-25. doi: 10.1093/humupd/dmm030.

14. The Rotterdam ESHRE/ASRM-sponsored PCOS consensus workshop group. Revised 2003 consensus on diagnostic criteria and long-term health risks related to polycystic ovary syndrome (PCOS). *Human Reproduction* 2004 Jan 1 [cited 2021 Nov 6];19(1). Available from: https://academic.oup.com/humrep/article/19/1/41/690226

15. Dokras A, Stener-Victorin E, Yildiz BO, Li R, Ottey S, Shah D, et al. Androgen Excess- Polycystic Ovary Syndrome Society: position statement on depression, anxiety, quality of life, and eating disorders in polycystic ovary syndrome. *Fertility and Sterility* 2018; 109(5): 888-899. doi: 10.1016/j.fertnstert.2018.01.038.

Chapter 20: Healing the war with your body – Disordered eating in PCOS

1. The Rotterdam ESHRE/ASRM-sponsored PCOS consensus workshop group. Revised 2003 consensus on diagnostic criteria and long-term health risks related to polycystic ovary syndrome (PCOS). *Human Reproduction* 2004 Jan 1 [cited 2021 Nov 6];19(1). Available from: https://academic.oup.com/humrep/article/19/1/41/690226

2. Thannickal A, Brutocao C, Alsawas M, Morrow A, Zaiem F, Murad MH, Chattha AJ. Eating, sleeping and sexual function disorders in women with polycystic ovary syndrome (PCOS): A systematic review and meta-analysis. *Clinical Endocrinology* 2020; 92(4): 338-349. doi: 10.1111/cen.14153.

3. Krug I, Giles S, Paganini C. Binge eating in patients with polycystic ovary syndrome: prevalence, causes, and management strategies. *Neuropsychiatric Disease and Treatment* 2019; 15: 1273-1285. doi: 10.2147/NDT.S168944

4. Lee I, Cooney LG, Saini S, Smith ME, Sammel MD, Allison KC, et al. Increased risk of disordered eating in polycystic ovary syndrome. *Fertility and Sterility* 2017; 107(3): 796-802. doi: 10.1016/j.fertnstert.2016.12.014

5. Naessén S, Carlström K, Garoff L, Glant R, Hirschberg AL. Polycystic ovary syndrome in bulimic women – an evaluation based on the new diagnostic criteria. *Gynecological Endocrinology* 2006; 22(7): 388-394. doi: 10.1080/09513590600847421

6. Morgan J, Scholtz S, Lacey H, Conway G. The prevalence of eating disorders in women with facial hirsutism: An epidemiological cohort study. *International Journal of Eating Disorders* 2008; 41(5): 427-431. doi: 10.1002/eat.20527

7. Krug I, Giles S, Paganini C. Binge eating in patients with polycystic ovary syndrome: prevalence, causes, and management strategies. *Neuropsychiatric Disease and Treatment* 2019; 15: 1273-1285. doi: 10.2147/NDT.S168944

8. National Institute for Health and Care Excellence. Eating disorders: recognition and treatment [Internet]. 2017 [cited 2021 Nov 12]. Available from: www.nice.org.uk/guidance/ng69/resources/ eating-disorders-recognition-and-treatment-pdf-1837582159813

Chapter 21: From counting sheep to a good night's sleep – Disturbed sleep

1. Conway G, Dewailly D, Diamanti-Kandarakis E, Escobar-Morreale HF, Franks S, Gambineri A, et al. The polycystic ovary syndrome: a position statement from the European Society of Endocrinology. *European Journal of Endocrinology* 2014; 171(4): P1-P29. doi: 10.1530/EJE-14-0253

2. Vgontzas AN, Legro RS, Bixler EO, Grayev A, Kales A, Chrousos GP. Polycystic Ovary Syndrome Is Associated with Obstructive Sleep Apnea and Daytime Sleepiness: Role of Insulin Resistance. *Journal of Clinical Endocrinology & Metabolism* 2001; 86(2): 517–520. doi: 10.1210/jcem.86.2.7185.

3. Tasali E, van Cauter E, Hoffman L, Ehrmann DA. Impact of Obstructive Sleep Apnea on Insulin Resistance and Glucose Tolerance in Women with Polycystic Ovary Syndrome. *Journal of Clinical Endocrinology & Metabolism* 2008; 93(10): 3878–3884. doi: 10.1210/jc.2008-0925

4. Royal College of Obstetricians and Gynaecologists. Long-Term Consequences of Polycystic ovary syndrome. 2014 [cited 2021 Nov 4]; Available from: www.rcog.org.uk/globalassets/documents/guidelines/gtg_33.pdf

5. Tasali E, van Cauter E, Ehrmann DA. Relationships between Sleep Disordered Breathing and Glucose Metabolism in Polycystic Ovary Syndrome. *Journal of Clinical Endocrinology & Metabolism* 2006; 91(1): 36-42. doi: 10.1210/jc.2005-1084

6. Helvaci N, Karabulut E, Demir AU, Yildiz BO. Polycystic ovary syndrome and the risk of obstructive sleep apnea: a meta-analysis and review of the literature. *Endocrine Connections* 2017; 6(7): 437-445. doi: 10.1530/EC-17-0129

7. Barbieri R, Ehrmann D. Clinical manifestations of polycystic ovary syndrome in adults. *UpToDate* www.uptodate.com/contents/ clinical-manifestations-of-polycystic-ovary-syndrome-in-adults

8. Mitchell MD, Gehrman P, Perlis M, Umscheid CA. Comparative effectiveness of cognitive behavioral therapy for insomnia: a systematic review. *BMC Family Practice* 2012; 13(1): 40. www.biomedcentral.com/1471-2296/13/40
9. National Institute for Health and Care Excellence (NICE). Polycystic ovary syndrome. Last revised September 2018. https://cks.nice.org.uk/topics/polycystic-ovary-syndrome/

Chapter 22: It's getting hot in here – PCOS and menopause

1. The Rotterdam ESHRE/ASRM-sponsored PCOS consensus workshop group. Revised 2003 consensus on diagnostic criteria and long-term health risks related to polycystic ovary syndrome (PCOS). Human Reproduction [Internet]. 2004 Jan 1 [cited 2021 Nov 6];19(1). Available from: https://academic.oup.com/humrep/article/19/1/41/690226
2. Collier CN, Harper JC, Cantrell WC, Wang W, Foster KW, Elewski BE. The prevalence of acne in adults 20 years and older. *Journal of the American Academy of Dermatology* 2008; 58(1): 56-59. doi: 10.1016/j.jaad.2007.06.045.
3. Elting MW, Korsen TJM, Rekers-Mombarg LTM, Schoemaker J. Women with polycystic ovary syndrome gain regular menstrual cycles when ageing. *Human Reproduction* 2000; 15(1): 24-28. doi: 10.1093/humrep/15.1.24
4. Elting M, Kwee J, Korsen TJM, Rekers-Mombarg LTM, Scoemaker J. Aging women with polycystic ovary syndrome who achieve regular menstrual cycles have a smaller follicle cohort than those who continue to have irregular cycles. *Fertility and Sterility* 2003; 79(5): 1154-1160. doi: 10.1016/s0015-0282(03)00152-3.
5. Schmidt J, Brännström M, Landin-Wilhelmsen K, Dahlgren E. Reproductive Hormone Levels and Anthropometry in Postmenopausal Women with Polycystic Ovary Syndrome (PCOS): A 21-Year Follow-Up Study of Women Diagnosed with PCOS around 50 Years Ago and Their Age-Matched Controls. *Journal of Clinical Endocrinology & Metabolism* 2011; 96(7): 2178-2185. doi: 10.1210/jc.2010-2959
6. Forslund M, Schmidt J, Brännström M, Landin-Wilhelmsen K, Dahlgren E. Reproductive Hormones and Anthropometry: A Follow-Up of PCOS and Controls From Perimenopause to Older Than 80 Years. *Journal of Clinical Endocrinology & Metabolism* 2021; 106(2): 421-430. doi.org/10.1210/clinem/dgaa840
7. Li J, Eriksson M, Czene K, Hall P, Rodriguez-Wallberg KA. Common diseases as determinants of menopausal age. *Human Reproduction* 2016; 31(12): 2856-2864. doi: 10.1093/humrep/dew264
8. Tehrani RF, Solaymani-Dodaran M, Hedayati M, Azizi F. Is polycystic ovary syndrome an exception for reproductive aging? *Human Reproduction* 2010; 25(7): 1775-1781. doi: 10.1093/humrep/deq088
9. Carmina E, Campagna AM, Lobo RA. A 20-Year Follow-up of Young Women With Polycystic Ovary Syndrome. *Obstetrics & Gynecology* 2012; 119(2, Part 1): 263-269. doi: 10.1097/AOG.0b013e31823f7135
10. Markopoulos MC, Rizos D, Valsamakis G, Deligeoroglou E, Grigoriou O, Chrousos GP, et al. Hyperandrogenism in Women with Polycystic Ovary

Syndrome Persists after Menopause. *Journal of Clinical Endocrinology & Metabolism* 2011; 96(3): 623-631. doi: 10.1210/jc.2010-0130

11. Pierpoint T, McKeigue PM, Isaacs AJ, Wild SH, Jacobs HS. Mortality of Women with Polycystic Ovary Syndrome at Long-term Follow-up. *Journal of Clinical Epidemiology* 1998; 51(7): 581-586. doi: 10.1016/s0895-4356(98)00035-3

Chapter 23: Living longer, living better – Long-term consequences of PCOS

1. National Institute for Health and Care Excellence (NICE). Polycystic ovary syndrome: What are the complications? [Internet]. 2018 [cited 2021 Nov 13]. Available from: https://cks.nice.org.uk/topics/polycystic-ovary-syndrome/background-information/complications/

2. Centers for Disease Control and Prevention (CDC). PCOS (Polycystic Ovary Syndrome) and Diabetes [Internet]. [cited 2021 Nov 13]. Available from: www.cdc.gov/diabetes/basics/pcos.html

3. Royal College of Obstetricians and Gynaecologists. Long-Term Consequences of Polycystic ovary syndrome. 2014 [cited 2021 Nov 4]; Available from: www.rcog.org.uk/globalassets/documents/guidelines/gtg_33.pdf

4. Monash University MA. PCOS Evidence-Based guidelines [Internet]. 2018 [cited 2021 Nov 4]. Available from: www.monash.edu/__data/assets/pdf_file/0004/1412644/PCOS_Evidence-Based-Guidelines_20181009.pdf

5. Barbieri R, Ehrmann D. Diagnosis of polycystic ovary syndrome in adults [Internet]. UpToDate. [cited 2021 Nov 13]. Available from: www.uptodate.com/contents/diagnosis-of-polycystic-ovary-syndrome-in-adults

6. Royal College of Obstetricians and Gynaecologists (RCOG UK). RCOG statement on new research on drinking during pregnancy. 2017 [cited 2021 Nov 7]; Available from: www.rcog.org.uk/en/news/rcog-statement-on-new-research-on-drinking-during-pregnancy/

7. Zhang G-Q, Chen J-L, Liu Q, Zhang Y, Zeng H, Zhao Y. Soy Intake Is Associated With Lower Endometrial Cancer Risk. *Medicine* 2015; 94(50): e2281. doi: 10.1097/MD.0000000000002281

8. Xu WH, Zheng W, Xiang YB, Ruan ZX, Cheng JR, Dai Q, et al. Soya food intake and risk of endometrial cancer among Chinese women in Shanghai: population based case-control study. *BMJ* 2004; 328(7451): 1285. doi: 10.1136/bmj.38093.646215.AE.

9. Kluzek S, Rubin KH, Sanchez-Santos M, O'Hanlon MS, Andersen M, Glintborg D, et al. Accelerated osteoarthritis in women with polycystic ovary syndrome: a prospective nationwide registry-based cohort study. *Arthritis Research & Therapy* 2021; 23(1): 225. doi: 10.1186/s13075-021-02604-w

10. Kyrou I, Karteris E, Robbins T, Chatha K, Drenos F, Randeva HS. Polycystic ovary syndrome (PCOS) and COVID-19: an overlooked female patient population at potentially higher risk during the COVID-19 pandemic. *BMC Medicine* 2020; 18(1): 220. doi: 10.1186/s12916-020-01697-5.

11. Subramanian A, Anand A, Adderley NJ, Okoth K, Toulis KA, Gokhale K, et al. Increased COVID-19 infections in women with polycystic ovary syndrome: a

population-based study. *European Journal of Endocrinology* 2021; 184(5): 637-645. doi: 10.1530/EJE-20-1163

Part Four: Introduction – How to live PCOS free

1. Umberson D, Karas Montez J. Social Relationships and Health: A Flashpoint for Health Policy. *Journal of Health and Social Behavior* 2010; 51(1_suppl): S54-S66. doi: 10.1177/0022146510383501
2. Conversano C, Rotondo A, Lensi E, della Vista O, Arpone F, Reda MA. Optimism and Its Impact on Mental and Physical Well-Being. *Clinical Practice & Epidemiology in Mental Health* 2010; 6(1): 25-29. doi: 10.2174/1745017901006010025
3. Campbell-Sills L, Barlow DH, Brown TA, Hofmann SG. Effects of suppression and acceptance on emotional responses of individuals with anxiety and mood disorders. *Behaviour Research and Therapy* 2006; 44(9): 1251-1263. doi: 10.1016/j.brat.2005.10.001
4. Way KL, Hackett DA, Baker MK, Johnson NA. The Effect of Regular Exercise on Insulin Sensitivity in Type 2 Diabetes Mellitus: A Systematic Review and Meta-Analysis. *Diabetes & Metabolism Journal* 2016; 40(4): 253-271. doi: 10.4093/dmj.2016.40.4.253

Chapter 24: Mind the gap – How to transition to a plant-based way of eating

1. Orlich MJ, Fraser GE. Vegetarian diets in the Adventist Health Study 2: a review of initial published findings. *American Journal of Clinical Nutrition* 2014; 100(1): 353S-358S. doi: 10.3945/ajcn.113.071233
2. Hu Y, Ding M, Sampson L, Willett WC, Manson JE, Wang M, et al. Intake of whole grain foods and risk of type 2 diabetes: results from three prospective cohort studies. *BMJ* 2020; 370: m2206. doi: 10.1136/bmj.m2206
3. Zong G, Lebwohl B, Hu FB, Sampson L, Dougherty LW, Willett WC, et al. Gluten intake and risk of type 2 diabetes in three large prospective cohort studies of US men and women. *Diabetologia* 2018; 61(10): 2164–2173. doi: 10.1007/s00125-018-4697-9
4. Singh P, Arora A, Strand TA, Leffler DA, Catassi C, Green PH, et al. Global Prevalence of Celiac Disease: Systematic Review and Meta-analysis. *Clinical Gastroenterology and Hepatology* 2018; 16(6): 823-836.e2. doi: 10.1016/j.cgh.2017.06.037.
5. Kuscu NK, Akcali S, Kucukmetin NT. Celiac disease and polycystic ovary syndrome. *International Journal of Gynaecology & Obstetrics* 2002; 79(2): 149–150. doi: 10.1016/s0020-7292(02)00241-2
6. Niland B, Cash BD. Health Benefits and Adverse Effects of a Gluten-Free Diet in Non-Celiac Disease Patients. *Gastroenterology & Hepatology* 2018; 14(2): 82–91.

7. Mansueto P, Seidita A, D'Alcamo A, Carroccio A. Non-Celiac Gluten Sensitivity: Literature Review. *Journal of the American College of Nutrition* 2014 Feb 17;33(1):39–54. doi: 10.1080/07315724.2014.869996

8. Roszkowska A, Pawlicka M, Mroczek A, Bałabuszek K, Nieradko-Iwanicka B. Non-Celiac Gluten Sensitivity: A Review. Medicina. 2019 May 28;55(6):222. doi: 10.3390/medicina55060222.

9. Thompson T. Folate, Iron, and Dietary Fiber Contents of the Gluten-free Diet. *Journal of the American Dietetic Association* 2000; 100(11): 1389–1396.

10. Konczak I, Zhang W. Anthocyanins—More Than Nature's Colours. *Journal of Biomedicine and Biotechnology* 2004; 2004(5): 239-240.

11. Fraser GE, Sabate J, Beeson WL, Strahan TM. A Possible Protective Effect of Nut Consumption on Risk of Coronary Heart Disease. The Adventist Health Study. *Archives of Internal Medicine* 1992; 152(7): 1416-1424.

12. Mathur R, Ko A, Hwang LJ, Low K, Azziz R, Pimentel M. Polycystic Ovary Syndrome Is Associated with an Increased Prevalence of Irritable Bowel Syndrome. *Digestive Diseases and Sciences* 2010; 55(4): 1085-1089. doi: 10.1007/s10620-009-0890-5

13. Nkhata SG, Ayua E, Kamau EH, Shingiro J-B. Fermentation and germination improve nutritional value of cereals and legumes through activation of endogenous enzymes. *Food Science & Nutrition* 2018; 6(8): 2446-2458. doi: 10.1002/fsn3.846

Chapter 25: Skip the SOS for PCOS – Salt, oil and sugar

1. Bates BCLMN et al. *National Diet and Nutrition Survey: assessment of dietary sodium. Adults (19 to 64 years) in England, 2014.* MRC: Human Nutrition Research [Internet]. 2016 [cited 2021 Nov 11]. Available from: https://assets.publishing.service.gov.uk/government/uploads/system/uploads/attachment_data/file/773836/Sodium_study_2014_England_Text_final.pdf

2. Kellesarian S v, Malignaggi VR, Kellesarian T v, Al-Kheraif AA, Alwageet MM, Malmstrom H, et al. Association between periodontal disease and polycystic ovary syndrome: a systematic review. *International Journal of Impotence Research* 2017; 29(3): 89-95. doi.org/10.1038/ijir.2017.7

3. Lula ECO, Ribeiro CCC, Hugo FN, Alves CM, Silva AAM. Added sugars and periodontal disease in young adults: an analysis of NHANES III data. *American Journal of Clinical Nutrition* 2014; 100(4): 1182-1187. doi: 10.3945/ajcn.114.089656

4. Räikkönen K, Martikainen S, Pesonen AK, et al. Maternal Licorice Consumption During Pregnancy and Pubertal, Cognitive, and Psychiatric Outcomes in Children. *American Journal of Epidemiology* 2017; 185(5): 317–328. doi.org/10.1093/aje/kww172)

5. Shishehbor F, Mansoori A, Shirani F. Vinegar consumption can attenuate postprandial glucose and insulin responses; a systematic review and meta-analysis of clinical trials. *Diabetes Research and Clinical Practice* 2017; 127: 1–9. doi.org/10.1016/j.diabres.2017.01.021

Chapter 26: Soya: healthy or not? – The role of soya in PCOS

1. Mariotti F, Gardner CD. Dietary Protein and Amino Acids in Vegetarian Diets—A Review. *Nutrients* 2019; 11(11): 2661. doi: 10.3390/nu11112661
2. Young VR. Soy protein in relation to human protein and amino acid nutrition. *Journal of the American Dietetic Association* 1991; 91(7): 828–835. PMID: 2071798
3. Messina M. Soy and Health Update: Evaluation of the Clinical and Epidemiologic Literature. *Nutrients* 2016; 8(12): 754. doi: 10.3390/nu8120754.
4. K'ížová L, Dadáková K, Kašparovská J, Kašparovský T. Isoflavones. *Molecules* 2019; 24(6): 1076. doi: 10.3390/molecules24061076
5. Setchell KDR, Cole SJ. Method of Defining Equol-Producer Status and Its Frequency among Vegetarians. *Journal of Nutrition* 2006; 136(8): 2188-2193. doi: 10.1093/jn/136.8.2188
6. Strom BL, Schinnar R, Ziegler EE, et al. Exposure to Soy-Based Formula in Infancy and Endocrinological and Reproductive Outcomes in Young Adulthood. *JAMA* 2001; 286(7): 807-814. doi: 10.1001/jama.286.7.807.
7. Vanegas JC, Afeiche MC, Gaskins AJ, Mínguez-Alarcón L, Williams PL, Wright DL, et al. Soy food intake and treatment outcomes of women undergoing assisted reproductive technology. *Fertility and Sterility* 2015; 103(3): 749-755. doi: 10.1016/j.fertnstert.2014.12.104
8. Hamilton-Reeves JM, Vazquez G, Duval SJ, Phipps WR, Kurzer MS, Messina MJ. Clinical studies show no effects of soy protein or isoflavones on reproductive hormones in men: results of a meta-analysis. *Fertility and Sterility* 2010; 94(3): 997-1007.
9. Karamali M, Kashanian M, Alaeinasab S, Asemi Z. The effect of dietary soy intake on weight loss, glycaemic control, lipid profiles and biomarkers of inflammation and oxidative stress in women with polycystic ovary syndrome: a randomised clinical trial. *Journal of Human Nutrition and Dietetics* 2018; 31(4): 533-543. doi: 10.1111/jhn.12545
10. Khani B, Mehrabian F, Khalesi E, Eshraghi A. Effect of soy phytoestrogen on metabolic and hormonal disturbance of women with polycystic ovary syndrome. *Journal of Research in Medical Sciences* 2011; 16(3): 297-302. PMID: 22091248
11. Barrett JR. The Science of Soy: What Do We Really Know? *Environmental Health Perspectives* 2006; 114(6): A352-A358. doi: 10.1289/ehp.114-a352
12. Sathyapalan T, Aye M, Rigby AS, Fraser WD, Thatcher NJ, Kilpatrick ES, et al. Soy Reduces Bone Turnover Markers in Women During Early Menopause: A Randomized Controlled Trial. *Journal of Bone and Mineral Research* 2017; 32(1): 157-164. doi: 10.1002/jbmr.2927
13. Messina M. Insights Gained from 20 Years of Soy Research. *Journal of Nutrition* 2010; 140(12): 2289S-2295S. doi: 10.3945/jn.110.124107
14. Ahnan-Winarno AD, Cordeiro L, Winarno FG, Gibbons J, Xiao H. Tempeh: A semicentennial review on its health benefits, fermentation, safety, processing, sustainability, and affordability. *Comprehensive Reviews in Food Science and Food Safety* 2021; 20(2): 1717–1767. doi.org/10.1111/1541-4337.12710

15. Cutler DA, Pride SM, Cheung AP. Low intakes of dietary fiber and magnesium are associated with insulin resistance and hyperandrogenism in polycystic ovary syndrome: A cohort study. *Food Science & Nutrition* 2019; 7(4): 1426-1437. doi: 10.1002/fsn3.977.
16. Hooper L, Ryder JJ, Kurzer MS, Lampe JW, Messina MJ, Phipps WR, et al. Effects of soy protein and isoflavones on circulating hormone concentrations in pre- and post-menopausal women: a systematic review and meta-analysis. *Human Reproduction Update* 2009; 15(4): 423-440. doi: 10.1093/humupd/dmp010.
17. Bitzer ZT, Wopperer AL, Chrisfield BJ, Tao L, Cooper TK, Vanamala J, et al. Soy protein concentrate mitigates markers of colonic inflammation and loss of gut barrier function in vitro and in vivo. *Journal of Nutritional Biochemistry* 2017; 40: 201-208. doi.org/10.1016/j.jnutbio.2016.11.012
18. Messina M, Messina V. The Role of Soy in Vegetarian Diets. *Nutrients* 2010; 2(8): 855-888. doi: 10.3390/nu2080855
19. Harvard T.H. Chan School of Public Health. The Nutrition Source: Straight Talk About Soy [Internet]. [cited 2021 Nov 13]. Available from: www.hsph.harvard.edu/nutritionsource/soy/
20. Dewell A, Weidner G, Sumner MD, Barnard RJ, Marlin RO, Daubenmier JJ, et al. Relationship of Dietary Protein and Soy Isoflavones to Serum IGF-1 and IGF Binding Proteins in the Prostate Cancer Lifestyle Trial. *Nutrition and Cancer* 2007; 58(1): 35-42. doi: 10.1080/01635580701308034
21. Kattan JD, Cocco RR, Järvinen KM. Milk and Soy Allergy. *Pediatric Clinics of North America* 2011; 58(2): 407-426. doi: 10.1016/j.pcl.2011.02.005
22. Baic S. Soya and health – the basics. Food Fact Sheet. British Dietetic Association. 2017. Available at: www.bda.uk.com/uploads/assets/a4f4b414-ecd8-4cc4-91e3f5309d211a9f/Soya-food-fact-sheet.pdf
23. Garber JR, Cobin RH, Gharib H, Hennessey J v., Klein I, Mechanick JI, et al. Clinical Practice Guidelines for Hypothyroidism in Adults: Cosponsored by the American Association of Clinical Endocrinologists and the American Thyroid Association. *Endocrine Practice* 2012; 18(6): 988-1028. doi: 10.4158/EP12280.GL
24. Messina M, Mejia SB, Cassidy A, Duncan A, Kurzer M, Nagato C, et al. Neither soyfoods nor isoflavones warrant classification as endocrine disruptors: a technical review of the observational and clinical data. *Critical Reviews in Food Science and Nutrition* 2021; 1-57. doi: 10.1080/10408398.2021.1895054.

Chapter 27: Food first approach – The role of supplements in PCOS

1. Irani M, Merhi Z. Role of vitamin D in ovarian physiology and its implication in reproduction: a systematic review. *Fertility and Sterility* 2014; 102(2): 460-468. e3.
2. Lin M-W, Wu M-H. The role of vitamin D in polycystic ovary syndrome. *Indian Journal of Medical Research* 2015; 142(3): 238.
3. Du D, Li X. The relationship between thyroiditis and polycystic ovary syndrome: a meta-analysis. *International Journal of Clinical and Experimental Medicine* 2013; 6(10): 880–889.

References

4. British Dietetic Association (BDA). Omega-3: Food Fact Sheet [Internet]. [cited 2021 Nov 19]. Available from: www.bda.uk.com/resource/omega-3.html

5. Middleton P, Gomersall JC, Gould JF, Shepherd E, Olsen SF, Makrides M. Omega-3 fatty acid addition during pregnancy. *Cochrane Database of Systematic Reviews* 2018; 11(11): CD003402. doi: 10.1002/14651858.CD003402.pub3

6. Ebrahimi F, Samimi M, Foroozanfard F, Jamilian M, Akbari H, Rahmani E, et al. The Effects of Omega-3 Fatty Acids and Vitamin E Co-Supplementation on Indices of Insulin Resistance and Hormonal Parameters in Patients with Polycystic Ovary Syndrome: A Randomized, Double-Blind, Placebo-Controlled Trial. *Experimental and Clinical Endocrinology & Diabetes* 2017; 125(06): 353–359.

7. Royal College of Obstetricians and Gynaecologists. Long-Term Consequences of Polycystic ovary syndrome. 2014 [cited 2021 Nov 4]; Available from: www.rcog.org.uk/globalassets/documents/guidelines/gtg_33.pdf

8. Günalan E, Yaba A, Yılmaz B. The Effect of Nutrient Supplementation in Management of Polycystic Ovary Syndrome Associated Metabolic Dysfunctions: A Critical Review. *Journal of the Turkish-German Gynecological Association* 2018; 19(4): 220-232. doi: 10.4274/jtgga.2018.0077.

9. Balk EM, Tatsioni A, Lichtenstein AH, Lau J, Pittas AG. Effect of chromium supplementation on glucose metabolism and lipids: a systematic review of randomized controlled trials. *Diabetes Care* 2007; 30(8): 2154–2163.

10. Unfer V, Facchinetti F, Orrù B, Giordani B, Nestler J. Myo-inositol effects in women with PCOS: a meta-analysis of randomized controlled trials. *Endocrine Connections* 2017; 6(8): 647–658.

11. Tang T, Glanville J, Hayden CJ, White D, Barth JH, Balen AH. Combined lifestyle modification and metformin in obese patients with polycystic ovary syndrome. A randomized, placebo-controlled, double-blind multicentre study. *Human Reproduction* 2006; 21(1): 80–89.

12. Pundir J, Psaroudakis D, Savnur P, Bhide P, Sabatini L, Teede H, et al. Inositol treatment of anovulation in women with polycystic ovary syndrome: a meta-analysis of randomised trials. *BJOG: An International Journal of Obstetrics & Gynaecology* 2018; 125(3): 299–308.

13. Monash University MA. PCOS Evidence-Based guidelines [Internet]. 2018 [cited 2021 Nov 4]. Available from: www.monash.edu/__data/assets/pdf_file/0004/1412644/PCOS_Evidence-Based-Guidelines_20181009.pdf

13a. Wakeman M. A Review of the Effects of Oral Contraceptives on Nutrient Status, with Especial Consideration to Folate in UK. *Journal of Advances in Medicine and Medical Research* 2019; 30(2): 1-17. doi.org/10.9734/jammr/2019/v30i230168

14. Arentz S, Abbott JA, Smith CA, Bensoussan A. Herbal medicine for the management of polycystic ovary syndrome (PCOS) and associated oligo/amenorrhoea and hyperandrogenism; a review of the laboratory evidence for effects with corroborative clinical findings. *BMC Complementary and Alternative Medicine* 2014; 14(1): 511.

15. Royal College of Obstetricians and Gynaecologists (RCOG). Healthy eating and vitamin supplements in pregnancy [Internet]. 2014 [cited 2021 Nov 19]. Available from: www.rcog.org.uk/globalassets/documents/patients/

patient-information-leaflets/pregnancy/pi-healthy-eating-and-vitamin-supplements-in-pregnancy.pdf

16. Gould JF, Smithers LG, Makrides M. The effect of maternal omega-3 (n-3) LCPUFA supplementation during pregnancy on early childhood cognitive and visual development: a systematic review and meta-analysis of randomized controlled trials. *American Journal of Clinical Nutrition* 2013; 97(3): 531–544.

17. Barbieri RL, Ehrmann DA. Clinical manifestations of polycystic ovary syndrome in adults. *UpToDate* Available at: https://www.uptodate.com/contents/clinical-manifestations-of-polycystic-ovary-syndrome-in-adults

Chapter 28: Daily affirmations for PCOS

1. Cascio CN, O'Donnell MB, Tinney FJ, Lieberman MD, Taylor SE, Strecher VJ, et al. Self-affirmation activates brain systems associated with self-related processing and reward and is reinforced by future orientation. *Social Cognitive and Affective Neuroscience* 2016; 11(4): 621-629. doi: 10.1093/scan/nsv136.

2. Bazarganipour F, Ziaei S, Montazeri A, et al. Body image satisfaction and self-esteem status among the patients with polycystic ovary syndrome. *Iranian Journal of Reproductive Medicine* 2013; 11(10): 829-836. pubmed.ncbi.nlm.nih.gov/24639704/

Chapter 29: Self-care activities

1. Riegel B, Dunbar SB, Fitzsimons D, Freedland KE, Lee CS, Middleton S, et al. Self-care research: Where are we now? Where are we going? *International Journal of Nursing Studies* 2021; 116: 103402. doi: 10.1016/j.ijnurstu.2019.103402.

2. International Self-Care Foundation. Pillar 1 Knowledge & Health Literacy [Internet]. [cited 2021 Nov 12]. Available from: https://isfglobal.org/practise-self-care/pillar-1-knowledge-health-literacy/

3. Godfrey CM, Harrison MB, Lysaght R, Lamb M, Graham ID, Oakley P. The experience of self-care: a systematic review. *JBI Database of Systematic Reviews and Implementation Reports* 2010; 8(34): 1351-1460. doi: 10.11124/01938924-201008340-00001.

Chapter 30: Forms of movement

1. Angel S. Movement perceived as chores or a source of joy: a phenomenological-hermeneutic study of physical activity and health. *International Journal of Qualitative Studies on Health and Well-being* 2018; 13(1): 1516088. doi: 10.1080/17482631.2018.1516088

Chapter 32: The 21-day programme for living PCOS free

1. Kahleova H, Belinova L, Malinska H, Oliyarnyk O, Trnovska J, Skop V, et al. Eating two larger meals a day (breakfast and lunch) is more effective than six smaller meals in a reduced-energy regimen for patients with type 2 diabetes: a randomised crossover study. *Diabetologia* 2014; 57(8): 1552-1560. doi: 10.1007/s00125-014-3253-5.

Chapter 33: Recipes for living PCOS free

1. Birt DF, Boylston T, Hendrich S, Jane J-L, Hollis J, Li L, et al. Resistant Starch: Promise for Improving Human Health. *Advances in Nutrition* 2013; 4(6): 587-601. doi: 10.3945/an.113.004325
2. Calado A, Neves PM, Santos T, Ravasco P. The Effect of Flaxseed in Breast Cancer: A Literature Review. *Frontiers in Nutrition* 2018; 5: 4. doi.org/10.3389/fnut.2018.00004
3. Wastyk HC, Fragiadakis GK, Perelman D, Dahan D, Merrill BD, Yu FB, et al. Gut-microbiota-targeted diets modulate human immune status. *Cell* 2021; 184(16): 4137-4153.e14. doi: 10.1016/j.cell.2021.06.019.
4. Shishehbor F, Mansoori A, Shirani F. Vinegar consumption can attenuate postprandial glucose and insulin responses; a systematic review and meta-analysis of clinical trials. *Diabetes Research and Clinical Practice* 2017; 127: 1–9. doi.org/10.1016/j.diabres.2017.01.021)
5. Stanaway L, Rutherfurd-Markwick K, Page R, Ali A. Performance and Health Benefits of Dietary Nitrate Supplementation in Older Adults: A Systematic Review. Nutrients 2017; 9(11): 1171. doi: 10.3390/nu9111171

Chapter 34: It is never too late – What we eat is bigger than just personal

1. Poore J, Nemecek T. Reducing food's environmental impacts through producers and consumers. *Science* 2018; 360(6392): 987-992. doi: 10.1126/science.aaq0216
2. Willett W, Rockström J, Loken B, et al. Food in the Anthropocene: the EAT-Lancet Commission on healthy diets from sustainable food systems. *Lancet* 2019; 393(10170): 447–492. doi.org/10.1016/S0140-6736(18)31788-4
3. Slade J, Alleyne E. The Psychological Impact of Slaughterhouse Employment: A Systematic Literature Review. *Trauma, Violence, & Abuse* 2021; doi.org/10.1177/15248380211030243
4. World Health Organization. No time to Wait: Securing the future from drug-resistant infections: Report to the Secretary-General of the United Nations [Internet]. 2019 [cited 2021 Nov 12]. Available from: www.who.int/publications/i/item/no-time-to-wait-securing-the-future-from-drug-resistant-infections

Index

*Glossary entries shown in bold.

Index

*Glossary entries shown in bold.

*Glossary entries shown in bold.

*Glossary entries shown in bold.

Index

Index

*Glossary entries shown in bold.

Index

*Glossary entries shown in bold.

*Glossary entries shown in bold.